iga

Psychological Aspects of Reconstructive and Cosmetic Plastic Surgery

Psychological Aspects of Reconstructive and Cosmetic Plastic Surgery
Clinical, Empirical, and Ethical Perspectives

EDITORS

David B. Sarwer, PhD
Associate Professor of Psychology
in Psychiatry and Surgery
University of Pennsylvania School of Medicine
The Edwin and Fannie Gray Hall
Center for Human Appearance
Philadelphia, Pennsylvania

Thomas Pruzinsky, PhD
Professor
Department of Psychology
Quinnipiac University
Hamden, Connecticut

Thomas F. Cash, PhD
University Professor
Department of Psychology
Old Dominion University
Norfolk, Virginia

Robert M. Goldwyn, MD
Clinical Professor of Surgery
Harvard Medical School
Boston, Massachusetts

John A. Persing, MD
Professor and Chief
Plastic Surgery
Yale University School of Medicine
New Haven, Connecticut

Linton A. Whitaker, MD
Professor of Surgery (Plastic)
University of Pennsylvania School of Medicine
Director, The Edwin and Fannie Gray Hall
Center for Human Appearance
Philadelphia, Pennsylvania

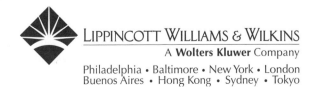

LIPPINCOTT WILLIAMS & WILKINS
A **Wolters Kluwer** Company

Philadelphia • Baltimore • New York • London
Buenos Aires • Hong Kong • Sydney • Tokyo

Acquisitions Editor: Brian Brown
Developmental Editor: Louise Bierig
Managing Editor: Julia Seto
Project Manager: Fran Gunning
Design Coordinator: Teresa Mallon
Marketing Manager: Adam Glazer
Production Services: Schawk, Inc.
Printer: Edwards Brothers, Inc.

© 2006 by Lippincott Williams & Wilkins
530 Walnut Street
Philadelphia, Pennsylvania 19106 USA
351 West Camden Street
Baltimore, Maryland 21201-2436 USA
LWW.com

Printed in the USA

Library of Congress Cataloging-in-Publication Data
Psychological aspects of reconstructive and cosmetic plastic surgery: clinical, empirical, and ethical perspectives/editors. David B. Sarwer, Thomas Pruzinsky
    p.; cm.
  Includes bibliographical references and index
  ISBN 0-7817-5362-7 (alk. paper)
  1. Surgery, Plastic—Psychological aspects. 2. Surgery, Plastic—Moral and ethical aspects. 3. Surgery, Plastic—Social aspects. I. Sarwer, David B. II. Pruzinsky, Thomas.
  [DNLM: 1. Reconstructive Surgical Procedures—psychology. 2. Ethics. Professional. 3. Surgery, Plastic—psychology. WO 600 P974 2005]
RD118.5.P79 2005
617.9'5—dc22

2005016508

The publishers have made every effort to trace copyright holders for borrowed material. If they have inadvertently overlooked any, they will be pleased to make the necessary arrangements at the first opportunity. To purchase additional copies of this book, call our customer service department at (800) 638-3030 or fax orders to (301) 824-7390. Lippincott Williams & Wilkins customer service representatives are available from 8:30 am to 6:30 pm, EST, Monday through Friday, for telephone access.

International customers shoud call (301)-714-2324. For other book services, including chapter reprints and large quantity sales, ask for the Special Sales department. Visit Lippincott Williams & Wilkins on the Internet: http://www.lww.com

10 9 8 7 6 5 4 3 2 1

CONTRIBUTORS

Barbara L. Andersen, PhD
Professor
Department of Psychology
Department of Obstetrics and Gynecology
The Ohio State University
Columbus, Ohio

Jeffrey T. Barth, PhD
Professor
Department of Psychiatric Medicine and
    Department of Neurological Surgery
University of Virginia Medical School
Charlottesville, Virginia

Patricia Blakeney, PhD
Clinical Professor
Department of Surgery
University of Texas Medical Branch
Galveston, Texas

Walter O. Bockting, PhD
Associate Professor
Program in Human Sexuality
Department of Family Medicine and Community Health
Coordinator of Transgender Health Services
University of Minnesota Medical School
Minneapolis, Minnesota

Thomas F. Cash, PhD
University Professor
Department of Psychology
Old Dominion University
Norfolk, Virginia

Canice E. Crerand, PhD
Instructor
Department of Psychiatry
University of Pennsylvania School of Medicine
Philadelphia, Pennsylvania

Elizabeth R. Didie, PhD
Clinical Psychology Post-doctoral Fellow
Department of Psychiatry and Human Behavior
Brown University/Butler Hospital
Providence, Rhode Island

Milton T. Edgerton, MD
Emeritus Professor of Plastic Surgery
University of Virginia Health Sciences Center
Charlottesville, Virginia

James A. Fauerbach, PhD
Associate Professor
Department of Psychiatry and Behavioral Sciences and
    Physical Medicine and Rehabilitation
The Johns Hopkins School of Medicine
Baltimore, Maryland

Carla Fenson, MEd
Human Services Planner/Evaluator III
Frank Porter Graham Child Development Institute
University of North Carolina at Chapel Hill
Carrboro, North Carolina

Georita M. Frierson, PhD
Centers for Behavioral and Preventive Medicine
Miriam Hospital
Brown University School of Medicine
Providence, Rhode Island

Leo C.T. Fung, MD
Associate Professor of Urologic Surgery and Pediatrics
Director of Pediatric Urology
University of Minnesota Medical School
Minneapolis, Minnesota

Lauren M. Gibbons, BA
Department of Psychiatry
University of Pennsylvania School of Medicine
Philadelphia, Pennsylvania

Robert M. Goldwyn, MD
Clinical Professor of Surgery
Harvard Medical School
Boston, Massachusetts

Mark Gorney, MD
The Doctor's Company
Napa, California

Brad K. Grunert, PhD
Associate Professor
Department of Plastic Surgery and
    Department of Psychiatry and Behavioral Medicine
Medical College of Wisconsin
Milwaukee, Wisconsin

Kathleen A. Kapp-Simon, PhD
Associate Professor
Department of Surgery
Northwestern University Feinberg School of Medicine
Chicago, Illinois

H. Asuman Kiyak, MA, PhD
Professor
Department of Oral & Maxillofacial Surgery
University of Washington School of Medicine
Seattle, Washington

Alice M. Laneader, MBe
Senior Regulatory Advisor
Office of Human Research
University of Pennsylvania School of Medicine
Philadelphia, Pennsylvania

Elie Levine, MD
Fellow, Division of Plastic Surgery
Department of Plastic Surgery
Mount Sinai Medical Center
New York, New York

Leanne Magee, BA
Doctoral Student
Department of Psychology
Temple University
Philadelphia, Pennsylvania

Robert Obrecht, PhD, LCDR/MSC/USN
Head
Neuropsychological Assessment Division
Naval Medical Center
San Diego, California

David R. Patterson, PhD
Professor
Department of Rehabilitation Medicine
University of Washington School of Medicine
Seattle, Washington

John A. Persing, MD
Professor and Chief
Plastic Surgery
Yale University School of Medicine
New Haven, Connecticut

Thomas Pruzinsky, PhD
Professor
Department of Psychology
Quinnipiac University
Hamden, Connecticut

Mary Rose, PsyD
Assistant Professor
Department of Medicine, Pulmonary and Critical Care
   Section
Baylor College of Medicine
Houston, Texas

David B. Sarwer, PhD
Associate Professor of Psychology
Department of Psychiatry and Surgery
University of Pennsylvania School of Medicine
The Edwin and Fannie Gray Hall
   Center for Human Appearance
Philadelphia, Pennsylvania

Robert J. Spence, MD
Associate Professor
Department of Surgery
The Johns Hopkins School of Medicine
Baltimore, Maryland

Margot B. Stein, PhD
Associate Clinical Professor
Department of Dental Ecology
UNC School of Dentistry
University of North Carolina at Chapel Hill
Chapel Hill, North Carolina

Ronald P. Strauss, DMD, PhD
Dental Friends Distinguished Professor and Chair
Department of Dental Ecology and
   Department of Social Medicine
UNC School of Dentistry and UNC School of Medicine
University of North Carolina at Chapel Hill
Chapel Hill, North Carolina

Marla E. Watson, MA
Research Assistant
BodyAesthetic Plastic Surgery & Skincare Center
St. Louis, Missouri

Linton A. Whitaker, MD
Professor of Surgery (Plastic)
University of Pennsylvania School of Medicine
Director, The Edwin and Fannie Gray Hall
   Center for Human Appearance
Philadelphia, Pennsylvania

Paul Root Wolpe, PhD
Senior Fellow
Center for Bioethics
University of Pennsylvania
Philadelphia, Pennsylvania

V. Leroy Young, MD
Chief of Surgical Services
Barnes-Jewish West County Hospital
St. Louis, Missouri

Milton Edgerton, Jr., MD

This book will be of great assistance to plastic surgeons as they evaluate and treat their patients. It also will give valuable help to nurses, psychologists, psychiatrists, and other professionals who are involved in the care of plastic surgery patients. The editors and authors are long-standing students of their subjects and many have pioneered research in the psychological aspects of plastic surgery.

Dr. David Sarwer has been a pioneer in uncovering many of the psychological aspects of cosmetic surgery. Drs. Tom Cash and Tom Pruzinsky are national leaders in the study of body image. Drs. Robert Goldwyn and John Persing are wise and experienced surgeons who have contributed much to this subject over many years. Dr. Goldwyn has advised all of us who are plastic surgeons to get to know ourselves, our biases, and how we make decisions. Dr. Persing has brought psychological issues to the attention of craniofacial surgeons. Dr. Linton Whitaker's Edwin and Fannie Gray Hall Center for Human Appearance houses a multidisciplinary group of professionals who have made extensive contributions to our understanding of the care of patients with appearance concerns. The experience and productivity of the editorial team deserves your attention. The last textbook on this important subject, written by Drs. John and Marcia Goin, was published 25 years ago. A great deal has been learned since then.

Every human develops a body image early in life. Some of that image comes from looking in mirrors; and some of it is shaped by the reactions of others to our physical appearance. If one is pleased with this image, personal relationships are approached with confidence and a more satisfying life often follows. If congenital or posttraumatic deformities occur, the body image may suffer and that individual may find it hard to approach life's challenges with strong self-confidence and in an uninhibited fashion. Many such individuals turn to plastic surgeons for help.

Strengthening an individual's self-image is often the principal purpose and benefit of plastic surgery. This is true of both reconstructive and cosmetic surgery. Thus, it is critical that plastic surgeons understand the psychological variables involved in changing (or refusing to change) a patient's appearance. In the case of cosmetic surgery, the *only* indication for surgery is the likelihood that it will improve the *emotional* health of the patient. Any physical change should be aimed at that goal.

Only a few training programs in plastic surgery devote sufficient effort to the education of their residents in the basic psychological aspects of appearance and deformity. This is unfortunate. As a result, many plastic surgeons have minimal understanding of some of the important issues that are involved in the proper choice and timing of surgical procedures. Not surprisingly, unhappy patients and unexpected reactions may follow apparently well-executed surgical procedures. The surgeon may be surprised and disappointed that the patient is unhappy with the operative results. Alternatively, some plastic surgeons categorically refuse to operate on any patient with evident emotional disturbance, simply because the surgeon is uncertain as to how that patient will respond to the operation.

Fortunately, a number of plastic surgeons and mental health professionals have begun to address these issues. Improved (and often multidisciplined) evaluation of patients seeking plastic surgery has revealed some major surprises. For example, often the amount of anatomical change is *not* correlated with the amount of psychological impact seen postoperatively. Many individuals with tiny abnormalities may be psychologically crippled, while others live with severe deformity and feel no need for plastic surgery.

The plastic surgeon is now learning that he or she should not let "experienced" aesthetic judgment trump the sometimes strange anatomical change that is specifically requested by the patient. The surgeon must listen carefully to the *exact* changes desired by each patient and resist the temptation to persuade the patient to let him or her add other changes for which the patient shows little enthusiasm.

Patients presenting with severe emotional disturbances require preoperative evaluation by a qualified mental health professional. That consultation will have little value unless that professional has had clinical experience with preoperative and postoperative plastic surgery patients. To the surprise of many, we have learned that a number of such disturbed patients may be helped by surgery *if* the plastic surgeon proceeds carefully, and when indicated, combine surgery with pre- and postoperative psychotherapeutic assistance.

The timing of surgery and the amount of physical change may be more effective if the plastic surgeon has a solid understanding of clinical psychology. In 1953, I was fortunate enough to have Dr. Eugene "Bill" Meyer as a friend and collaborator in the study of "disturbed" plastic surgery patients. As head of the Division of Psychosomatic Medicine at the Johns Hopkins Hospital, he would see such patients before and after surgery to help me assess the value (if any) of operating on each patient. He acknowledged that most psychiatrists had little or no experience with plastic surgery patients, other than the occasional disastrous result referred to them after an unwise operation. His open mind allowed him to appreciate the power of surgery as a method of improving emotional health. At the same time, he taught me much about how to evaluate the psychological strengths and weaknesses of my patients. Later, Drs. Wayne Jacobson, Norman Knorr, and other psychiatrists joined the faculty. In recent years Drs. Tom Pruzinsky and Ina Langman have made great contributions to the program. Every plastic surgeon would profit from such a close relationship with an interested behavioral scientist. The surgeon who has not developed such a working partnership with a clinical psychologist or psychiatrist will find him or herself ill-equipped to manage those patients with serious psychological disorders who seek relief through surgical changes. They should know to refer such patients to a plastic surgeon who is part of an experienced, multidisciplinary team.

We now know that "deformity," when not associated with functional limitations, is a disease ("dis-ease") *only* when it damages the individual's confidence in his or her body image. The surgeon must change this body image perception if he or she is to help the patient. To do so, he or she may, at times, have to make anatomical changes that might *not* seem entirely reasonable to others.

There are some who handle significant deformity without apparent loss in social effectiveness. Somehow, they manage to maintain a positive image. How do they do this? Dr. Cash has developed a program that teaches patients how they may develop a more positive body image. Could such a program be used *in place of,* or perhaps as a *complement* to, plastic surgery? Patients often tell their plastic surgeons that they just want "to seem lovable" (to others)—perhaps this desire is just another way of saying that they want a more satisfying body image.

Clinical observation has suggested the curious hypothesis that among patients coming to plastic surgeons, those with similar physical deformities often have similar types of psychological disturbances. Examples include patients with severe acne scarring, large port-wine facial angiomas, women with micromastia, or men with nasal deformities. Those within each group tend to show similar psychological profiles. How can we explain this? Does a given deformity lead to a particular emotional disturbance? Or does a given emotional disturbance tend to cause an individual to focus on a particular anatomical feature? So much more needs to be learned.

This book will produce a heightened awareness of the questions that plastic surgeons and behavioral scientists must ask of themselves and their patients. I would predict that the specialties of psychiatry and psychology will turn out an increasing number of individuals (like many of those contributing to this book) who will be available to collaborate with plastic surgeons. The resulting teams will come to better understand the sometimes magical transformations that result from surgical alterations of the face, body, or limbs. Patients who seek plastic surgery will profit from that knowledge.

The editors set out to produce a "must have" book for plastic surgeons. They have done an outstanding job!

Milton T. Edgerton, MD
Emeritus Professor of Plastic Surgery
University of Virginia Health Sciences Center
Charlottesville, VA 22901

PREFACE

This book has one primary goal: to summarize what is currently known about the psychological experience of reconstructive and cosmetic surgery patients so that plastic surgeons can more effectively help patients reduce their emotional distress and attain the highest quality of life possible.

Plastic surgeons recognize, at least on some level, that the ultimate purpose of their work is to address the psychological needs of their patients—to reduce emotional distress and enhance quality of life. The means by which surgeons pursue this purpose is, of course, through surgery. However, surgeons can expand their effectiveness as physicians by complementing their surgical skills with a deeper understanding of the psychosocial functioning of their patients.

This book places into the hands of plastic surgeons, and other medical and mental health professionals, a comprehensive, yet practical summary of the scientific and clinical literature on the psychological aspects of plastic surgery. The editorial team is comprised of three psychologists and three plastic surgeons with over 150 years of combined professional experience. Chapter authors were specifically chosen because of their long-term clinical experience and extensive research contributions in their particular subspecialties. This book distills the wisdom of many decades of experience with literally thousands of patients and research participants into a readily accessible form.

Detailed questionnaires related to the topics of study appear at the end of many of the chapters. We encourage you (with the express permission of the publisher) to copy and distribute the questionnaires in the book to your patients and to use them as a starting point for discussing their perceptions of their appearance and related experiences as well as their response to surgery. We are convinced that such a dialogue can be very helpful to you, the members of the treatment team, and the patient's loved ones.

The book is constructed to achieve four objectives:

1. To articulate the relationships among physical appearance, body image, and psychosocial functioning essential to understanding the experiences and motivations of individuals who seek out the care of plastic surgeons.
2. To provide a comprehensive and critical review of the empirical literature evaluating the psychological functioning of reconstructive and cosmetic surgical patients.
3. To give clear, concise, and clinically effective recommendations for plastic surgeons (and their staffs) to better care for the psychological needs of patients.
4. To provide a review of the critical ethical and professional issues that plastic surgeons encounter.

This book is organized into four major sections, which follow a foreword by Dr. Milton Edgerton. Over the course of his distinguished career, Dr. Edgerton wrote many of the seminal articles on the psychological aspects of cosmetic surgery. Directly and indirectly, he has influenced the interests of the editorial team as well as much of the research discussed in the individual chapters of this volume. His foreword is a particularly meaningful contribution to the book.

Section I: Understanding the Psychology of Plastic Surgery

The book begins with an introductory chapter written by the editors. This chapter provides a historical and conceptual context for building a bridge between plastic surgery and psychology. The second chapter of this section, authored by Goldwyn, provides the plastic surgeon's perspective on addressing the psychological issues in caring for plastic surgery patients. In the following chapter, Sarwer and Magee review the role of physical appearance in society (i.e., the "outside" view of physical appearance) and explore the relationship between this body of research and the pursuit of plastic surgery. In the final chapter of this section, Cash provides a detailed review of the literature on body image (i.e., the "inside" view of physical appearance) and its integral relationship to plastic surgery.

Section II: Psychological Perspectives on Reconstructive Surgery

This section of the book presents a comprehensive review of psychological perspectives on reconstructive surgical procedures. The first chapter, by Kapp-Simon, reviews the clinical and scientific literature specifically relevant to individuals with congenital craniofacial conditions. The following four chapters, on pediatric burn injury (Rose and Blakeney), adult burn injury (Fauerbach, Spence, and Patterson), facial disfigurement acquired through trauma or cancer (Pruzinsky, Levine, Persing, Barth, and Obrecht), and traumatic hand injury (Grunert) all address issues specific to patients with acquired disfigurement. The last four chapters in this section, on orthognathic surgery (Kiyak), breast reconstruction (Frierson and Andersen), breast reduction (Young and Watson), and genital reconstruction (Bockting and Fung), describe a broad range of psychological concerns in patients who undergo plastic surgical and adjunctive treatments to address objective clinical problems. These chapters are written by professionals who are recognized experts in these subspecialties, and, therefore presents readers with the most comprehensive discussion of the relevant psychosocial issues possible.

Section III: Psychological Perspectives on Cosmetic Surgery

The first two chapters of this section review the literature on the psychological aspects of cosmetic surgery of the face (Crerand, Cash, and Whitaker) and body (Sarwer, Didie, and Gibbons). The final chapter of this section by Sarwer discusses the psychological assessment of cosmetic surgery patients as performed by both the plastic surgeon and mental health professional.

Section IV: Ethical and Professional Issues in Plastic Surgery

The final section of the book begins with a chapter by Strauss, Stein, and Fenson on the bioethical issues in reconstructive craniofacial surgery. Laneader and Wolpe provide a discussion of similar issues in cosmetic surgery. In the final chapter of the book, Gorney shares with the reader the plastic surgeon's perspective on professional and legal issues in cosmetic surgery.

The editors strongly believe that the clinical and scientific knowledge presented in this unique volume can lead to a higher standard of care for both reconstructive and cosmetic surgery patients. Our hope is that it will result in the greatest possible reductions of distress and attainment of the most satisfying quality of life possible for each patient.

ACKNOWLEDGMENTS

The editors would like to acknowledge numerous individuals who, in a variety of ways, have contributed to this book. First, we would like to express our gratitude and respect to our chapter authors. We consider ourselves very fortunate to have enlisted the help of these recognized experts. They have provided just what we hoped for and envisioned—clear reviews of the scientific literature combined with the clinical insight that can only be gained through many years of providing compassionate clinical care. We are exceptionally confident that the readers of this book, and their patients, will greatly benefit from the wisdom they have shared in these pages.

The three psychologist editors also want to acknowledge our exceptional good fortune for the opportunity to work with our plastic surgeon colleagues; Drs. Robert Goldwyn, John Persing, and Linton Whitaker. They have brought to this project over 100 years of unparalleled contributions to their field as well as a unique dedication to improving the surgical and psychological care of plastic surgery patients. We thank them for all they have done to help build bridges between the professions of plastic surgery and psychology.

This book was a true team effort. As with many scholarly endeavors, some of the most important contributions came from individuals who did not necessarily author chapters in this book. Our work on this project would not be complete if we did not individually recognize the colleagues, peers, friends, and family members who, in some cases, contributed to the creation of this book even before the first word was typed.

David Sarwer—First and foremost, I would like to thank my coeditors. As the "rookie" on the team, I leaned heavily on their experience and expertise to bring this book together. Even prior to the development of the book, each of them provided me with opportunities to develop my professional interests in this area. While he would never admit it, Tom Pruzinsky is one of the "founding fathers" of the interface between plastic surgery and psychology. This book would not exist without his belief that the field needed such a comprehensive resource. Tom Cash has made innumerable contributions to the study of body image and physical appearance. His scholarship is unparalleled, and without him, the field simply would not be where it is today. After working together on this project, I am honored to consider both of them colleagues, and more importantly, friends.

In 1995, Linton Whitaker recruited me to join the Center for Human Appearance at the University of Pennsylvania School of Medicine with the task of developing a body of research on the psychological aspects of plastic surgery. He provided me with my first job and countless other opportunities over the past decade to meet this goal. I have a very deep sense of gratitude for his support.

The other members of the Center for Human Appearance, in particular those in the Division of Plastic Surgery, have been incredibly supportive of my research. From providing me with access to patients to collaborating on manuscripts, I am deeply grateful to them. I also would like to acknowledge my colleagues and friends in the Department of Psychiatry. In particular, Dr. Thomas Wadden, Professor of Psychology and Director of the Weight and Eating Disorders Program, has made immeasurable contributions to my professional development as an academic clinical psychologist. I also would like to acknowledge my current and former students, several of whom have contributed to this book. Their enthusiasm and energy have greatly enhanced the quality of our research.

Finally, my deepest gratitude and love goes to Miranda and Ethan. The joy that you bring to my life each and every day brings even greater meaning to my professional accomplishments.

Tom Pruzinsky—It is a great joy to express my heartfelt gratitude to Drs. Milton Edgerton and Ina Langman of the University of Virginia Health Sciences Center for so generously giving me a priceless education, for making my entire career possible, and for countless opportunities which I could never repay. It was unquestionably a privilege to witness how they selflessly and tirelessly helped so many people through decades of service devoted to understanding and reducing the suffering of plastic surgery patients.

Drs. Edgerton and Langman also made it possible for me to have the good fortune of working with the truly remarkable colleagues who collaborated on this book, including each of the editors and contributors. I am especially grateful to David Sarwer for all of his hard work and his unceasing dedication to making this book the best possible piece of scholarship we could create; to John Persing who I have been privileged to know for 20 years and for whom I have the greatest respect and admiration; and to Tom Cash, who is surely the best colleague and friend one could imagine. I also consider it a great honor to have collaborated on this book with Drs. Goldwyn and Whitaker, both of whom have made many exceptional contributions to our understanding of the psychological experience of plastic surgery patients.

My deep appreciation also goes to Dr. Joseph McCarthy at the New York University Medical School Institute of Reconstructive Plastic Surgery (NYU-IRPS), who graciously and generously opened many doors of opportunity for me. It is a particularly special pleasure to express my deep gratitude and respect for Patricia Chibbaro, RN (NYU-IRPS) who is a paragon of selfless service to those in need. May her generosity be repaid a thousandfold! Thank you also to the Quinnipiac University Research Committee for granting me time to work on this project.

I also very much want to acknowledge my brother Chris, who died during the completion of this book. He gave the world many wonderful gifts, including his magnificent sense of humor. May he and all who loved him be at peace. It is not possible to thank my parents enough for all they have given me. They gave both Chris and me all the love and care that two sons could ever hope for.

My deepest thanks go to my precious wife—the best friend and companion anyone could ever hope for. Without her patience, support, and love, there is absolutely no way I would have the career I have been privileged to pursue. If you think I am exaggerating or just being nice by saying this, you would be mistaken. This is the truth.

Tom Cash—Over the course of my 32-year career as a clinical and research psychologist, there have been many people who have contributed to the pleasure and productivity of my professional life. I will always be grateful to Paul Dokecki, my graduate school mentor at George Peabody College of Vanderbilt Univerity, who convinced me, against my naïve resistance, to conduct my dissertation research on how physical appearance influences interpersonal interactions. I'm one of those fortunate academics whose first job was a keeper. My faculty colleagues in the Department of Psychology at Old Dominion University have provided a friendly and supportive organizational climate enabling me to "do my thing." I am indebted to the many graduate and undergraduate students with whom I have worked and learned and enjoyed the challenges of psychological science. Without

these wonderful, motivating students, my work would have just been work.

I offer my heartfelt thanks to three psychologists who are modern-day pioneers in the field of human appearance and body image. First, Tom Pruzinsky is a true friend and one of the most genuine and selfless people I know. This is the third book on which he and I have collaborated. He always brings a synthesis of devotion to detail, freshness of perspective, and contagious enthusiasm to whatever we are working on. It was Tom who, many years ago, taught me to see the significance of the interface of body image and medical/health specialties. Second, I am sincerely grateful to Kevin Thompson at the University of South Florida. My friend Kevin is a prolific and imaginative body image researcher, who's been at it nearly as long as I have. He contributes substantially to the field and has inspired me greatly. Finally, I am forever thankful to David Sarwer. This volume reflects his unbelievably hard work to make it the best that it can be. As you will see in reading the book, David's contributions to a contemporary scientific understanding of the psychological aspects of plastic surgery are unsurpassed. Those of us in the field who are beginning to contemplate retirement are reassured that, as a young, innovative scientist, he will continue to be "the captain of the ship."

As always, I thank my sons, TC and Ben. Who they are and the lives they live give me greater satisfaction than anything I've ever done professionally.

We would be remiss if we neglected to thank our editorial team at Lippincott Williams & Wilkins. Brian Brown, Joanne Bersin, Karen Carter, Michelle LaPlante, and James Mulligan have all contributed to the development of this project. Julia Seto and Fran Gunning joined the project toward the end and did a fantastic job bringing the book together. Rebecca Dodson and Cathy Tounsend, Sue McKinnon, Linda Attman, and Kristen Kriesant at Schawk Publishing Solutions made rounding the chapters into shape look easy. To all of the individuals named here, and countless others, we thank you for your help in bringing this book to the fields of plastic surgery and psychology.

CONTENTS

Understanding the Psychology of Plastic Surgery

Chapter 1

Multiple Perspectives on the Psychology of Plastic Surgery

Thomas Pruzinsky, PhD, David B. Sarwer, PhD, Thomas F. Cash, PhD, Robert M. Goldwyn, MD, John A. Persing, MD, and Linton A. Whitaker, MD

Patients entering the offices and operating rooms of plastic surgeons desire to change their physical appearance and/or physical functioning. Although patients may not explicitly articulate the thought, they understand that the ultimate goal of surgery is to bring about psychological change. From the patients' perspective, they undergo plastic surgery to reduce distress and maximize quality of life.

From the plastic surgeon's perspective, the primary goal of surgery is to provide the patient with the best possible aesthetic and functional outcome. Surgeons often recognize the psychological motivations for, and effects of, surgery, but usually contemplate these only when significant emotional problems become evident. However, by cultivating a deeper understanding of the many causes and consequences of patients' psychological distress, plastic surgeons may come to recognize that surgery alone may not always be the only method to relieve that distress.

Mental health professionals can help bridge the gap between the patient's psychological motivations for, and response to, surgery and the surgeon's tentative understanding of the patient's psychological experiences. This book is based on the premise that by integrating a well-developed psychological understanding of the plastic surgery patient into a surgeon's routine clinical practice, significant improvements in the quality of patient care will occur—improvements that cannot be achieved by surgery alone.

This chapter highlights historical and contemporary developments that shape our current understanding of the psychology of plastic surgery. The chapter also makes clear that such understanding must include an appreciation for the psychological challenges faced by both reconstructive and cosmetic surgery patients and the complementary roles of clinical experience and scientific research in enhancing our knowledge.

HISTORICAL PERSPECTIVES ON THE PSYCHOLOGY OF PLASTIC SURGERY

Attempts to recognize and comprehend the psychological aspects of plastic surgery have a long history. The often-used quotation from the renowned 16th century plastic surgeon, Gaspari Tagliacozzi, asserts a noble aspiration of plastic surgeons: "We restore, repair, and make whole those parts which fortune has taken away, not so much that they delight the eyes but that they may buoy up the spirit and help the mind of the beset."

This quotation captures the heart of the intention of this book. A plastic surgeon's increased psychological understanding of patients can greatly contribute to the surgeon's skills.

The Contributions of Milton Edgerton

The genesis of this book was strongly influenced by the work of Milton Edgerton, who wrote the Foreword. Any book on the psychology of plastic surgery would be neither credible nor complete without making clear his many contributions to the field.

Edgerton cultivated his interest in, and knowledge of, the psychological aspects of plastic surgery from the earliest stages of his career at Johns Hopkins University in the 1950s and through his long tenure at the University of Virginia Medical Center. He and his colleagues published scores of papers on a wide range of psychological topics over five decades. These include, but are not limited to, pioneering descriptions of the motivations for breast augmentation (1–2), rhinoplasty (3), and rhytidectomy (4–5). Presciently, Edgerton et al. also described the psychological characteristics of the "minimal deformity" (6) and "insatiable" patient (7), which are likely the first descriptions of plastic surgery patients who are now believed to have body dysmorphic disorder and are discussed at length in the cosmetic surgery section of this book. Edgerton and his colleagues also illuminated the unique psychological characteristics of male (8) and adolescent patients (9). They provided what are now classic descriptions of distinct patterns of psychological motivation for surgery (10–11), as well as, some of the earliest discussion of patients with factitious wounds (12). He certainly appreciated the crucial role of body image in understanding plastic surgery patients (13). Many of his papers were the first formal investigations of these patient groups and were catalysts for much of the subsequent scientific work discussed throughout this book.

Edgerton's compassion was evinced by his deep commitment to understanding the psychological experience of his patients. Over five decades of practice, he spent countless hours in extended clinical consultations learning to empathize with a patient's experience of deformity as "dis-ease" (14). He discerned a core clinical truth of plastic surgery—namely, that having a deformity, either real or perceived, causes great emotional distress ("dis-ease") and that treating this psychological suffering is the heart of the plastic surgeon's work.

Throughout his career, Edgerton's courage was evident in his willingness to treat many patients who suffered greatly but who were often shunned by colleagues. These patients included transsexuals (15–19) and persons with particularly severe forms of psychopathology. Often, other plastic surgeons looked askance at his persistent willingness to help these uncared for individuals. Despite the resistance, he continually stressed "the plastic surgeon's obligation to the emotionally disturbed patient" (20) and explored just how far the healing powers of plastic surgery could be stretched to reduce patient unhappiness and to enhance quality of life. He collaborated closely with a series of mental health colleagues over the span of his career, setting the standard for how to improve clinical and scientific understanding of plastic surgery patients (21–23).

The Contributions of John and Marcia Goin

The plastic surgeon–psychiatrist team of John and Maria Goin embodied the integration of surgical and psychiatric perspectives. Their collaborative research covered a wide range of topics (24–30) and offered informative perspectives on such critical issues as a patient's psychological reactions while under local anesthesia (27) and the psychological experience of tissue expansion (30). Among the Goins' many insights were that a substantial number of facelift patients experienced a period of postoperative depression that was associated with preoperative depressive symptoms (24) and that some reduction mammaplasty patients experienced negative postoperative psychological adjustment reactions not routinely detected by the plastic surgeon (26). The Goins are particularly well-known for their informative text, *Changing the Body: Psychological Effects of Plastic Surgery* (31). The book was the only resource of its kind for over two decades and provided a foundation on which this book was built.

Other Contributions

Several other books over the past decade have directly or indirectly touched on the psychological issues in plastic surgery. Sander Gilman has written two books, *Making the Body Beautiful* (32) and *Creating Beauty to Cure the Soul: Race and Psychology in the Shaping of Aesthetic Surgery* (33), which discuss the relationship between cosmetic surgery and psychology against the larger historical backdrop of race and culture. Elizabeth Haiken's (34) *Venus Envy: A History of Cosmetic Surgery* touches on similar themes. Kathy Davis's *Reshaping the Female Body: The Dilemma of Cosmetic Surgery* (35) and *Dubious Equalities and Embodied Differences: Cultural Studies on Cosmetic Surgery* (36), as well as Virginia Blum's *Flesh Wounds: The Culture of Cosmetic Surgery* (37) all look at the evolution of cosmetic surgery in relation to cultural influences. Although not specifically focused on plastic surgery, Marilyn Yalom's *The History of the Breast* (38) and Nancy Etcoff's *Survival of the Prettiest: The Science of Beauty* (39) are also helpful in understanding of the psychology of physical appearance.

PLASTIC SURGERY IN 2005

The explosion in the popularity of plastic surgery and cosmetic surgery, in particular, underscores the timeliness of this book. According to the American Society of Plastic Surgeons (ASPS), over 13.5 million plastic surgical procedures were performed in 2004 (40). As seen in Table 1-1, the majority of procedures were minimally invasive cosmetic procedures, many of which did not exist in 1992 when the ASPS started tracking procedures. Cosmetic surgical procedures have grown in popularity over the past decade, leveling off in the past several years. Table 1-2 presents the number of reconstructive procedures performed in 2004, 2000, and 1992.

These statistics, while familiar to many plastic surgeons, are often staggering to lay persons who have little idea of the frequency with which Americans now look to medicine to enhance their appearance. Nevertheless, these numbers are likely an underestimate of the number of procedures performed annually, as they do not account for the increasing number of non-plastic surgeon physicians who now offer these treatments.

How can we understand the dramatic increase in the popularity of cosmetic surgery? The answer likely comes from at least three different areas (41–42). As noted throughout this book, changes in the medical and surgical community—from improved safety and wound care to direct-to-consumer marketing—have likely contributed to the growth. The mass media and entertainment industries have long championed plastic surgery, perhaps no more so than during the current era of "reality-based" cosmetic surgery television programs and Golden Globe winning fictional dramas about the profession. As discussed in Chapter 3, the relentless bombardment of mass media ideals of beauty has likely contributed as well. Chapter 4 points to evidence of a growing discontent over several decades that many people, especially women, have experienced with respect to their physical appearance. Finally, our society's increasing acceptance of the use of medicine to enhance appearance, coupled, perhaps, with a greater awareness of the importance of physical appearance in daily life, has potentially fueled cosmetic surgery's increase in popularity.

▶ TABLE 1-1 Cosmetic Surgical and Minimally Invasive Procedures Performed in 2004, 2002, and 1992

COSMETIC PROCEDURES	2004	2002	1992	Percent Change 2002 vs 2004
Breast augmentation	264,041	212,500	32,607	24%
Breast implant removals[a]	35,208	40,787	18,297	−14%
Breast lift (Mastopexy)	75,805	52,836	7,963	43%
Breast reduction in men (Gynecomastia)	13,963	20,351	4,997	−31%
Buttock lift	3,496	1,356	291	158%
Cheek implants	9,318	10,427	1,741	−11%
Chin augmentation	15,822	26,924	4,115	−41%
Dermabrasion	54,018	42,218	13,457	28%
Ear surgery (Otoplasty)	25,915	36,295	6,371	−29%
Eyelid surgery (Blepharoplasty)	233,334	327,514	59,461	−29%
Facelift	114,279	133,856	40,077	−15%
Forehead lift	54,993	120,971	13,501	−55%
Hair transplantation	48,925	44,694	1,955	9%
Lip augmentation (other than injectables)	26,730	18,589	—	44%
Lipoplasty (liposuction)	324,891	354,015	47,212	−8%
Lower body lift	8,926	207	—	4212%
Nose reshaping (Rhinoplasty)	305,475	389,155	50,175	−22%
Thigh lift[b]	8,123	5,303	1,023	53%
Tummy tuck (Abdominoplasty)	107,019	62,713	16,810	71%
Upper arm lift[b]	9,955	338	434	2845%
TOTAL COSMETIC SURGICAL PROCEDURES	1,740,236	1,901,049	320,487	−8%
Botox® injection[c]	2,992,607	786,911	—	280%
Cellulite treatment	44,569	23,952	—	86%
Chemical peel	1,090,523	1,149,457	19,049	−5%
Laser hair removal	573,970	735,996	—	−22%
Laser skin resurfacing	164,451	170,951	—	−4%
Laser treatment of leg veins	103,460	245,424	—	−58%
Microdermabrasion	858,867	868,315	—	−1%
Sclerotherapy	544,898	866,555	—	−37%
Soft tissue fillers:				
Calcium hydroxylapatite (Radiance™)	56,631	—	—	N/A
Collagen	521,769	587,615	41,623	−11%
Fat	56,377	65,270	—	−14%
Hyaluronic acid (Hylaform®, Restylane®)	461,397	—	—	N/A
TOTAL COSMETIC MINIMALLY- INVASIVE PROCEDURES	7,470,391	5,500,446	60,672	36%
TOTAL COSMETIC PROCEDURES	9,210,627	7,401,495	413,208	24%

Statistical data courtesy of the American Society of Plastic Surgeons (ASPS).
N/A = Not available (was not asked in prior survey).
[a] 70% of breast implant removals in 2004 were replaced.
[b] 76% of total 2004 thigh and upper arm lifts were after massive weight loss.
[c] The number reported for 2004 Botox injections is the number of anatomic sites injected.
Final figures are projected to reflect nationwide statistics and represent procedures performed by ASPS member plastic surgeons certified by the American Board of Plastic Surgery® as well as other physicians certified by American Board of Medical Specialties-recognized boards.

▶ TABLE 1-2 Reconstructive Surgical Procedures Performed in 2004, 2002, and 1992

RECONSTRUCTIVE PROCEDURES	2004	2002	1992	Percent Change 2002 vs 2004
Animal bite repair	44,801	43,089	10,376	4%
Birth defect reconstruction	38,583	40,076	33,501	−4%
Breast implant removals[a]	16,424	16,806	18,297	−2%
Breast reconstruction	62,930	80,908	29,607	−22%
Breast reduction	105,592	84,780	39,639	25%
Burn care	35,720	31,058	17,552	15%
Hand surgery	179,046	208,878	138,233	−14%
Laceration repair	314,844	358,666	135,494	−12%
Maxillofacial surgery	84,469	79,331	22,095	6%
Microsurgery	34,584	32,037	19,405	8%
Scar revision	187,386	221,858	52,647	−16%
Tumor removal	4,084,651	4,609,882	502,567	−11%
Other reconstructive procedures	386,157	376,270	116,737	3%
TOTAL RECONSTRUCTIVE PROCEDURES	5,575,187	6,183,639	1,127,690	−10%

Statistical data courtesy of the American Society of Plastic Surgeons (ASPS)
[a] 28% of reconstructive breast implants removed in 2004 were replaced
Final figures are projected to reflect nationwide statistics and represent procedures performed by ASPS member plastic surgeons certified by the American Board of Plastic Surgery® as well as other physicians certified by American Board of Medical Specialties-recognized boards.

SURGICAL AND PSYCHOLOGICAL PERSPECTIVES

This book seeks to build a bridge between the perspectives of plastic surgery and psychology. Indeed, by no accident, the editors of this volume are three psychologists and three plastic surgeons. In building this bridge between the two disciplines, we wish to emphasize three points. First, we do not believe that plastic surgeons need to become de facto mental health professionals to appropriately treat their patients. Second, we also do not believe that all plastic surgery patients require formal psychological evaluation or treatment prior to plastic surgery. Third, we do believe that an increased understanding of the psychological aspects of plastic surgery can surely enhance the quality of patient care.

Plastic surgeons typically have not been provided with adequate training in how to better understand the emotional and interpersonal aspects of patient functioning, a point amplified in Chapters 2 and 19. Nevertheless, many surgeons could benefit from an opportunity to develop these skills. To obtain such training and integrate these skills into their everyday practice adds to the already demanding burdens that all surgeons experience. However, compared to their investments in developing surgical skills, the amount of time and effort needed to develop a deeper understanding of the psychological functioning of their patients is relatively small. Yet, this investment can have a payoff—including higher rates of patient satisfaction, reduced patient distress, and higher levels of patient quality of life.

Psychologists and other mental health providers also can benefit from an increased understanding of the psychological aspects of plastic surgery. Given the large numbers of individuals undergoing plastic surgery, it is increasingly likely that all mental health professionals will encounter people who have undergone or who are contemplating undergoing a plastic surgical procedure. As evident throughout this book, there is a need for mental health professionals to develop specialized clinical competencies for selected patient populations. Furthermore, it is primarily through the collaboration of plastic surgeons and mental health professionals that progress will be made in scientific understanding of the motivations for, and outcomes of, all types of plastic surgery.

Just as there continues to be important, steady advances in surgical techniques, there have been many important advances in our understanding of the psychological functioning of plastic surgery patients. In particular, a great deal of progress has been made in clarifying and specifying the relationship between an individual's body image and interest in, and reactions to, plastic surgery. Many chapters in this book review the substantial value of a cognitive-behavioral model for understanding body image, psychological assessment, and treatment in the care of plastic surgery patients. Both mental health professionals and plastic surgeons can greatly benefit from learning how this model can be used to provide effective and cost-efficient services for the full spectrum of patients.

RECONSTRUCTIVE AND COSMETIC PERSPECTIVES

Quite often, attempts to understand psychological issues in plastic surgery have come from inquiries into the motives and responses of cosmetic surgery patients. There is much to learn, however, about the psychological experience of reconstructive surgery patients. In fact, the reader of this volume will note that there are twice as many chapters on reconstructive surgery than on cosmetic surgery.

The two groups of patients share many commonalities, including concerns that are best understood in terms of body image functioning, a recurrent theme throughout this text. However, reconstructive surgery patients often experience different psychological motivations for, and responses to, surgery. For example, they may have to cope with the social responses to their disfigurement. Some patients who undergo reconstructive surgery (including those with burn injuries, facial trauma, or hand trauma) may experience symptoms of post-traumatic stress disorder. Because of the nature of their disease or injury, reconstructive surgery patients most commonly have less "choice" than cosmetic surgery patients regarding the need for surgery. Often, their life has been (and still may be) threatened by their condition. They also may be going through extended periods of rehabilitation with uncertain outcomes.

Cosmetic surgery patients, on the other hand, have decided of their own volition to enhance their appearance through surgery. In most instances, there is minimal direct social pressure to undergo treatment. They anticipate that surgery will result in a better life and have specific hoped-for changes. Though many do not experience blatant psychopathology, some do suffer from depression, anxiety, and, in some cases, body dysmorphic disorder.

The skilled plastic surgeon will learn how to meet the different psychological needs of these diverse patient groups. One of the first steps in this process is to understand the typical psychological responses of patients. Thus, the vast majority of the chapters in this book focus on specific groups of patients. The chapter authors provide a detailed discussion of the sometimes unique psychological issues of these patients.

CLINICAL AND EMPIRICAL PERSPECTIVES

The professions of plastic surgery and psychology both share a deeply held commitment to the ideal of integrating clinical experience and scientific knowledge as the primary way to improve the quality of patient care. Most chapters in the book provide a comprehensive review of the extant scholarly psychological literature pertinent to the topic at hand. Many chapters also offer practical, concrete, and experienced guidance for the plastic surgeon. Clinical cases are often used to illustrate the psychological management of both routine and challenging patients. In addition, chapters 4–13 and 16 include brief questionnaires that can be used to more effectively assess patients' psychological concerns. Although some of these questionnaires have not been subjected to rigorous psychometric evaluation, they will, without question, provide helpful clinical information to the plastic surgery team. These patient psychological self-reports can serve as foundations for more detailed discussions during surgical consultations.

Many of the chapters provide clear suggestions on how plastic surgeons can effectively refer patients to mental health professionals. This skill is not frequently taught, but it is easily learned. By mastering the skills of psychological screening and effective patient referral, the plastic surgeon can appropriately handle more challenging situations and provide these individuals with the most appropriate care.

FUTURE DEVELOPMENTS IN THE PSYCHOLOGY OF PLASTIC SURGERY

This book is a testament to the progress already made in our understanding of the psychological aspects of plastic surgery. However, there is still much clinical understanding to be gained and scientific research to be conducted if the goal is to attain the highest standards of care possible.

The contributors to this book have, in many cases, proposed clear standards of care to address patients' psychological needs. These standards have been created on the foundation of systematic research. This is clearly true for craniofacial surgery and also quite evident in pediatric and adult burn care, though surely much remains to be learned about the lives of these individuals. Clinical understanding and research on hand trauma, breast reduction, and breast reconstruction also have achieved some significant advances. However, there is less known in the area of acquired facial disfigurement and adjustment to genital disorders.

Taken *in toto,* the clinical and scientific knowledge regarding how psychology can be applied to, and integrated with, the practice of plastic surgery is developmentally in early adolescence. Each chapter in this book provides a solid foundation on which future knowledge will be built. However, many important questions remain. These include, but are not limited to, the following:

- What is the best way to train plastic surgeons to integrate knowledge regarding the psychology of plastic surgery into their routine clinical practice? Can the development of these skills be made a routine part of resident training?
- Is it possible to establish standards of care in plastic surgery to address psychological issues? (Precedent exists in the areas of craniofacial surgery, gender identity disorders, and, to a significant degree, in burn care.)
- How can we integrate what is known about body image assessment and treatment into the routine evaluation and care of plastic surgery patients?
- In the course of everyday clinical practice, what is the most efficient and effective way to identify patients in need of psychological assessment or treatment?
- What needs to occur to create more frequent and closer collaborations in clinical practice between plastic surgeons and mental health professionals?
- What are the best ways of providing psychological therapy and rehabilitation interventions? Can we provide scientific documentation of their effectiveness?
- How can standards of psychological care be raised while also addressing the issue of cost to the patient and/or third-party reimbursement?
- How can we establish an extensive collaborative network between plastic surgeons and psychological researchers to collect ongoing systematic data on important questions about optimizing patient care?

Perhaps the most significant barrier to progress in raising treatment standards in which patients' psychological concerns are systematically assessed and addressed has been the lack of a clear, well-delineated body of clinical and scientific knowledge.

Hopefully, with the publication of this book, this barrier has been removed and the next generation of treatment innovations and research advances will become clearer.

SUMMARY

After reading this book, we hope that plastic surgeons, along with their nursing and other health care colleagues, can walk into their next patient consultation with a renewed and deepened appreciation and understanding of the psychological experience of that patient. To use this book for the purposes for which it was created, the reader may wish to choose a patient care chapter that is of greatest interest, read it, and contemplate how you might approach your next patient consultation in a slightly different way than you typically would. What could you do differently, in terms of how you listen, how you observe, and what you ask?

By returning to the text and reviewing its many other topics, all members of the plastic surgery team can steadily develop their psychological knowledge and skills in patient care. If reading this book does not lead to a change in the manner in which patients are cared for, then it will have failed its ultimate purpose—to help reduce patient distress and improve patient quality of life. Both of these goals can be accomplished in many ways; perhaps one of the most important of which is helping patients to feel that their psychological experiences—their body image concerns, their hopes, and anxieties—have been truly heard and understood.

REFERENCES

1. Edgerton MT, McClary AR. Augmentation mammaplasty: psychiatric implications and surgical indications. *Plast Reconstr Surg* 1958;21:279–305.
2. Edgerton MT, Jacobson WE, Meyer E. Augmentation mammaplasty II: further surgical and psychiatric consideration. *Plast Reconstr Surg* 1961;27:279–302.
3. Jacobson WE, Meyer E, Edgerton MT, et al. Screening of rhinoplasty patients from the psychologic point of view. *Plast Reconstr Surg* 1961;28:279–281.
4. Edgerton MT, Webb WL, Slaughter R, et al. Surgical results and psychosocial changes following rhytidectomy. *Plast Reconstr Surg* 1964;33:503–521.
5. Webb WL Jr, Slaughter R, Meyer E, et al. Mechanisms of psychosocial adjustment in patients seeking "face lift" operation. *Psychosom Med* 1965;27:183–192.
6. Edgerton MT, Jacobson WE, Meyer E. Surgical-psychiatric study of patients seeking plastic (cosmetic) surgery: ninety-eight patients with minimal deformity. *Br J Plast Surg* 1960;13:136–145.
7. Knorr NJ, Edgerton MT, Hoopes JE. The "insatiable" cosmetic surgery patient. *Plast Reconstr Surg* 1967;40:285–288.
8. Jacobson WE, Edgerton MT, Meyer E, et al. Psychiatric evaluation of male patients seeking cosmetic surgery. *Plast Reconstr Surg* 1960;26:356–372.
9. Knorr NJ, Hoopes JE, Edgerton MT. Psychiatric-surgical approach to adolescent disturbance in self image. *Plast Reconstr Surg* 1968;41:248–253.
10. Meyer E, Jacobson WE, Edgerton MT, et al. Motivational patterns in patients seeking elective plastic surgery (women who seek rhinoplasty). *Psychosom Med* 1960;22:193–203.
11. Edgerton MT, Knorr NJ. Motivational patterns of patients seeking cosmetic (esthetic) surgery. *Plast Reconstr Surg* 1971;48:551–557.
12. Drinker H, Knorr NJ, Edgerton MT Jr. Factitious wounds. A psychiatric and surgical dilemma. *Plast Reconstr Surg* 1972;50:458–461.
13. Pruzinsky T, Edgerton MT. Body-image change and cosmetic plastic surgery. In: Cash TF, Pruzinsky T, eds. *Body Images: Development, Deviance, and Change.* New York: Guilford Press, 1990:217–236.
14. Edgerton MT. Deformity is a disease. *Trans Stud Coll Physicians Phila* 1973;41:124–130.
15. Edgerton MT, Knorr NJ, Callison JR. The surgical treatment of transsexual patients. Limitations and indications. *Plast Reconstr Surg* 1970;45:38–46.
16. Edgerton MT, Meyer JK. Surgical and psychiatric aspects of transsexualism. In: Horton C, ed. *Plastic and Reconstructive Surgery of the Genital Area.* Boston: Little, Brown and Company, 1973:117–161.
17. Edgerton MT, Langman MW, Schmidt JS, et al. Psychological considerations of gender reassignment surgery. *Clin Plast Surg* 1982;9:355–366.
18. Pauly IB, Edgerton MT. The gender identity movement: a growing surgical psychiatric liaison. *Arch Sex Behav* 1986;15:315–329.
19. Edgerton MT, Kenney JG, Langman MW. Gender reassignment surgery. In: Georgiade NG, Georgiade GS, Riefkohl R, Barwick WJ, eds. *Essentials of Plastic, Maxillofacial, and Reconstructive Surgery.* Baltimore: Williams & Wilkins, 1987:780–796.

20. Edgerton MT. The plastic surgeon's obligation to the emotionally disturbed patient. *Plast Reconstr Surg* 1975;55:81–83.
21. Thomson JA Jr, Knorr NJ, Edgerton MT Jr. Cosmetic surgery: the psychiatric perspective. *Psychosomatics* 1978;19:7–15.
22. Pruzinsky T, Edgerton MT, Barth JT. Medical psychotherapy and plastic surgery: collaboration, specialization and cost-effectiveness. In: Anchor K, ed. *The Handbook of Medical Psychotherapy.* Toronto: Hans Huber Publishers, 1991:101–122.
23. Pruzinsky T, Edgerton MT. Psychological understanding and management of the plastic surgery patient. In: Georgiade NG, Georgiade GS, Riefkohl R, Barwick WJ, eds. *Essentials of Plastic, Maxillofacial, and Reconstructive Surgery.* Baltimore: Williams & Wilkins, 1997:1189–1197.
24. Goin MK, Burgoyne RW, Goin JM. Face-lift operation: the patient's secret motivations and reactions to "informed consent." *Plast Reconstr Surg* 1976;58:273–279.
25. Goin MK. Psychological understanding and management of rhinoplasty patients. *Clin Plast Surg* 1977;4:3–7.
26. Goin MK, Goin JM, Gianini MH. The psychic consequences of a reduction mammaplasty. *Plast Reconstr Surg* 1977;59:530–534.
27. Burgoyne RW, Goin JM, Goin MK. Intraoperative psychological reactions in face-lift patients under local anesthesia. *Plast Reconstr Surg* 1977;60:582–588.
28. Goin MK, Goin JM. Midlife reactions to mastectomy and subsequent breast reconstruction. *Arch Gen Psychiatry* 1981;38:225–227.
29. Goin MK, Goin JM. Psychological reactions to prophylactic mastectomy synchronous with contralateral breast reconstruction. *Plast Reconstr Surg* 1982;70:355–359.
30. Goin MK, Goin JM. Growing pains: the psychological experience of breast reconstruction with tissue expansion. *Ann Plast Surg* 1988;21:217–222.
31. Goin JM, Goin MK. *Changing the Body: Psychological Effects of Plastic Surgery.* Baltimore: Williams & Wilkins, 1981.
32. Gilman SL. *Making the Body Beautiful: A Cultural History of Aesthetic Surgery.* Princeton, NJ: Princeton University Press, 1999.
33. Gilman SL. *Creating Beauty to Cure the Soul: Race and Psychology in the Shaping of Aesthetic Surgery.* Durham, NC: Duke University Press, 1998.
34. Haiken E. *Venus Envy: A History of Cosmetic Surgery.* Baltimore: The Johns Hopkins University Press, 1999.
35. Davis K. *Reshaping the Female Body: The Dilemma of Cosmetic Surgery.* New York: Routledge, 1995.
36. Davis K. *Dubious Equalities and Embodied Differences: Cultural Studies on Cosmetic Surgery.* Lanham, MD: Rowman & Littlefield, 2003.
37. Blum VL. *Flesh Wounds: The Culture of Cosmetic Surgery.* Berkeley, CA: University of California Press, 2003.
38. Yalom M. *A History of the Breast.* New York: Ballantine Books, 1998.
39. Etcoff N. *Survival of the Prettiest: The Science of Beauty.* New York: Anchor, 1999.
40. *2005 Report of the 2004 National Clearinghouse of Plastic Surgery Statistics.* Arlington Heights, IL: American Society of Plastic Surgeons, 2005.
41. Sarwer DB, Crerand CE. Body image and cosmetic medical treatments. *Body Image: An International Journal of Research* 2004;1:99–111.
42. Sarwer DB, Magee L, Crerand CE. Cosmetic surgery and cosmetic medical treatments. In: Thompson JK, ed. *Handbook of Eating Disorders and Obesity.* Hoboken, NJ: John Wiley and Sons, 2004:718–737.

Chapter 2

Psychological Aspects of Plastic Surgery: A Surgeon's Observations and Reflections

Robert M. Goldwyn, MD

Like any physician, the plastic surgeon can greatly benefit from developing a reasonable set of psychological skills that he or she can use in providing the highest level of care. This is a necessity not a luxury, because it can mean the difference between a successful or unsuccessful outcome, for both the patient and the surgeon. For example, the plastic surgeon performing a cosmetic procedure must realize that a technically well-performed operation does not guarantee a satisfied patient (1). It is quite often the case that understanding the patient's motivations and personality can be as crucial to the ultimate outcome as undertaking the actual surgical procedure. Similarly, surgeons should be aware of their own motivations and attitudes toward their practice. It is important that each plastic surgeon have a willingness and capacity to engage in introspection.

This chapter provides a plastic surgeon's view of the psychological aspects of plastic surgery. It begins with a general discussion of basic preoperative considerations. Several specific patient types associated with an increased likelihood of a poor postoperative outcome are highlighted. Postoperative considerations, particularly as they relate to issues of patient satisfaction, are also reviewed. This chapter concludes by addressing the question: "Can plastic surgeons enhance their psychological skills?"

PREOPERATIVE CONSIDERATIONS

From the plastic surgeon's point of view, the major objective of the initial consultation is likely the proper selection of the patient. The patient's medical history and current status determine whether the patient is medically appropriate for a given procedure. Cosmetic surgery is almost always elective, and patients are almost always in good health. The patient, however, is willing to risk this good health (at least to a limited extent) in order to experience improvements in physical appearance, and perhaps more importantly, self-esteem, body image, and quality of life. In this context, the plastic surgeon is in the somewhat odd position of making a healthy patient "ill" in order to help him or her feel better about himself or herself.

Perhaps as a result of this, the initial consultation in plastic surgery is more important than any other visit. The consultation with a cosmetic surgeon is different from other surgical consultations in at least one respect. In cosmetic surgery, the patient is, more often than not, hoping that the surgeon will recommend surgery. By contrast, in the case of neurosurgery or orthopedics, for example, the patient is likely hoping that the surgeon will not recommend surgery. In some respects, this difference places a greater emphasis on the nature of the surgeon–patient interpersonal relationship than is likely found in other surgical specialties.

The initial consultation brings together a patient and surgeon who have probably never known each other. Each brings with them an established personality with behavior patterns evolved from innumerable responses to countless previous social interactions and life events stimuli (2). In theory, the patient and the surgeon could interact in infinite ways in this initial meeting. In reality, they do not. Rather, both likely behave in a manner more or less consistent with typical sociocultural roles. What happens is remarkably circumscribed. The patient is there to decide whether or not to receive care from the surgeon or to convince the surgeon to comply with his or her desire to have surgery. In turn, the surgeon is making a decision concerning whether or not to accept that person as a patient. This evaluative process puts the personality characteristics of both individuals on display.

The patient can recognize arrogance, hostility, and other negative personality traits even when the surgeon believes that these traits are well hidden (or is unaware of them). Similarly, the patient who has been kept waiting an inordinately long time will recognize and appreciate a sincere apology and not one that is perfunctory. As much as possible, it is useful for the surgeon to imagine himself or herself in the role of the patient. By doing so, the surgeon will find it easier to understand the patient's perspective and, perhaps, the patient's motivations and emotions. This awareness will likely have a positive impact on rapport.

By imagining themselves in the position of the patient, surgeons may have a better understanding of the guilt and embarrassment experienced by some cosmetic surgery patients who may be at least mildly ashamed about seeking surgery to improve appearance. Cosmetic surgery involves the elusive objective of happiness, which is an implied outcome of a successful postoperative result. Again, this is in contrast to other areas of medicine, where the efficacy of therapy is usually measured in terms of the reduction or elimination of symptoms or improved function. The prolonged recoveries often observed in other surgical specialties are seen with far less frequency in cosmetic surgery. Patients who experience complications that result in an unexpectedly long recovery are often disappointed and angry. As discussed later in this chapter and also in Chapter 19, the quality of the surgeon–patient relationship becomes critically important in these situations.

POTENTIALLY PROBLEMATIC PATIENTS FROM A PSYCHOLOGICAL PERSPECTIVE

Individuals with a variety of personality types are believed to be potentially problematic patients in a plastic surgery practice (2–5). (Several of these patient types are also discussed in the context of patient selection from a legal perspective in Chapter 19.) Persons with these characteristics require careful evaluation by the surgeon, and often by a qualified mental health professional, before being accepted as a surgical patient. Although not formally studied, mental health professionals would likely diagnose these individuals with personality or other disorders. Several chapters throughout this book discuss the formal psychiatric diagnoses likely to be seen within select groups of plastic surgery patients.

The VIP Patient

The VIP patient may be a local or national celebrity, professionally successful, or simply an individual who believes that he or she warrants special treatment from the surgeon and staff. These patients' strong sense of entitlement leads them to expect special treatment and not to be held to the same rules as others. A VIP patient's renown, wealth, or power does not change anatomy or physiology and certainly does not eliminate the hazards of undergoing any procedure.

The danger with this type of individual is that surgical judgment may be in deference to fame or self-importance. Without realizing it, and without the patient demanding it, the surgeon may make medical decisions for the VIP patient that he or she would not make for others. Departure from the surgeon's routine office practice, standards of care, or personal comfort zone may increase the likelihood of an undesirable result (3). As highlighted in Chapter 16, members of the office or nursing staff may be the first to recognize these patients. They may be on their best behavior with the surgeon, but treat the staff with a lack of respect or decency. Surgeons should encourage staff to alert them about such behavior.

The VIP patient often has difficulty dealing with routine office procedures. Some refuse to accept the next available appointment and will try to bypass the secretary to be seen earlier. Others may herald their initial visit with a letter or phone call that is not simply providing information but is also pleading their case for surgery and appealing to the surgeon's ego (as discussed below). Generally such letters contain an obsessively described saga of repeated dissatisfaction following multiple treatments of a condition that may be objectively less major than the patient believes. In these cases, as well as others where there is concern about a patient's previous surgical treatment history, previous medical records should be obtained.

During the consultation, some patients may become overly friendly with the surgeon. Some may address a doctor on a first name basis without asking. Occasionally, surgeons may find themselves in consultation with patients who have made themselves overly comfortable in the office or consultation room. The patient may look through papers or remove books from the shelves. In my experience, this patient is less curious than aggressive and wishes to assume control of his or her care by establishing an immediate intimacy. This behavior may reflect some underlying anxiety about dependency and perhaps the patient is trying to allay uneasiness by dominating the situation.

When these VIP patient behaviors force the surgeon to practice outside of a typical comfort zone, it may be useful to call to the patient's attention that they seem to be having a difficult time being a patient. The surgeon may even consider disclosing an understanding of the problem, because he or she, as a physician, also has difficulty being a patient. In fact, sometimes this kind of patient is a physician.

The Patient Who Appeals to the Surgeon's Ego

Some patients understand that few surgeons, like most people, can resist flattery. This patient may plump the surgeon's ego with praise, saying, "I heard you are the best in town/in the country/in the world." In reality, the patient usually has no valid frame of reference for this opinion and may be responding to a flattering newspaper story or word of mouth from friends. Such adulation should not persuade the surgeon to perform an operation that will never satisfy the patient.

Some patients may appeal to the surgeon's ego through flirtation. In these instances, the surgeon must immediately restructure the interaction to stop this inappropriate behavior. This often can be done by speaking to the patient in a serious, matter-of-fact tone and avoiding intimate conversation and playful banter. The surgeon should likewise monitor the use of unnecessary personal touch as well as more flippant ("Honey, you will look beautiful") or sexual language ("You will look really hot after surgery"). When interacting with patients of the opposite sex, particularly when they are undressed, it is advisable to have a nurse or staff member of the patient's sex in the room.

The out-of-town patient, who comes from a great distance, may directly or indirectly appeal to the surgeon's ego. As a surgeon's reputation grows, so will the radius of referrals. Surgeons may feel a glow when a patient comes from afar to get their opinion or receive their care. However, this situation poses several potential problems. The first is that both the patient and the surgeon may feel pressured to decide immediately on a course of treatment. Frequently, a patient may have been tentatively scheduled for an operation even before being seen, a situation that is not optimal but occasionally unavoidable. It is much harder to refuse to operate on the patient under those circumstances. Another problem with the patient from faraway is that communication with the referring physician is not always easy. Most importantly, however, is that should something go wrong, these patients are not near their usual support of family and friends. Sometimes a postoperative patient returning home may have difficulty obtaining surgical follow-up should it be necessary. The patient from afar should certainly be given an opportunity to be a patient, but the surgeon should be aware that someone who experiences a complication or is dissatisfied with the result can best be managed if living minutes, not hours, away.

The Perfectionistic Patient

The perfectionistic patient can present for surgery in many forms. The "minimal deformity" patient reports an excessive degree of preoccupation with a comparatively modest deviation from a "normal" appearance (6). The "insatiable" patient (also described as the "Surgiholic Patient" in Chapter 19) may return to the same or often different surgeons with complaints that a given feature is "just not right" despite a series of revision procedures (7). As discussed in Chapters 14 and 16, descriptions of these patients are consistent with present-day descriptions of persons with body dysmorphic disorder.

Other patients may simply have a perfectionistic or obsessive-compulsive interpersonal style that colors most, if not all, of their interpersonal encounters. This patient presents for cosmetic surgery with some frequency. This is not particularly surprising when we recall that the goal of cosmetic surgery is to enhance an otherwise normal appearance. Some degree of striving for physical improvement, if not perfection, is essentially a prerequisite for cosmetic surgery. These patients, however, may be impossible to satisfy because they are seldom satisfied in other areas of life, expecting perfection of themselves and others (8). When the surgeon is overly concerned about a patient's expectations of perfection, it may be useful to say: "I am afraid that you wish a result that I doubt I can give you. I am not sure whether anyone else can. Of course, you may consult anyone you want, but be careful if that surgeon promises you something perfect." Just because something can be "done" for the patient, does not necessarily mean that it is in the patient's best interest for the surgeon to undertake the procedure.

The Patient Under Psychiatric Care

The management of the cosmetic surgery patient with a psychiatric history has been discussed in the literature for decades. As reviewed by Sarwer et al. elsewhere (9–12), and in Chapters 14 and 15 of this book, the literature has painted an inconsistent picture of the degree and extent of psychopathology among cosmetic surgery patients. Many of the early studies suggested high rates of psychopathology. More recent studies, with more scientifically sound methodology, have found significantly lower rates. With the exception of body dysmorphic disorder (Chapter 14), the base rate of most forms of psychopathology among cosmetic surgery patients is unknown. Nevertheless, a recent study found that 18% of cosmetic surgery patients reported a history of mental health treatment at the time of their initial consultation and 17% reported using a psychiatric medication, primarily antidepressant medications (13). Both rates were significantly higher than the 4% of reconstructive surgery patients who reported a history of current or past psychiatric treatment.

Most cosmetic surgeons would probably agree that a cosmetic procedure, like most other medical procedures, should not be performed on a patient who is psychotic, actively abusing substances, or experiencing a major depressive episode. Nevertheless, a history of past or current psychiatric treatment should not likely serve as an absolute contraindication to a cosmetic procedure for patients who are experiencing less significant forms of psychopathology. As suggested by the study by Sarwer et al. (13), this would rule out a sizable minority of cosmetic surgery patients. Patients experiencing depression or anxiety disorders may be appropriate candidates for surgery, if their symptoms are well managed and treatment is coordinated with a mental health professional.

In cases where a patient is under psychiatric care, the plastic surgeon should communicate directly with mental health professional. Occasionally, the patient has sought the surgeon's opinion without having discussed it first with his or her therapist. In this situation, a phone call, letter, or e-mail to the mental health professional is recommended. The letter should communicate the reason for the consultation and the surgeon's recommendation for treatment. It also should ask for the mental health professional's opinion on the appropriateness of treatment at this time.

The Patient Thought to Be in Need of Psychiatric Care

Few, if any, plastic surgeons insist that every prospective patient be seen for a mental health evaluation prior to treatment. Although perhaps ideal, most surgeons and patients would likely find it impractical. As discussed throughout this book, plastic surgeons will often encounter the patient in need of psychiatric consultation or treatment. Chapter 16 provides pointed recommendations on how to screen patients for common psychiatric disorders as well as other suggestions on how to communicate with mental health professionals. Both Chapters 16 and 19 highlight the importance of these strategies from a professional, risk management perspective.

Unfortunately, most patients resent the plastic surgeon's suggestion that they undergo a psychiatric consultation prior to treatment. Nevertheless, it is appropriate for surgeons to give the patient an honest opinion about the patient's psychological appropriateness for surgery. In these situations, the surgeon may say: "While I think that you might be helped by plastic surgery *(if this is true)*, I do not think that I would like to undertake it or that you should undergo it at this time. I sense you are having some personal/emotional problems or issues that could get worse if I operated on you now." It may be useful to add: "I know you are likely to be offended by my suggestion. Seeing a therapist is not unusual these days, but not seeing one when needed would be shortsighted. I would really like to see you work these difficulties out. I can give you the name of a professional who I respect and can help us determine if this is an appropriate time for surgery."

Most plastic surgeons do not practice within the context of a formal team that includes a mental health professional. These surgeons should identify a trusted mental health professional in their community who understands plastic surgery and will see a patient promptly. Some mental health professionals, especially those with a more traditional psychoanalytic orientation, may view the request for cosmetic surgery as itself a reflection of psychopathology. Their opinions may be of limited use in helping the surgeon determine the patient's appropriateness for surgery. The most appropriate consultants are those who have an informed understanding of the psychological aspects of plastic surgery and body image. Chapter 4 describes a cognitive-behavioral approach that has been found to be effective in helping persons with a range of body image and other problems.

The plastic surgeon also should keep in mind that while a person can elect to pursue a cosmetic procedure, that does not mean that the surgeon must agree to perform it. On occasion, a patient's spouse or partner may place undo influence on the patient's decision to seek surgery. In some cases, the partner may be pushing the patient to have surgery; in others, the partner may be strongly against surgery. For example, this may occur when a displeasing aspect of appearance to the wife may serve as an important fulcrum for emotional leverage for the husband. In this situation, the wife may have a negative body image or poor self-esteem, and this fact is exploited by the husband in order to maintain some power or control in the marital relationship. For that reason, the husband does not want his wife to have the operation, lest it change the dynamic of their relationship. In other cases, the wife may be interested in surgery as a last attempt to save a failing marriage. In both examples, referral to a mental health professional is warranted.

Unfortunately, some surgeons are unwilling to spend the necessary time to understand and ultimately help the patient struggling with psychological issues. Some surgeons may quote a patient an outlandish fee in the hope that he or she will refuse and leave. This, however, is not a behavior of a true physician. Although it may extricate the plastic surgeon from that situation, it is not in the best interests of the patient, which should always be the surgeon's objective. Again, a referral to a mental health professional is the most appropriate way to handle this patient. If a patient interested in a cosmetic procedure was a poor candidate because of incipient heart failure, a plastic surgeon would not hesitate to refer that patient to a cardiologist. The patient with a psychiatric problem should be treated in the same fashion.

Patients Who Display Other "Red Flag" Behavior

Other patients may display a variety of atypical behavior that leads the surgeon to question their appropriateness for surgery. On occasion, the surgeon may suspect the patient of lying. In some instances, a patient's medical or surgical history does not make intuitive sense or contradicts reality. For example, patients deny previous cosmetic procedures but clearly have the scars of a facelift. Other patients may describe occupational or social histories that have an unconvincing fictional quality. In these examples, the surgeon should calmly confront the inconsistencies of the history with the current presentation. Ultimately, the surgeon may find it difficult to trust the patient. Absolute candor, from the patient and surgeon, is necessary for the development of a trusting, professional relationship.

Understandably, few people like to disrobe before a doctor or a nurse, particularly one of the opposite sex. However, if a patient absolutely refuses to submit to a proper examination, it is impossible to recommend treatment. In such a situation, it is important to inquire directly about the patient's hesitancy. In some instances, the patient's concerns can be alleviated. For example, the patient may fear that photographs will be used for educational or promotional purposes without proper consent. The surgeon can easily reassure a patient about this and other issues.

Some patients may arrive at an initial consultation trying to "play the part" of a cosmetic surgery patient. They may be flawlessly groomed and dressed in their most stylish clothes. Many cosmetic surgery patients are understandably invested in their appearance. Other patients may arrive for their consultation with a disheveled appearance. This atypical presentation should be met with questions about the patient's current and past psychiatric history.

Infrequently, the surgeon will encounter a patient whose personality clashes with his or her own. The patient might be rude, aggressive, or insulting. After the conclusion of the initial consultation, it may be useful to say: "For some reason, you and I do not seem to be getting along. I sense the friction; perhaps you do, too. I do not think I should operate on you. You would be better with someone else." As also discussed in Chapter 19, performing an elective, cosmetic procedure on a patient whom the surgeon does not like reflects an unnecessary risk rarely worth taking.

POSTOPERATIVE CONSIDERATIONS

A patient who is dissatisfied with the postoperative result requires all the psychological skills that a surgeon can muster (14). The patient who is unhappy with the result often occupies an inordinate portion of the surgeon's mental landscape. Surgeons are trained to help patients. Dealing with a patient who the surgeon has not only failed to help but possibly made worse is distressing. Instead of being grateful, these patients may be hostile, accusatory, and possibly litigious. Unfortunately, the only way to avoid the stressful reality of the dissatisfied patient is by retirement.

The first step in caring for the dissatisfied patient is obvious—find out the reason for the dissatisfaction. Usually, the patient will remove all ambiguity by a strong, un-equivocal statement of complaint. If this is not forthcoming, the surgeon should be alert to veiled discontent—sullenness, irritability, or passive-aggressive behavior, such as not keeping a follow-up appointment or not paying the bill. It certainly would be easier for the surgeon to have such a patient leave one's practice without deter-mining the basis of the discontent. However, sooner or later, the surgeon will likely have to confront the problem. A helpful comment to open dialogue in such circum-stances might be "You don't seem too happy today. Is there something troubling you?"

In some situations, patient's dissatisfaction may be alleviated with reassurance, but only if it is justified by reality. For example, the patient who is depressed and concerned about swelling ten days after a facelift can be told with some confidence that the swelling will subside as healing progresses over the next several weeks and months. No surgeon, however, should promise that result.

In other cases, the patient's unhappiness may be the result of unmet postoperative expectations. Some patients expect that the change in appearance will lead to signif-icant improvement in self-confidence or in the social reactions from family and friends. Often, this dissatisfaction is a byproduct of unrealistic expectations that were not discussed or identified prior to surgery. The patient might be second-guessing the surgical results because some family member has become critical of the results or of the patient's decision to have had the surgery. Such outcomes underscore the impor-tance of inquiring about the patient's motivations and expectations during the initial consultation, as detailed in Chapter 16. Even a technically successful operation can alter the patient's life in unanticipated ways, occasionally putting the patient in a position to face new circumstances and challenges that may be accompanied by untoward and unexpected psychological reactions.

Fortunately, most patients comply with most of the surgeon's recommendations for postoperative care. Others, however, do not comply and, as a result, have com-plications that bring with them dissatisfaction. In these situations, it is tactically and morally wrong to blame a patient for having an unfavorable result. Even when pa-tients have not complied with recommendations for postoperative care, such as when a patient returns to smoking the day after a facelift, they should not be casti-gated for resulting complications. Another reprehensible behavior on the part of the surgeon is to tell a cosmetic patient that the complication is "nothing compared to what a cancer patient has to endure." Not only is that type of remark unsympathetic and insulting, but it is guaranteed to worsen the relationship with the patient.

When a patient is angry and the surgeon retaliates, both regress together. Anger directed toward a patient does no good but much harm. When the patient looks to the healer for guidance and comfort, and he or she is met with defensiveness and anger, the patient's fear and anxiety are heightened. To the dissatisfied and hostile patient, it is often helpful to say, "I know you are angry. I would be, too, if I were in your position. However, it is important for us to work through this together; but I need your support and I can assure you that you will have mine."

The surgeon may have the urge to avoid the dissatisfied patient. However, this is not what the surgeon should do. The dilemma is that the unhappy patient needs more attention while the surgeon feels less inclined to give it. The surgeon must em-pathize with the patient and take the time and make the effort to imagine oneself in that patient's position. It may be useful to imagine, "would we be cheerful and happy if an adverse result happened to us or a member of our family?" Medical–legal considerations aside, it is inappropriate for a professional to retreat when the pa-tient's suffering is greatest.

The dissatisfied patient's unhappiness can worsen in the presence of ambiguity. Therefore, whenever possible, the patient should be provided with a treatment plan to address any existing problems. This can be useful, even if a specific timetable for full recovery cannot be offered. A common pitfall to avoid is to offer false security by saying that "everything will come out fine," when this, in fact, may not occur. That, in essence, is lying and the patient consequently loses any remaining trust in the surgeon.

It is remarkable how reluctant some plastic surgeons are to refer a patient to a trusted colleague when they know that the patient is questioning their judgment or when the surgeon is uncertain about what to do next. A surgeon should be sufficiently sensitive to realize when a patient wants a second opinion. The surgeon should facilitate such a consultation with a telephone call or letter, not resist it. Some patients, however, may be suspicious and reluctant to go to the recommended surgeon. In this situation, it is helpful to refer the patient to anyone he or she wishes.

The dissatisfied patient can often benefit from social and emotional support from family and close friends. The surgeon should involve family members in the patient's care as much as possible. For the patient with extreme or lingering dissatisfaction, a referral to a trusted mental health professional may be appropriate. The objective of this referral is not to suggest that the patient's problem is in his or her head or to hand over the patient's care to another professional. Rather, the mental health professional may be able to provide additional emotional support to the dissatisfied patient.

Finally, the plastic surgeon must remember that the cosmetic patient has usually paid a large fee in the expectation of a satisfying enhancement and now must confront a frustrating complication. In addition to the disappointment and anger, there is the reality of the financial loss potentially made worse by additional expenses to correct an unanticipated problem. The surgeon also must keep in mind that the patient may have to be out of work longer than planned, thereby increasing the economic stress. Patients understandably become angry when the surgeon charges for treating a complication. Thus, surgical fees should not be charged in these situations.

CAN PLASTIC SURGEONS ENHANCE THEIR PSYCHOLOGICAL SKILLS?

The simple answer to this question is "Yes." If I, the other editors, and the contributors to this book believed that plastic surgeons could not enhance their psychological skills, there would be no reason for this book. That being said, the reality is that plastic surgeons, like people in most professions, differ in their psychological sensitivity. Although medical schools usually seek to admit those who they think would be mindful of the feelings and motivations of patients, the fact is that some doctors are inept at handling the doctor–patient relationship. They also might struggle in their interactions with their spouse, children, friends, and colleagues. Realizing their inadequacies, some may choose a medical career with less patient contact. Even then, their lack of interpersonal competence can be a serious detriment, not only to their career, but to their happiness. Psychological skills depend greatly upon the person's early and late role models: parents, siblings, friends, or teachers. Formal training instruction in communications skills should be required in medical school and during residency. A trainee in plastic surgery will learn helpful behavior if he or she is fortunate to have a mentor who is empathetic, compassionate, and psychologically attuned. Not having such teachers, however, does not necessarily condemn someone to remain psychologically clueless. These skills also can be learned by astutely observing colleagues with particularly well-developed interpersonal skills.

Just as we learn or should learn to improve our surgical skills throughout our professional life, we must also try to better our performance in the psychological arena (15). The plastic surgeon must take the opportunity and make the effort toward self-appraisal. If a patient's psychological diagnosis is missed, then we should learn from it, just as we would if we had missed a physical diagnosis or performed the wrong operation (16). Unlike knowing how to make a better incision, knowing how to improve our ability to understand another person's motivations and expectations for surgery can benefit our life beyond the operating room or the office.

Unfortunately, given the current rapid pace of contemporary medical practice, too few surgeons take the time necessary to understand a patient's psychological needs. Yet, that should not be an excuse for not trying. This issue is particularly problematic when the training of surgical residents is considered. The reality of same day surgery and rapid discharge leave little time for surgery residents to interact with the patient, who is, more often than not, unconscious when the resident first sees him or her. The resident is put in the difficult situation of meeting the patient, if not under anesthesia, then immediately prior to the operation or later, groggy in the recovery room. Thus, the practitioner is provided with precious little time to get to know the patient as a person.

As more and more patients are seen in less and less time, optimal care is harder to achieve. In the mistaken assumption that proper psychological assessment takes too much time, it is the first thing to be relegated to lower importance. This kind of shortcut seldom saves time and is ultimately counterproductive. As highlighted in Chapter 19, it can also have devastating consequences.

All plastic surgeons, including residents and the most senior among us, can and should make a professional commitment to developing and refining those skills that will help us to better understand the psychological dynamics that are always present in our interactions with patients. We should promote and take advantage of continuing education opportunities in the psychological understanding and management of our patients. Giving steady and concerted attention to developing these skills over the course of a career will lead to greater professional satisfaction and to greater reduction in patients' suffering as well as improvement in the quality of their lives and ours.

REFERENCES

1. Borah G, Rankin M, Wey P. Psychological complications in 281 plastic surgery practices. *Plast Reconstr Surg* 1999;104:1241–1246.
2. Goldwyn RM. *The Patient and the Plastic Surgeon.* 2nd ed. Boston: Little, Brown and Company; 1991.
3. Goldwyn RM, Cohen MN, eds. *The Unfavorable Result in Plastic Surgery: Avoidance and Treatment.* 3rd ed. Philadelphia: Lippincott Williams & Wilkins, 2001.
4. Gorney M. Claims prevention for the aesthetic surgeon: preparing for the less-than-perfect outcome. *Facial Plast Surg* 2002;18:135–142.
5. Gorney M, Martello J. Patient selection criteria. *Clin Plast Surg* 1999;26:37–40.
6. Edgerton MT, Jacobson WE, Meyer E. Surgical-psychiatric study of patients seeking plastic (cosmetic) surgery: ninety-eight consecutive patients with minimal deformity. *Br J Plast Surg* 1960;13:136–145.
7. Knorr NJ, Edgerton MT, Hoopes JE. The "insatiable" cosmetic surgery patient. *Plast Reconstr Surg* 1967;40:285–289.
8. Hewitt PL, Sherry SB, Flett GL, Shick R. Perfectionism and cosmetic surgery. *Plast Reconstr Surg* 2003;112:346.
9. Sarwer DB. Psychological considerations in cosmetic surgery. In: Goldwyn RM, Cohen MN, eds. *The Unfavorable Result in Plastic Surgery: Avoidance and Treatment.* 3rd ed. Philadelphia: Lippincott Williams & Wilkins, 2001:14–23.
10. Sarwer DB, Crerand CE. Body image and cosmetic medical treatments. *Body Image: An International Journal of Research* 2004;1:99–111.
11. Sarwer DB, Pertschuk MJ, Wadden TA, Whitaker LA. Psychological investigations of cosmetic surgery patients: a look back and a look ahead. *Plast Reconstr Surg* 1998;101:1136–1142.
12. Sarwer DB, Wadden TA, Pertschuk MJ, Whitaker LA. The psychology of cosmetic surgery: a review and reconceptualization. *Clin Psychol Rev* 1998;18:1–22.
13. Sarwer DB, Zanville HA, LaRossa D, et al. Mental health histories and psychiatric medication usage among persons who sought cosmetic surgery. *Plast Reconstr Surg* 2004;114:1927–1933.
14. Goldwyn RM. The dissatisfied patient. In: Goldwyn RM, Cohen MN, eds. *The Unfavorable Result in Plastic Surgery: Avoidance and Treatment.* 3rd ed. Philadelphia: Lippincott Williams & Wilkins, 2001:8–13.
15. Rohrich RJ. The who, what, when and why of cosmetic surgery: do our patients need a preoperative psychiatric evaluation? *Plast Reconstr Surg* 2000;106:1605–1607.
16. Goldwyn RM. Why we fail. In: Goldwyn RM, Cohen MN, eds. *The Unfavorable Result in Plastic Surgery: Avoidance and Treatment.* 3rd ed. Philadelphia: Lippincott Williams & Wilkins, 2001:1–8.

Chapter 3

Physical Appearance and Society

David B. Sarwer, PhD, and Leanne Magee, BA

This chapter reviews the evolutionary and psychological literatures on the role of physical appearance in contemporary society and its relationship with plastic surgery. The discussion begins with a review of physiological influences on appearance and perceptions of attractiveness and it draws from both human and animal research and focuses on characteristics of attractiveness such as youthfulness, symmetry, and averageness. The review then turns to sociocultural influences on physical appearance, focusing on research investigating the importance of physical appearance throughout the life span. Included in this section is a discussion of the role of the mass media in the development and promotion of standards of beauty. Throughout the chapter, we discuss how these factors contribute to the "beauty bias" so prevalent in today's society, as well as the resulting pursuit of plastic surgery.

PHYSIOLOGICAL INFLUENCES ON PHYSICAL ATTRACTIVENESS

Darwin's conceptualization of natural selection is one of the earliest discussions of importance of physical appearance (1). According to the theory of natural selection, the goal of all species is survival and successful reproduction. Identifying a mate who can successfully contribute to reproduction is a central part of that process. Through natural selection, specific physical characteristics have evolved in ways to signal an animal's (or human's) reproductive availability (2). As a result, these characteristics typically serve as the foundation for what is considered "attractive" in another individual. Thus, the notion that a healthy physical appearance, whether defined by facial or bodily characteristics, is considered attractive is not surprising.

In the animal world (and to a certain extent in the human world) a desirable characteristic, such as bright color, might draw the attention of potential mates; but it may also draw the attention of potential predators who might interfere with reproduction. Darwin's explanation of the development of these "attention-grabbing" characteristics was sexual selection. Although these traits potentially may interfere with survival, they evolve to provide surviving animals with a distinct reproductive advantage over those without these characteristics.

This chapter was supported, in part, by funding from National Institute of Diabetes and Digestive and Kidney Diseases (Grant #K23 DK60023-03) to Dr. Sarwer.

Facial Appearance

Facial appearance is likely the predominant marker of chronological age. Features such as clear skin, bright eyes, and lustrous hair are typically equated with a youthful appearance and are desirable for both men and women in many cultures throughout the world (3). Thus, they are important characteristics of attractiveness, particularly when they develop in symmetry. The development of an "average" facial appearance also may suggest reproductive health.

Youthfulness

The development of adult facial features at puberty signals reproductive potential. Increased testosterone contributes to the development of a large mandible, prominent eyebrow ridges, and cheekbones characteristic of an adult male. High levels of estrogen in females are associated with the development of facial features such as prominent cheekbones and clear, smooth skin (4–5).

These characteristics also may convey a message of health (6–7). Testosterone production at puberty suppresses immune functioning and, thus, increases susceptibility to disease producing pathogens (8). The physical characteristics of adult males, therefore, may actually communicate that the male has been sufficiently resistant to illness to produce those features. As such, the features suggest reproductive quality (9). Supporting this theory, Mueller and Mazur found that college men with broad chins reported more girlfriends and more frequent sexual intercourse (10). Estrogen works in a similar fashion, in that the byproducts of estrogen can be toxic to the body. Like testosterone for men, the physical expressions of high estrogen may serve as markers that the individual's immune system is healthy and strong, thereby communicating reproductive potential (5).

Some research indirectly supports the notion that attractiveness signals health and resistance to illness. In cultures with high pathogen prevalence (i.e., Nigeria, Zambia, and India), as compared to those cultures with low pathogen prevalence (i.e., Germany, Sweden, and Norway), men and women rated physical attractiveness as a more important trait in long-term mate selection as compared to other personality characteristics (11). Nevertheless, there is as yet no empirical evidence to suggest that more attractive humans are healthier or experience greater resistance to illness. Of course, the physical appearance (and attractiveness) of ill or dying persons often deteriorates as testimony to their physical vulnerability.

While a youthful appearance is considered attractive, aging is not. For women and men, ratings of youthfulness and facial attractiveness are highly correlated (12–14). Women are rated as less feminine as they grow older, whereas men's ratings of masculinity do not vary with age (15). As noted above, age signals reproductive potential. With increasing age, fertility declines for females of many mammalian species, but has little impact on male fertility (16).

A woman's youthful appearance may trump her chronological age in terms of perceptions of attractiveness. Younger looking faces were judged by men from five different populations as more attractive as compared to age-appropriate or older faces (17). Similarly, digitally altering facial features to make them appear more youthful results in higher ratings of attractiveness (12). Repeated evidence that women's standards of attractiveness are more closely tied with youthfulness than they are for men is consistent with evolutionary theories of sexual selection (18).

Symmetry

Like youthfulness, symmetry of facial and body features is thought to phenotypically demonstrate pathogen resistance (19). In the absence of illness, paired body features are thought to develop in concert, leading to an increasingly symmetrical and, thus, more attractive appearance. Evolutionary theorists have proposed that the ability to develop symmetrically in environmentally harsh conditions will be conferred upon only the healthiest and hardiest of a given population (20).

Numerous studies have confirmed the reproductive advantages of symmetrical over asymmetrical animals in a variety of species (21–24). The relationship between symmetry and physical attractiveness also has been supported by some (6,19,25), but not all (4), studies of humans. Men and women with more symmetrical facial features are judged as more attractive (6,19,25). Furthermore, attractiveness ratings of faces were increased when digital technology was employed to enhance symmetry (26). Both men and women preferred symmetric faces, although the preference was stronger for men (7,19). The degree of facial symmetry also appears to influence behavior. Men with more symmetrical features, as compared to those who are less symmetrical, have reported an earlier onset of sexual activity and increased number of sexual experiences (7).

Averageness

Intuitively, an "average" appearance is not associated with beauty (27). However, averageness may actually signal reproductive health, and, therefore, serve as a marker of attractiveness. Those who fall near the mean of the population distribution are probably less likely to be bearers of potentially harmful or mutated genes than those who fall at the extremes of the distribution (28–29).

Studies of human faces have supported the notion that averageness is characterized as attractive. Several investigations have used digital imaging techniques to "breed" or combine faces of varying facial appearance (28). The bred composite faces of the opposite sex were judged as more attractive for both men and women than the individual faces that comprised the composite (30). The more faces used to make the composite, the more attractive the composite face was rated (28). Nevertheless, some experts believe that symmetry is a more salient feature of attractiveness than averageness (6).

Though the average composite faces were judged as more attractive, the most beautiful of the digitally combined faces were far from average, in terms of both the specific facial features and overall facial structure (31–32). The highest rated composite for females was that of a petite face with a smaller than average mouth and jawline, paired with full lips as well as pronounced eyes and cheekbones (32–33). Preferences for attractive faces appear to occur quite early in life. Three-month-old to 6-month-old infants have been found to be more attentive to attractive versus unattractive female faces (34–35). Additionally, 6-month-old infants were found to prefer mathematically averaged prototypical faces in the same way that adults do (36). Three-year-old children show consensus with adults in their ratings of attractiveness of other children (34). Such discriminative abilities are likely present prior to significant socialization and exposure to sociocultural standards of beauty, suggesting that preferences for attractive faces are innate (37). Studies also have suggested that preferences for attractive faces are relatively consistent across race, nationality, and age (33,38). Both sets of findings lend further support to the evolutionary influence on perceptions of attractiveness.

Body Appearance

The waist-hip ratio (WHR) is a measure of the circumference of the waist relative to the hips. It reflects the distribution of fat between the upper and lower body relative to the amount of abdominal fat and is thought to signal physical beauty and reproductive potential (39). Prepubertal males and females have comparable WHRs. During puberty, increased estrogen in females contributes to the addition of fat deposits in the breasts and hips. For males, increased testosterone levels stimulate fat deposits in abdominal regions while inhibiting fat deposits in the hips and thighs.

Women with a WHR lower than 0.8 (a waist that is less than 80% the size of the hips) have been rated by men as more attractive, younger, healthier, and more feminine looking as compared to those with a higher WHR (39–41). A WHR of 0.6 to 0.8 (a waist that is 60% to 80% the size of the hips) is typically representative of healthy, fertile women (42). However, waist and hip size are not the only body characteristics that influence determinants of female attractiveness. When WHR is held constant, women with larger breasts were rated as more attractive then women with smaller breasts (43). WHR may similarly influence ratings of attractiveness for men. Healthy men have WHRs between 0.85 and 0.95 (44). Women typically consider men with such ratios as more attractive as compared to men with larger or smaller WHRs (40). However, a male's status also influenced female judgments of male attactiveness, which bestows reproductive advantages by providing both short-term and long-term access to the male's social and economic resources. Thus, women rated men who have WHRs between 0.85 and 0.95, as well as higher financial status, as the most attractive of potential partners (45). These ratios appear to be related to reproductive behavior. Males with a high shoulder to hip ratio and women with a low WHR were found to report sexual intercourse at an earlier age, more sexual partners, and more sexual experiences outside of an ongoing relationship (46).

Like several of the facial characteristics discussed above, the relationship between WHR, reproductive status, and judgments of attractiveness may be moderated by health. For women with a WHR greater than 0.8, and men with a WHR greater than 1.0, the risk of obesity-related comorbidities (such as type II diabetes and hypertension) increases (47). For females, increasing body fat distribution, as indicated by WHR, is negatively associated with the probability of conception. WHR is believed to have a greater impact on likelihood of conception than either age or obesity (48).

Gender Differences

Although men and women the world over agree that certain facial and bodily characteristics define attractiveness, there may be a considerable gender difference in what is considered most attractive in a potential mate (49–50). Men seem particularly drawn to features that signal reproductive potential. This may be a function of the relatively time-limited commitment that males need for reproduction. A male need only be present during conception in order to fulfill his evolutionary destiny of promoting his genetic material to the next generation. As such, he can reproduce with many women in a short period of time, concerning himself with those aspects of appearance that signal reproductive health.

Women are similarly attracted to those physical characteristics that indicate reproductive potential. However, evolutionarily speaking, women have a greater investment in reproduction and, thus, must also consider a potential mate's long-term abilities to obtain resources and provide protection for both her and the offspring. This suggests that, at least from a physical perspective, females would find muscular and athletic males most attractive because of their abilities to protect and provide. In contemporary society, financial and social strength, to an extent, have supplanted physical strength as characteristics women find attractive in men. Across many cultures, women rated financial strength as more important than physical characteristics when indicating traits desired in a potential mate (3,51). The observations that women were influenced by both a mate's potential to provide as well as his physical attractiveness, whereas men were swayed more by physical beauty alone, may reflect fundamental biological differences that serve an adaptive, evolutionary purpose as much as they reflect gender differences shaped by years of socialization (27).

The Relationship to Plastic Surgery

Research of evolutionary biologists and psychologists suggests that specific facial and bodily characteristics indicate reproductive potential and therefore, are considered attractive. Thus, they have a specific evolutionary purpose. These characteristics not only impact our preferences for the appearance of others, but likely impact efforts to improve our appearance through a variety of means, including plastic surgery.

Within the past decade, there has been an expanding market of products from moisturizers to toothpastes designed to turn back the hands of time on aging faces. Some of the most popular cosmetic surgical procedures, such as facelifts and blepharoplasties, are anti-aging techniques designed to restore one's facial appearance to a more youthful state (52). Perhaps even more reflective of the desire for a youthful appearance is the explosion in popularity of botulinum toxin (Botox®) injection treatments for facial wrinkles. Injections such as these were the most commonly performed surgical or minimally-invasive treatment in the United States in 2004 (52).

Two of the most popular cosmetic surgical procedures, liposuction and abdominoplasty, can alter WHR. As a result, they may improve perceptions of attractiveness, although this has yet to be empirically demonstrated. While breast size does not directly influence WHR, women with larger breasts are judged as more attractive and healthier looking compared to women with smaller breasts (43). Considering this finding, the popularity of breast enhancing brassieres and breast augmentation surgery is not surprising (53).

Intuitively, women's greater acceptance and use of appearance enhancing tools can explain the traditional 9:1 female to male ratio among cosmetic surgery patients (52). Perhaps the gender difference also can be understood in the context of evolutionary theory, which suggests that physical appearance is a more important characteristic for women than for men. At least two studies have suggested that female cosmetic surgery patients are strongly dedicated to health and fitness (54–55). As a result, for some individuals, it may make a great deal of sense from an evolutionary and psychological perspective to invest thousands of dollars in elective, cosmetic surgery on an otherwise healthy body (53).

SOCIOCULTURAL INFLUENCES ON PHYSICAL APPEARANCE

Although evolutionary determinants of reproductive status certainly impact perceptions of attractiveness, they unarguably occur within a powerful sociocultural environment. The impact of sociocultural influences on the development of physical appearance ideals has received a great deal of attention in both academic research and popular culture. From the research, it is safe to conclude that a variety of sources influence our perceptions of attractiveness. In turn, these sources likely influence the pursuit of plastic surgery as well. The discussion of these influences will be examined developmentally and then will turn to the unique influence of the mass media.

Childhood and Adolescence

Parental Influence

Parents may influence their children with their general attitudes and behaviors toward their own, and their children's, bodies (56–57). Both mothers and fathers have been found to place moderate amounts of importance on their children's attractiveness, however, mothers were significantly more likely to experience outside pressures from others to improve their children's appearance (58). While the mass media often indicts mothers in the development of their daughter's body image and eating disturbances, empirical findings have been rather inconsistent. Some studies have found a positive connection between mother and daughter concerns about eating and weight (59–63), while others have not (58,64–67). (Chapter 4 provides a more detailed discussion of the developmental influences on body image.)

Peer Influence

Peer interactions also play an important role in the development and maintenance of beliefs about attractiveness. Physical attractiveness has been linked to perceived and actual popularity, particularly for girls (68–73). Those who are less attractive may be more likely to experience more frequent appearance-related teasing than their attractive peers. Such teasing is positively correlated with body dissatisfaction (74–78).

As noted above, studies have found that infants as young as 2 to 3 months of age showed a preference for attractive faces (34,36–37). Adults displayed a reciprocal preference for attractive infants and were more likely to attribute characteristics as being smart, cheerful, healthy, responsive, and likable to attractive infants rather than unattractive ones (79). Such preferences for attractive individuals, regardless of age, have been reliably established (49). While these findings support the notion that our preference for attractive individuals is "hard-wired," this preference also influences subsequent self-esteem, social competence, and future ratings of attractiveness. The combination of attractiveness and academic competence predicted 53% of the variance in a child's self-esteem at age 8, but by age 11 physical attractiveness alone explained 43% of the variance (80). Unattractive sixth grade girls perceived themselves as less attractive, less satisfied with their body shape and size, and less popular in comparison to their attractive and average-looking peers (73). For high school age girls, but not boys, attractiveness predicted increased likelihood of getting married and also of marrying into a higher socioeconomic status group (50).

Physical attractiveness also plays a central role in the formation of childhood friendships (71). Attractiveness is considered a more important criterion than intelligence in the selection of friends (81). Regardless of a classmate's academic competence, students have shown preference for working with attractive classmates on school projects (69). Some of this may be a function of our beliefs about attractive individuals. Children between 3 and 6 years old were found to believe that attractive children are smarter, more friendly, and less aggressive (82–83). Furthermore, they believed that unattractive children would be more likely to scare and hurt other children without reason (82).

Appearance-related teasing and resulting body image dissatisfaction was once considered a benign "rite of passage" of childhood and adolescence. Recent evidence suggests that it can have long-lasting, often damaging effects. Appearance-related feedback such as peer teasing was associated with increased dieting behaviors and concerns about physical appearance (84). Girls typically believed that thinness increases likeability among their peer group (85). The strength of this belief was found to be a better predictor of weight and body image concerns than appearance-related feedback or participating in body-related activities (85). Many of these features may contribute to the development of eating disorders in adolescence or early adulthood (56,84).

Physical attractiveness also appears to influence relationships in the classroom. Teachers have been found to rate their attractive students as having better academic potential, higher intelligence, and more social skills, in addition to being more confident and popular than their unattractive classroom counterparts (86–88). Such perceptions are, in some cases, accurate. Attractive children have been found to be more popular than their peers. They also were ascribed more positive personality traits and were believed to be more intellectually competent and better adjusted than their unattractive classmates (72,89).

The impact of physical attractiveness in the classroom exists for a student's perceptions of teachers as well. First and sixth grade students believed they would learn best when taught by an attractive teacher rather than unattractive one (90). Similarly, middle school and high school students reported that they would be more likely to ask for help from an attractive college professor and to recommend the professor to other students (91). Despite the apparent beauty bias in the educational system, there is no evidence that attractive individuals are more intelligent than those who are less attractive (89).

Adulthood

The importance of physical appearance in social relationships is even more evident in adulthood. Employment decisions, experiences in the medical and legal professions, and romantic relationships are all influenced by physical appearance.

Employment

Although we would like to think otherwise, physical appearance affects our careers. Several studies have found that hiring decisions and promotions are influenced by physical appearance (92–98). More attractive applicants were more likely to receive job offers than less attractive applicants (97). Physical attractiveness also affects promotional opportunities. For example, attractive male attorneys were more likely to be promoted to early partnership than their less attractive peers (92). Interestingly, the opposite was found for attractive female lawyers; for beautiful female attorneys, attractiveness was related to lower rates of promotion to partnership (92). This is consistent with the "what-is-beautiful-is-sex-typed" stereotype, which suggests that attractive females are regarded as more feminine (and attractive males as more masculine) as they represent the "ideal" of their gender (99).

Numerous studies have suggested that more attractive individuals also earn more money than those who are less attractive (92,94–95,97–98). It is not clear why such a "beauty premium" exists. One possibility is that unattractive people receive a "plainness penalty" by which they earn even less than their average-looking coworkers (95). Others have proposed that attractive individuals are simply reaping the benefits from the positive attributes bestowed upon them by people in their professional environment. As others are more likely to perceive attractive individuals as more intellectually and occupationally competent, they may be more willing to do business with them (72,89).

Medical and Legal Systems

The physical appearance of patients impacts their treatment by medical professionals. Physicians have shown preference for working with more attractive patients and may even treat those who are less attractive differently. Unattractive patients were rated to be in worse health and as experiencing greater pain and distress than attractive patients. Several studies have documented the negative, indifferent, or demeaning behavior that unattractive, facially disfigured, or obese individuals have received from their physicians (101).

Not surprisingly, patients evaluate attractive and unattractive professionals differently. Patients reported that they would prefer to be treated by attractive mental health professionals (102–107). Over 50% of the variance in perceived effectiveness of the professional was explained by the counselors' appearances (106).

The legal system is not immune to the physical attractiveness bias. In their seminal text on physical appearance, Hatfield and Sprecher concluded that more attractive individuals were less likely to be caught committing a crime (108). Once in the legal system, attractive defendants seem to fare better than their less attractive counterparts (109–112). In mock trials and actual courtrooms, attractive defendants often received more lenient sentences. Attractive defendants lost this advantage when they were perceived to have used their beauty as part of the crime, as in extortion (112). The benefits of physical beauty apply to victims as well, as attractive victims appeared to be more successful in winning their legal cases (108).

Physical appearance also influences more general helping behaviors. Men will be more likely to help an attractive woman than an unattractive one with a variety of tasks (113). Whereas attractive individuals are more likely to receive help, they are less likely to be asked for help. We are more likely to ask less attractive friends and strangers for help when in need, perhaps out of fear of rejection or concern about looking helpless in front of a beautiful person (114).

Romantic Relationships

Attractiveness undoubtedly influences the development of romantic relationships. Frequently, the first information we receive about a potential romantic partner is their physical appearance. A positive response may spark our romantic interest and lead the relationship to flourish. This occurs, in part, because we are more likely to make positive personality attributions to those who are more attractive (108). From an evolutionary perspective, it makes sense that both men and women would seek out the most attractive partner possible. However, in the real world, the desire for the most attractive partner is balanced by the fear of rejection, and personality characteristics such as intelligence, sense of humor, and loyalty play a more significant role in the selection of romantic partners. Additionally, similarity of physical attractiveness within romantic partners is important. Couples who were more closely matched on physical attractiveness, in addition to other desirable personality characteristics, were found to be more satisfied with their relationships (108).

As discussed above, men place greater importance on having an attractive mate than do women (115–116). Men preferred attractive women over unattractive women regardless of profession and financial status (117). In contrast, women indicated increased preference for average or unattractive men who are financially successful over attractive men in low-paying professions. Nevertheless, for both men and women, the preference for attractive romantic partners appears to have increased over the past half century (115).

Mass Media Influences

This increase in the preference of attractive individuals may be a function of our increased exposure to the mass media (27). The beauty ideals found in the mass media have shifted from the voluptuous figures of the first half of the 20th century to the often strikingly lean and fit figures of more contemporary society. Marilyn Monroe, the definitive beauty ideal of her time, would be considered overweight by today's standards, although her measurements are similar to those of today's average American woman (118). Similarly, beauty icons such as Miss America and *Playboy* centerfolds have grown increasingly lean over the past decades (119–120). The average body weights of both groups of women are currently at low levels and are consistent with weights of women with anorexia nervosa (121–123). Similar trends toward increasing thinness have been found in models pictured in popular women's magazines (124–125).

This trend toward a thinner ideal, when combined with increased height, is in direct contradiction to the positive correlation of weight and height found in most women. While large breasts have always been a popular feature of many beauty icons, they, like height, are correlated with overall body fat, not thinness (20). More recently, muscularity has been added to the list of desired physical traits for beauty icons. As a result, one of the present dominant images of female beauty is that of a thin, muscular, yet large-breasted woman. This body type, however, does not often occur naturally without restrictive dieting, excessive exercise, and cosmetic surgery (118).

Increasingly, the mass media has shifted focus to include idealization of male appearance as well. An extremely muscular physique was popularized in the 1980s and 1990s through movies, television, and print advertisements. Much like the idealized female physique, the ideal for males is often attainable only through the use of endless exercise and extreme dieting. When such methods are not enough to reach the ideal, many men turn to the use of illegal steroids and other supplements (126). The recent "metrosexual" phenomenon, referring to the noticeable increase of predominantly young, urban males who invest a great deal of time, energy, and money in their physical appearance, underscores the prominence of male attractiveness in contemporary society. Increasingly, men who devote time and effort to caring for their bodies are viewed as engaging in healthy pursuits of self-fulfillment, rather than being seen as vain or out of the ordinary, as they once were (126). On the extreme end of this spectrum lies what has come to be called muscle dysmorphia, a preoccupation with being insufficiently large and muscular (127). (Chapter 15 offers a more detailed discussion of muscle dysmorphia.)

The Relationship to Plastic Surgery

These sociocultural influences shape our interest in appearance-enhancing behaviors in many ways. The most direct way is likely through the development of body image dissatisfaction, as detailed in Chapter 4. As further discussed in Chapters 14 and 15, body image dissatisfaction is thought to play a central role in the pursuit of cosmetic surgery, as well as many appearance-related pursuits, such as weight loss and cosmetics use.

Interactions with our parents and peers likely influence not only our attitudes toward cosmetic surgery, but also our experiences. A recent study of over 550 college-age women found that 5% had undergone cosmetic surgery (128). Approximately, one-third of all women surveyed indicated that a family member had undergone surgery. A parent who undergoes a cosmetic procedure sends a strong message to his or her child about the importance of appearance. For most adolescents and young adults interested in cosmetic surgery, parents yield the greatest influence of all in two forms—informed consent and the checkbook.

Interactions with childhood and adolescent peers may influence the pursuit of plastic surgery in other ways. According to the ASPS, over 326,000 individuals 18 years and younger underwent a cosmetic surgical or minimally-invasive procedure in 2004 (52). Many more young women appear to hold relatively favorable views about cosmetic surgery. Forty percent of college-aged women indicated that they would consider having a cosmetic procedure in the near future; 48% said they would consider it in middle age (128).

Perhaps this awareness and interest in cosmetic surgery among young women is not all that surprising. In the popular press, there is almost endless speculation about whether any number of Hollywood celebrities who appeal to younger audiences have undergone cosmetic surgery. Anecdotal reports suggest that cosmetic procedures such as rhinoplasty or breast augmentation are relatively common Sweet Sixteen or high school graduation presents for young women in select suburbs of many American cities.

The experience of appearance-related teasing also may play a role in the decision to seek surgery. Breast augmentation candidates, as compared to small-breasted women not interested in surgery, reported more frequent appearance-related teasing during adolescence (129). Thus, the negative experience of being teased may influence the decision to pursue surgery. At least two studies have suggested that following rhinoplasty, most patients are seen as more physically attractive and are judged more positively on a variety of personality characteristics (130–131). It is unclear, however, if these improvements change the way patients are treated by others. Patients who seek plastic surgery for the potential secondary gains of improved social relationships are thought to be less likely to meet their postoperative surgical goals (118) (also see Chapter 16). It may be that the greatest benefits from surgery are improvements in psychological characteristics, such as body image and not specifically interactions with others (132).

As discussed above, a large body of research over the last decade has confirmed the "beauty bias" in our society. Not only are physically attractive individuals judged more favorably, but they also appear to receive preferential treatment in a range of interpersonal situations across the life span. In contrast, those with an abnormal facial appearance are seen not only as less attractive, but as less honest and employable (133). Whether we like to admit it or not, our appearance does seem to matter. The possibility of improved social and professional interactions may motivate some people to seek plastic surgery (53). In some respects, it is no different than what motivates most people to exercise regularly—improved appearance (134). Why do billions of people across so many cultures routinely engage in appearance managing and enhancing behaviors to be more attractive or look their best? All things considered, it may make a great deal of sense to attempt to improve appearance through cosmetic surgery (53).

We have previously argued that the mass media and the promotion of specific beauty ideals have likely inspired women to pursue cosmetic surgery and related treatments for decades (53,118). Unfortunately, many laypersons may fail to remember and appreciate all of the "behind the scenes" work that goes into the perfect image of beauty on the cover of a magazine. While the model's physical beauty may, in part, be a function of wonderful genetics, she likely has a great deal of help cultivating her look—personal trainers, make-up artists, stylists, etc. All of this takes place before the hundreds of pictures are shot, inspected, and, ultimately, computer enhanced to create that flawless look that ultimately stares back at the reader. Figuratively and literally, we "buy" the image, and often the accompanying product. It is estimated that Americans spend at least $40 billion annually on weight loss products (135) and in 2004 they spent approximately $12.5 billion on surgeons' fees for cosmetic medical treatments (136). Americans are clearly comfortable spending large amounts of money to improve their physical appearance. We appear to have grown similarly comfortable with viewing our bodies as malleable entities (53). Decades ago, organ transplantation surgery was front-page news. Today, hospitals throughout the Western world perform these procedures on a daily basis to little fanfare. Many of us appear to have grown similarly comfortable with changing our outward appearance with cosmetic surgery.

Within the last few years, a new mass media influence on physical beauty has appeared—"reality-based" cosmetic surgery television programs. Shows such as *Extreme Makeover* and *The Swan*, as well as fictional programs such as *Nip/Tuck*, typically receive high ratings. More traditional depictions of cosmetic surgery, as often seen on the Discovery Channel, also air with great frequency. These shows, coupled with the long-standing popularity of articles on the most recent developments in cosmetic surgery in magazines, newspapers, and television news programs, have likely put cosmetic surgery on the minds of many more individuals than ever before. Whether or not this translates into a further increase in popularity in cosmetic surgery, or if these programs are simply "guilty pleasures" that are enjoyed but do not influence behavior, is yet to be seen.

SUMMARY

Our discussion of physiological and sociocultural influences on physical appearance has offered explanations and support for theories regarding how beauty standards are created and maintained. These influences have likely contributed to the relatively recent explosion of popularity in cosmetic surgery. The effects of thousands of years of evolution, years of individual experience, interactions with others, and our cultures all play roles in the establishment, maintenance, and propagation of beauty ideals. These influences impact the potential pursuit of cosmetic surgery to attain those ideals. Additional research on the psychology of physical appearance, and its relationship with cosmetic surgery, will help us gain a better understanding of why we hold this "beauty bias" and why we try so hard throughout the life span to seek beauty in ourselves and others.

REFERENCES

1. Darwin C. *The Origin of Species.* New York: Books, Inc., 1900.
2. Symons D. *The Evolution of Human Sexuality.* New York: Oxford University Press, 1979.
3. Buss DM, Abbot M, Angleitner A, et al. International preferences in selecting mates: a study of 37 cultures. *Journal of Cross-Cultural Psychology* 1990;35:5–47.
4. Fink B, Grammer K, Thornhill R. Human (homo sapiens) facial attractiveness in relation to skin texture and color. *J Comp Psychol* 2001;115:92–99.
5. Fink B, Penton-Voak I. Evolutionary psychology of facial attractiveness. *Current Directions in Psychological Science* 2002;11:154–158.
6. Grammer K, Thornhill R. Human facial attractiveness and sexual selection: The role of symmetry and averageness. *J Comp Psychol* 1994;108:233–242.
7. Thornhill R, Gangestad SW. Human fluctuating asymmetry and sexual behavior. *Psychol Sci* 1994;5: 297–302.
8. Hamilton W, Zuk M. Heritable true fitness and bright birds: a role for parasites. *Science* 1982;218:384–387.
9. Zahavi A, Zahavi A. *The Handicap Principle.* Oxford, London: Oxford University Press, 1997.
10. Mueller U, Mazur A. Facial dominance in *Homo sapiens* as honest signaling of male quality. *Behavioral Ecology* 1997;8:569–579.
11. Gangestad SW, Buss DM. Pathogen prevalence. *Ethol Sociobiol* 1993;14:89–96.
12. Jones D. *Physical Attractiveness and the Theory of Sexual Selection.* Ann Arbor, MI: Museum of Anthropology, University of Michigan; 1996.
13. McClellan B, McKelvie SJ. Effects of age and gender on perceived facial attractiveness. *Canadian Journal of Behavioural Sciences* 1993;25:135–142.
14. Zebrowitz LA, Olson K, Hoffman K. Stability of babyfaceness and attractiveness across the lifespan. *J Pers Soc Psychol* 1993;65:453–466.
15. Deutsch FM, Zalenski CM, Clark ME. Is there a double standard of aging? *J App Soc Psych* 1986;16:771–785.
16. Keefe DL. Reproductive aging is an evolutionarily programmed strategy that no longer provides adaptive value. *Fertil and Steril* 1998;70:204–206.
17. Cunningham MR. Measuring the physical in physical attractiveness: quasi-experiments on the sociobiology of female facial beauty. *J Pers Soc Psych* 1986;50:925–935.
18. Jones D. An evolutionary perspective on physical attractiveness. *Evolutionary Anthropology* 1996;5:97–109.
19. Thornhill R, Gangestad SW. Human facial beauty: averageness, symmetry, and parasite resistance. *Human Nature* 1993;4:237–269.
20. Grammer K, Fink B, Moller AP, Thornhill R. Darwinian aesthetics: sexual selection in the biology of beauty. *Bio Rev* 2003;78:385–407.
21. Moller AP. Female swallow preferences for symmetrical male sexual ornaments. *Nature* 1992;357:238–240.
22. Petrie M, Halliday TR, Sanders C. Peahens prefer peacocks with elaborate trains. *Anim Behav* 1991;41:323–331.
23. Swaddle JP, Cuthill IC. Preference for symmetric males by female zebra finches. *Nature* 1994;367:165–166.
24. Thornhill R. Fluctuating asymmetry and the mating system of the Japanese scorpionfly, *panorpa japonica. Anim Behav* 1992;44:867–879.
25. Gangestad SW, Thornhill R, Yeo R. Facial attractiveness, developmental stability and fluctuating asymmetry. *Ethol Sociobiol* 1994;15:73–85.
26. Rhodes G, Proffitt F, Grady M, Sumich A. Facial symmetry and the perception of beauty. *Psych Bull Rev* 1998;5:659–669.
27. Sarwer DB, Grossbart TA, Didie ER. Beauty and Society. In: Kaminer MS, Dover JS, Arndt KA, eds. *Atlas of Cosmetic Surgery.* Philadelphia: WB Saunders, 2002:48–59.
28. Langlois JH, Roggman LA, Musselman L. What is average and what is not average about attractive faces. *Psychol Sci* 1994;5:214–220.
29. Mitton JB, Grant MC. Associations among protein heterozygosity, growth rate and developmental homeostasis. *Annu Rev Ecol System* 1984;15:479–499.
30. Langlois JH, Roggman LA. Attractive faces are only average. *Psychol Sci* 1990;1:115–121.
31. Alley TR, Cunningham MR. Averaged faces are attractive but very attractive faces are not average. *Psychol Sci* 1991;2:123–125.
32. Johnston VS, Franklin M. Is beauty in the eye of the beholder? *Ethol Sociobiol* 1993;14:183–199.
33. Perrett DI, May KA, Yoshikawa S. Facial shape and judgment of female attractiveness. *Nature* 1994;386:239–242.
34. Langlois JH, Roggman LA, Casey RJ, et al. Infant preferences for attractive faces: rudiments of a stereotype. *Dev Psychol* 1987;23:363–369.
35. Slater AM, Von der Schulenburg C, Brown E, et al. Newborn infants prefer attractive faces. *Infant Behavior and Development* 1998;21:345–354.

36. Rubenstein AJ, Kalakanis L, Langlois JH. Infant preferences for attractive faces: a cognitive explanation. *Dev Psychol* 1999;35:848–855.

37. Langlois JH, Roggman LA, Reiser-Danner LA. Infants' differential social responses to attractive and unattractive faces. *Dev Psychol* 1990;26:153–159.

38. Thakerar JN, Iwawaki S. Cross-cultural comparisons in interpersonal attraction of females toward males. *J Soc Psychol* 1979;108:121–122.

39. Singh D. Adaptive significance of female physical attractiveness: role of waist-to-hip ratio. *J Pers Soc Psychol* 1993;65:456–466.

40. Singh D. Female health, attractiveness, and desirability for relationships: role of breast asymmetry and waist-to-hip ratio. *Ethol Sociobiol* 1995;16:465–481.

41. Streeter SA, McBurney DH. Waist-hip ratio and attractiveness: new evidence and a critique of "a critical test." *Evolution and Human Behavior* 2004;24:88–98.

42. Lanska DJ, Lanska MJ, Hartz AJ, Rimm AA. Factors influencing anatomic location of fat tissue in 52,953 women. *Int J Obes* 1985;9:29–38.

43. Singh D, Young RK. Body weight, waist-to-hip ratio, breasts, and hips: role is judgments of female attractiveness and desirability for relationships. *Ethol Sociobiol* 1995;16:483–507.

44. Jones PR, Hunt MJ, Brown TP, Norgan D. Waist-hip circumference ratio and its relation to age and over-weight in British men. *Hum Nutr Clin Nutr* 1986;40:239–247.

45. Singh D. Female judgment of male attractiveness and desirability for relationships: role of waist-to-hip ratio and financial status. *J Pers Soc Psychol* 1995;69:1089–1101.

46. Hughes SM, Gallup GG. Sex differences in morphological predictors of sexual behavior: should to hip and waist to hip ratios. *Evolution and Human Behavior* 2003;24:173–178.

47. Dalton M, Cameron AJ, Zimmet PZ, et al. Waist circumference, waist-hip ratio and body mass index and their correlation with cardiovascular disease risk factors in Australian adults. *J Intern Med* 2003;254:555–563.

48. Zaadstra BM, Seidell JC, Van Noord PAH, et al. Fat and female fecundity: prospective study of effect of body fat distribution on conception rates. *Br Med J* 1993;30:484–487.

49. Jackson LA. *Physical Appearance and Gender: Sociobiological and Sociocultural Perspectives*. Albany, NY: SUNY Press, 1992.

50. Etcoff, N. *Survival of the Prettiest*. New York: Doubleday, 1999.

51. Buss DM, Schmitt DP. Sexual strategies theory: an evolutionary perspective on human dating. *Psychol Rev* 1993;100:204–232.

52. *2005 Report of the 2004 National Clearinghouse of Plastic Surgery Statistics*. Arlington Heights, IL: American Society of Plastic Surgeons, 2005.

53. Sarwer DB, Magee L, Clark VL. Physical appearance and cosmetic medical treatments: physiological and sociocultural influences. *J Cos Derm* 2004;2:29–39.

54. Didie ER, Sarwer DB. Factors which influence the decision to undergo cosmetic breast surgery. *J Womens Health* 2003;12:241–253.

55. Sarwer DB, Wadden TA, Pertschuk MJ, Whitaker LA. Body image dissatisfaction and body dysmorphic disorder in 100 cosmetic surgery patients. *Plast Reconstr Surg* 1998;101:1644–1649.

56. Smolak L. Body image development in children. In: Cash TF, Pruzinsky T, eds. *Body Images: A Handbook of Theory, Research, and Clinical Practice*. New York: Guilford Press, 2002:65–73.

57. Thompson JK, Heinberg LJ, Altabe M, Tantleff-Dunn S. *Exacting Beauty: Theory, Assessment and Treatment of Body Image Disturbance*. Washington, DC: American Psychological Association, 1999.

58. Striegel-Moore R, Kearney-Cooke A. Exploring parents' attitudes and behaviors about their children's physical appearance. *Int J Eat Disord* 1994;15:377–385.

59. Benedikt R, Wertheim E, Love A. Eating attitudes and weight-loss attempts in female adolescents and their mothers. *J Youth Adol* 1998;27:43–57.

60. Hill AJ, Weaver C, Blundell JE. Dieting concerns of 10-year-old girls and their mothers. *Br J Clin Psychol* 1990;29:346–348.

61. Levinson R, Powell B, Steelman LC. Social location, significant others, and body image among adolescents. *Soc Psychol Q* 1986;49:330–337.

62. Pike K, Rodin J. Mothers, daughters, and disordered eating. *J Abnorm Psychol* 1991;100:198–204.

63. Rodin J, Silberstein LR, Striegel-Moore RH. Women and weight: A normative discontent. In: Sonderegger TB, ed. *Psychology and Gender: Nebraska Symposium on Motivation, 1984*. Lincoln, NE: University of Nebraska Press, 1985:267–307.

64. Attie I, Brooks-Gunn J. Development of eating problems in adolescent girls: a longitudinal study. *Dev Psychol* 1989;25:70–79.

65. Fisher M. Parents' views of adolescent health issues. *Pediatrics* 1992;90:335–341.

66. Saftner JL, Crowther JH, Crawford PA, Watts DD. Maternal influence (or lack thereof) on daughters' eating attitudes and behaviors. *Eating Disorders: The Journal of Treatment and Prevention* 1996;4:147–159.

67. Thelen MH, Cormier JF. Desire to be thinner and weight control among children and their parents. *Beh Ther* 1995;26:85–99.

68. Adams GR, Rooparnine JL. Physical attractiveness, social skills, and same-sex peer popularity. *Journal of Group Psychotherapy, Psychodrama, and Sociometry* 1994;47:15–35.

69. Boyatzis CJ, Baloff P, Durieux C. Effects of perceived attractiveness and academic success on early adolescent popularity. *J Genet Psychol* 1998;159:337–344.

70. Drewry DL, Clark ML. Factors important in the formation of preschoolers' friendships. *J Genet Psychol* 1985;146:37–44.

71. Krantz M. Physical attractiveness and popularity: a predictive study. *Psychol Rep* 1987;60:723–726.

72. Langlois JH, Kalakanis L, Rubenstein AJ, et al. Maxims or myths of beauty? A meta-analytic and theoretical review. *Psychol Bull* 2002;126:390–423.

73. Zakin DF, Blyth DA, Simmons RG. Physical attractiveness as a mediator of the impact of early pubertal changes for girls. *J Youth Adol* 1984;13:439–450.

74. Cash TF. Developmental teasing about physical appearance: retrospective descriptions and relationships with body image. *Soc Behav Pers* 1995;23:123–130.
75. Fabian LJ, Thompson JK. Body image and eating disturbance in young females. *Int J Eat Disord* 1989;8:63–74.
76. Grilo CM, Wilfley DE, Brownell KD, Rodin J. Teasing, body image, and self-esteem in a clinical sample of obese women. *Addict Behav* 1994;19:443–450.
77. Thompson JK, Psaltis K. Multiple aspects and correlates of body figure ratings: a replication and extension of Fallon and Rozin (1985). *Int J Eat Disord* 1988;7:813–818.
78. Rieves L, Cash TF. Social developmental factors and women's body image attitudes. *J Soc Beh Pers* 1996;11:63–78.
79. Stephan CW, Langlois JH. Baby beautiful: adult attributions of infant competence as a function of infant attractiveness. *Child Dev* 1984;55:576–585.
80. Muldoon OT. Social group membership and self-perceptions in northern Irish children: a longitudinal study. *Brit J Dev Psych* 2000;18:65–80.
81. Clark ML. Ayers M. The role of reciprocity and proximity in junior high school friendships. *J Youth Adol* 1988;17:403–411.
82. Dion KK. Young children's stereotyping of facial attractiveness. *Dev Psychol* 1973;9:183–188.
83. Langlois JH, Stephan CW. The effects of physical attractiveness and ethnicity on children's behavioral attributions and peer preferences. *Child Dev* 1977;48:1694–1698.
84. Tantleff-Dunn S, Gokee JL. Interpersonal influences on body image development. In: Cash TF, Pruzinksy T, eds. *Body Images: A Handbook of Theory, Research, and Clinical Practice.* New York: Guilford Press, 2002:108–116.
85. Oliver KK, Thelen MH. Children's perceptions of peer influence on eating concerns. *Beh Ther* 1996;27:25–39.
86. Kenealy P, Frude N, Shaw W. Influence of children's physical attractiveness on teachers' expectations. *J Soc Psychol* 1988;128:373–383.
87. Lerner RM, Delaney M, Hess LE, Jovanovic J. Early adolescent physical attractiveness and academic competence. *J Early Adol* 1990;10:4–20.
88. Ritts V, Patterson MI, Tubbs ME. Expectations, impressions, and judgments of physically attractive students: a review. *Rev Ed Res* 1992;62:413–426.
89. Jackson LA, Hunger JE, Hodge CN. Physical attractiveness and intellectual competence: a meta-analytic review. *Soc Psychol Q* 1995;58:108–122.
90. Hunsberger B, Cavanagh B. Physical attractiveness and children's expectations of potential teachers. *Psych Women Quarterly* 1988;25:70–74.
91. Romano ST, Bordieri JE. Physical attractiveness stereotypes and students' perceptions of college professors. *Psychol Rep* 1989;64:1099–1102.
92. Biddle JE, Hamermesh DS. Beauty, productivity, and discrimination: lawyers' looks and lucre. *J Labor Econ* 1998;16:172–201.
93. Cann A, Siegfried WD, Pearce L. Forced attention to specific applicant qualifications: impact on physical attractiveness and sex of applicant biases. *Personnel Psych* 1981;34:65–75.
94. Frieze IH, Olson JE, Russell J. Attractiveness and income for men and women in management. *J App Soc Psych* 1991;21:1039–1057.
95. Hamermesh DS, Biddle JE. Beauty and the labor market. *Am Econ Rev* 1994;84:1174–1194.
96. Kyle DJ, Mahler HIM. The effects of hair color and cosmetic use on perceptions of a female's ability. *Psych Women Quarterly* 1996;20:447–455.
97. Marlowe CM, Schneider SL, Nelson SE. Gender and attractiveness biases in hiring decisions: are more experienced managers less biased? *J App Psychol* 1996;81:11–21.
98. Umberton D, Hughes M. The impact of physical attractiveness on achievement and psychological well-being. *Soc Psychol Q* 1987;50:227–236.
99. Cash TF. The psychology of physical appearance: aesthetics, attributes, and images. In: Cash TF, Pruzinsky T, eds. *Body Images: Development, Deviance, and Change.* New York: Guilford Press, 1990:51–79.
100. Hadjistavropoulos HD, Ross MA, von Baeyer CL. Are physicians' ratings of pain affected by patients' physical attractiveness? *Soc Sci Med* 1990;31:69–72.
101. Puhl R, Brownell KD. Bias, discrimination, and obesity. *Obes Res* 2001;9:788–805.
102. Cash TF, Begley PJ, McCown DA, Weise BC. When counselors are heard but not seen: initial impact of physical attractiveness. *J Counseling Psych* 1975;22:273–279.
103. Cash TF, Kehr J. Influence of non-professional counselors' physical attractiveness and sex on perceptions of counselor behavior. *J Counseling Psych* 1977;25:336–342.
104. Green CF, Cunningham J, Yanico BJ. Effects of counselor and subject race and counselor physical attractiveness on impressions and expectations of a female counselor. *J Counseling Psych* 1986;33:349–352.
105. Lewis KN, Walsh WB. Physical attractiveness: its impact on the perception of a female counselor. *J Counseling Psych* 1978;25:210–216.
106. Vagra AM, Borokowski JG. Physical attractiveness: interactive effects of counselor and client on counseling processes. *J Counseling Psych* 1983;30:146–157.
107. Vagra AM, Borokowski JG. Physical attractiveness and counseling skills. *J Counseling Psych* 1982;29:246–255.
108. Hatfield E, Sprecher S. *Mirror, Mirror... The Importance of Looks in Everyday Life.* Albany, NY: SUNY Press, 1986.
109. DeSantis A, Kayson WA. Defendants' characteristics of attractiveness, race, sex and sentencing decisions. *Psychol Rep* 1997;81:679–683.
110. Mazzella R, Feingold A. The effects of physical attractiveness, race, socioeconomic status, and gender of defendants and victims on judgments of mock jurors: a meta-analysis. *J App Soc Psych* 1994;24:1315–1344.
111. Stewart JE. Appearance and punishment: the attraction-leniency. *J Soc Psychol* 1985;123:373–376.

112. Weunsch KL, Chia RC, Castellow WA, et al. Effects of physical attractiveness, sex, and type of crime on mock juror decisions: a replication with Chinese students. *Journal of Cross-Cultural Psychology* 1993;24: 414–427.
113. Benson PL, Karabenick SA, Lerner RM. Pretty pleases: the effects of physical attractiveness, race, and sex on receiving help. *J Exper Soc Psych* 1976;12:409–415.
114. Nadler A, Shapira R, Ben-Itzhak S. Good looks may help: effects of helpers' physical attractiveness and sex of helper on males' and females' help-seeking behavior. *J Pers Soc Psychol* 1982;42:90–99.
115. Buss DM, Shackelford TK, Kirkpatrick LA, Larsen RJ. A half century of mate preferences: the cultural evolution of values. *J Marital Fam Ther* 2001;63:491–503.
116. Feingold A. Gender differences in effects of physical attractiveness on romantic attraction: a comparison across five research paradigms. *J Pers Soc Psychol* 1990;59:981–993.
117. Townsend JM, Levy GD. Effects of potential partners' costume and physical attractiveness on sexuality and partner selection. *J Psychol* 1990;124:371–389.
118. Sarwer DB, Magee L, Crerand CE. Cosmetic surgery and cosmetic medical treatments. In: Thompson JK, ed. *Handbook of Eating Disorders and Obesity*. New York: John Wiley and Sons, 2004:718–737.
119. Garner DM, Garfield PE, Schwartz D. Cultural expectations of thinness in women. *Psychol Rep* 1980;47:483–491.
120. Mazur A. U.S. trends in feminine beauty and overadaption. *J Sex Res* 1986;22:281–303.
121. Katzmarzyk PT, Davis C. Thinness and body shape of *Playboy* centerfolds from 1978 to 1998. *Int J Obes* 2001;25:590–592.
122. Rubinstein S, Caballero B. Is Miss America an undernourished role model? *JAMA* 2001;283:1569.
123. Wiseman CV, Gray J, Mosimann JE, Aherns AH. Cultural expectations of thinness in women: an update. *Int J Eat Disord* 1992;11:85–89.
124. Morris A, Cooper T, Cooper PJ. The changing shape of female fashion models. *Int J Eat Disord* 1989;8: 593–596.
125. Silverstein B, Perdue L, Patterson B, Kelly E. The role of mass media in promoting a thin standard of bodily attractiveness for women. *Sex Roles* 1986;14:519–532.
126. Luciano L. *Looking Good: Male Body Image in Modern America.* New York: Hill and Wang, 2001.
127. Pope HG, Phillips KA, Olivardia R. *The Adonis Crisis: The Secret Crisis of Male Body Obsession.* New York: The Free Press, 2000.
128. Sarwer DB, Cash TF, Magee L, et al. Female college students and cosmetic surgery: An investigation of experiences, attitudes, and body image. *Plast Reconstr Surg* 2005;115:931–938.
129. Sarwer DB, LaRossa D, Bartlett SP, et al. Body image concerns of breast augmentation patients. *Plast Reconstr Surg* 2003;112:83–90.
130. Cash TF, Horton CE. Aesthetic surgery: effects of rhinoplasty on the social perceptions of patients by others. *Plast Reconstr Surg* 1983;72:543–550.
131. Kalick SM. Aesthetic surgery: how it affects the way patients are perceived by others. *Ann Plast Surg* 1979;2:128–134.
132. Sarwer DB, Wadden TA, Pertschuk MJ, Whitaker LA. The psychology of cosmetic surgery: a review and reconceptualization. *Clin Psychol Rev* 1998;18:1–22.
133. Rankin M, Borah GF. Perceived functional impact of abnormal facial appearance. *Plast Reconstr Surg* 2003;111:2140–2146.
134. Cash TF, Novy PL, Grant JR. Why do women exercise?: Factor analysis and further validation of the Reasons for Exercise Inventory. *Percept Mot Skills* 1994;78:539–544.
135. Wickelgren I. Obesity: how big a problem? *Science* 1998;280:1364–1367.
136. American Society for Aesthetic Plastic Surgery. *Cosmetic Surgery National Data Bank—2004 Statistics.* New York: American Society for Aesthetic Plastic Surgery, 2004.

Chapter 4

Body Image and Plastic Surgery

Thomas F. Cash, PhD

The psychology of physical appearance may be approached from two different perspectives—the "outside, body-in-society view" and the "inside, body-in-self view" (1). The first perspective considers how certain aspects of human appearance, such as physical attractiveness, weight, height, body shape, hair color, etc., affect interpersonal perceptions, cognitions, and behaviors. As Sarwer and Magee reviewed in the previous chapter, behavioral scientists have systematically studied appearance stereotyping and whether people who differ with regard to particular physical characteristics receive different social reactions and outcomes (1–5). Whether due to bioevolutionary "pre-wiring," cultural socialization, or people's interactions with each other, there is little doubt that physical appearance can exert both subtle and profound effects on human relations, from infancy to old age, and from the bedroom to the boardroom.

The second perspective is the body-in-self view of one's appearance, which essentially defines "body image" (6–8). Body image refers to the person's own experiences of embodiment, especially self-perceptions and self-attitudes toward one's appearance. Psychological scientists have investigated how body image develops, what physical and psychosocial factors shape this development, and, in turn, how body image affects other facets of the individual's functioning. People's experiences of their own appearance are often quite different from how others see and evaluate them. Good looks do not guarantee a subjectively positive body image nor is a plain or homely appearance necessarily associated with a problematic body image.

Plastic surgeons work at the intersection of these two perspectives on human appearance. With precision and skill, they alter and sometimes transform outward physical appearance—refining, reshaping, rejuvenating, restoring, or reconstructing to create an external change that looks "better," "more attractive," or "normal." At the same time, surgeons understand that it is the patient's perceptions and attitudes toward this change that will ultimately determine the outcome. Indeed, Edgerton has maintained that "Although aesthetic or cosmetic surgery is undertaken to improve the patient's appearance, the purpose of aesthetic surgery is to facilitate positive psychological changes. In fact, the *only* rationale for performing aesthetic plastic surgery is to improve the patient's psychological well being" (9). For most cosmetic surgery patients this desired improvement is specifically focused on body image but not necessarily on other aspects of psychosocial quality of life. That is, most cosmetic surgery patients seek to feel more positively about specific aspects of their appearance, but likely are not seeking to change, via surgery, broader aspects of their life. For others, however, the desired changes may be even more pervasive (e.g., to change one's overall self-concept). And, of course, a small minority of people look to cosmetic surgery for a "life transformation"—more often than not, a misguided and ineffective solution to their unhappiness.

Body image is central to plastic surgery, as nearly every chapter in this volume articulates. The extensive research on cosmetic surgery by Sarwer and colleagues has advanced the field considerably, moving us from an early era of unscientific and biased inquiry to a more sophisticated scrutiny of the motives for, and outcomes of, specific cosmetic procedures, armed with a contemporary conceptual framework and improved research methodology (10–15). Moreover, body image research has become increasingly relevant to reconstructive surgery for both congenital and acquired disfigurements (16–19).

The primary aim of this chapter is to clarify the meaning and importance of the multiple dimensions that define body image and, ultimately, its relationship to plastic surgery. The chapter provides a conceptual framework that organizes these dimensions and delineates their causal development as well as their consequences. It also identifies some of the best methods to measure these various aspects of body image, particularly among plastic surgery patients. The chapter concludes with the discussion of an empirically supported psychosocial approach to body image change, one that may be helpful as an adjunct or alternative to plastic surgical procedures. All facets of this chapter will inform the plastic surgeon about crucial issues in understanding body image.

A BRIEF HISTORICAL OVERVIEW OF BODY IMAGE

The study of body image, or "body schema," originated at the turn of the 20th century as physicians sought to understand the causes of certain neurological patients' strange bodily sensations, including such phenomena as "phantom limb," "autotopagnosia," "hemiasomatognosia," and "anosognosia" (20). From 1914 to 1940, Schilder broadened the focus from neuropathology to the attitudes and feelings patients had about their bodies. At the same time, psychoanalytic professionals expanded Freud's psychosexual theory to understand patients' perceptions of the body as the "boundary" between themselves and their external world (21), a boundary that takes on meaning especially with respect to one's largely unconscious feelings about the self. Subsequently, Fisher dedicated much of his career as a psychologist to the investigation of body image from a psychoanalytic viewpoint, publishing prolifically on the "body boundary" construct (21–23) Shontz (24) was critical of this psychodynamic perspective, drawing from his integration of theory and data from several areas of experimental psychology. He conceptualized body experience as multidimensional, and he applied research findings to understand and help individuals with physical disabilities (25).

Over the past several decades, clinical and empirical interests in body image have flourished, largely in response to the increasing prevalence of, and interest in, eating disorders. Numerous new assessments of body image have emerged and scientific knowledge has expanded (7–8,26–28). Despite these advances, such research has fostered a limited, perhaps myopic, view of body image (29–30). Body image and its measurement have focused intensively on weight/shape concerns among women and girls. The publication of body image research has been scattered across a range of scientific journals. A complete understanding of human experiences of embodiment must transcend so narrow a vision.

Cash and Pruzinsky (7) have argued that the future of body image scholarship lies at the interface of behavioral and medical/health sciences. In their edited volume, *Body Image: A Handbook of Theory, Research, and Clinical Practice*, there are eight chapters devoted to understanding body image issues in the specialties of dermatology (31), dental medicine (32), obstetrics and gynecology (33), urology (34), endocrinology (35), oncology (36), and rehabilitation medicine (37), as well as body image issues among persons with HIV/AIDS (38). Moreover, several chapters examine body image and its changes via cosmetic (11) and reconstructive surgery (16–18). As the volume's contents further attest, important developments are occurring in the prevention of body image problems, the growing recognition of body image issues among boys and men, and greater attention to the cultural and ethnic diversity of body images. Indeed, these themes are reflected in the mission of a new peer-reviewed scientific journal, *Body Image: An International Journal of Research*, that commenced publication in 2004. This journal is founded on the proposition that experiences and conditions of embodiment have far-reaching implications for human development and the quality of life.

DEFINING AND ASSESSING BODY IMAGE: CONTEMPORARY PERSPECTIVES

Body image is now typically viewed as a multidimensional construct consisting of two overarching components: *perceptions* and *attitudes* (6–8). The perceptual component of body image pertains to the extent to which a person is able to judge his or her appearance accurately on some physical dimension, usually body size. Researchers have developed instruments to assess individuals' degree of body-size distortion, whether based on perceptions of the whole body or discrete areas of the body (8,39–40). These methods range from simple figural stimuli (e.g., silhouettes) to more elaborate video technologies whereby persons adjust projected images of their own body to convey their body perceptions. However, among various scientific shortcomings of these perceptual assessments, they usually neglect self-perceived attributes of specific body features (e.g., facial characteristics, height, hair, muscularity, etc.).

Body image attitudes consist of individuals' thoughts, feelings, and behaviors related to their physical appearance. These attitudes are typically assessed by self-report questionnaires. Thompson et al. (8,41) provide an extensive listing of these instruments. Body image attitudes themselves are multidimensional, comprised of body-image evaluation/affect and body image investment. *Body-image evaluation* refers to one's level of body satisfaction or dissatisfaction and evaluative thoughts or beliefs about one's body (e.g., appearance). The degree of body satisfaction (or dissatisfaction) depends on the degree of congruence (or discrepancy) between self-views of the body or body parts and one's personal physical ideals. The Body-Image Ideals Questionnaire is one tool that assesses this self-ideal discrepancy dimension of the construct (42–43). Other examples of well-validated and widely used measures of body satisfaction pertinent to plastic surgery include the Body Esteem Scale (44) and the Multidimensional Body-Self Relations Questionnaire-Appearance Scales (MBSRQ-AS), which contains multiple subscales to measure particular attitudes toward one's appearance (45–47). Questionnaire 4-1 provides two of these MBSRQ scales—the Appearance Evaluation Scale has seven items and the Body Areas Satisfaction Scale has nine items.

Associated with these evaluations is *body image affect*, which refers to the emotional experiences that result from one's body image appraisals. For example, when a person evaluates his or her appearance unfavorably in some particular context, dysphoric emotions (e.g., anxiety, disgust, or shame) may result. The Situational Inventory of Body-Image Dysphoria (48) measures how often individuals experience negative body-image emotions in each of 20 situations (e.g., looking in the mirror, exercising, interacting with attractive people, etc.). This measure may be useful with plastic surgery patients, as it provides an assessment of negative emotional experiences across a range of interpersonal and other situations.

The attitudinal dimension of *body-image investment* refers to the extent to which one's attention, thoughts, and actions focus on one's looks, including the extent of reliance on physical appearance as a criterion for defining one's sense of self. Examples of measures of this facet of body image include the Appearance Orientation subscale of the MBSRQ-AS (46) and the Appearance Schemas Inventory-Revised (ASI-R) (49). The ASI-R assesses two somewhat different aspects of body image investment. The first aspect, *self-evaluative salience*, reflects the extent to which people define themselves by their physical appearance. The second aspect, *motivational salience*, refers to how much individuals attend to their appearance and engage in appearance-management behaviors. Self-evaluative salience constitutes a more pathogenic type of body image investment, because one's looks dictate one's self-worth. Motivational salience, on the other hand, is not inherently problematic, as it mostly entails taking care of or pride in one's appearance (49). In a recent study of 214 college women (50), those who were most invested in their appearance were most favorably predisposed toward cosmetic surgery. The relationship was stronger for self-evaluative salience than for motivational salience.

The Epidemiology of Body Image Discontent

Large sample surveys confirm that body image dissatisfaction is fairly commonplace in America. From a national *Psychology Today* magazine survey using the MBSRQ-AS, Cash et al. (51) sampled 2,000 individuals to represent the United States population, stratified by age and gender distributions. The results revealed that 38% of women and 34% of men were dissatisfied with their appearance in general. Although most respondents were content with their face and height, their body weight and middle torso were the foci of body dissatisfaction for most men and women. A representative survey of American women in 1993 (52) found that 48% of respondents were dissatisfied with their appearance, as well as, preoccupied with being or becoming overweight. A *Psychology Today* survey published in 1997 (53) revealed that 56% of the women and 43% of the men evaluated their overall appearance negatively, suggesting a possible increase in body image dissatisfaction across the population. Although such survey results are quite interesting, methodological problems particularly with the magazine surveys, including possible sample self-selection biases and the non-comparability of questions across the various studies, may have inflated dissatisfaction rates in the most recent survey data (54). Still, there is little doubt that a sizeable percentage of women and men find aspects of their physical appearance to be unacceptable.

A meta-analysis of 222 body-image studies from the past 50 years found a widening gender gap in body image, with continual increases in women's discontent (55). However, several recent studies suggest that, at least among college women, rates of body image dissatisfaction may have leveled off or actually declined in the past few years, despite their increase in body weight (56). Although numerous studies confirm significant gender differences in body satisfaction, differences extend beyond evaluative body image. For example, Muth and Cash (57) investigated body image evaluation, affect, and investment among college women and men. Relative to men, women reported greater self-ideal discrepancies, frequent negative body image emotions, and more cognitive and behavioral investment in their physical appearance. Thus, dissatisfaction with, and distress about, their looks are more common among women, who are also more invested in their appearance as a source of self-definition. Furthermore, gender differences in body image evaluation seem to be greatest during adolescence and early adulthood, when females are especially vulnerable to body image disturbances (55,58). Although Garner (53) did not observe greater discontent among young people in his 1996 survey, he noted the curious fact that with increasing body weight among older groups, women's body dissatisfaction did not worsen. Moreover, among cosmetic surgery patients, older women interested in rhytidectomy and/or blepharoplasty reported less dissatisfaction with their facial appearance as compared to younger women interested in rhinoplasty (59). Perhaps aging brings a shift in values and a more secure identity that facilitates divestment of youthful appearance standards (60–61).

Currently, there is a growing interest in male body image, especially in relation to issues concerning the cultural idealization of muscularity (62–65). (Chapter 15 discusses the relationship between muscularity and body contouring procedures.) Male cosmetic surgery patients, as compared to female patients, reported less investment in their appearance (as assessed by the Appearance Orientation scale of the MBSRQ-AS) but otherwise did not differ in their body image concerns (66).

In addition to age and gender differences, ethnicity is relevant to body satisfaction. In general, even at higher body weights African-American women hold more favorable body image evaluations than do European-American or Hispanic-American women (52,67). Because a thin female body size is idealized less within African-American culture, these women of color may experience less of a self-ideal discrepancy, even at heavier body weights (68–69). Relative to European-American women, they also have a higher threshold for perceiving a body as "fat" (68). Increasingly, researchers are also recognizing that there is substantial diversity of body image experiences within ethnic groups (67,70–71).

Body image experiences may also differ due to sexual orientation. However, the research findings are somewhat clearer for men than for women. Morrison et al. (72) conducted a meta-analysis of 27 extant body image studies that compared heterosexual and homosexual men and women. On average, gay men reported less body satisfaction relative to heterosexual men, whereas lesbian and heterosexual women's body images did not differ, except in those studies in which the two groups were comparable in body mass. In the latter research, lesbian participants expressed a more favorable body image evaluation. In many studies, lesbians have been found to be significantly heavier than heterosexual women (72–73), and this weight disparity may mask women's sexual orientation differences in body image. Most research on body image and sexual orientation has examined the evaluative aspect of body image, yet ignored body image investment. A few published studies have observed higher levels of appearance investment among gay men relative to heterosexual men (74–76).

In summary, contemporary researchers recognize that body image is truly multidimensional; it is not "one thing." Accordingly, numerous psychological assessment techniques have been developed to measure these various facets of body image. Such advances have enabled scientists and clinicians to understand body image with more precision and to elucidate many contributions to individual differences in body image experiences, such as gender, age, ethnicity, and sexual orientation.

BODY IMAGE: HISTORICAL AND DEVELOPMENT DETERMINANTS

According to a cognitive social learning perspective, body image develops as a complex function of various historical and concurrent influences (77–81). Figure 4-1 summarizes this model for understanding body image development and its operation in everyday life. Historical factors refer to past events, attributes, and experiences as well as developmental processes that shape how people come to think, feel, and behave with regard to their physical appearance. These historical/developmental determinants fall into several categories: (i) cultural socialization about the importance and meanings of human physical appearance and one's own body; (ii) interpersonal experiences (including both familial and peer influences), especially experiences during childhood and adolescence; (iii) actual physical characteristics and developmental changes in these attributes; and (iv) personality variables that affect how the individual construes his or her body. As a result of these influences, individuals acquire basic body image attitudes that, in turn, serve to predispose how they attend to, perceive, interpret, and react to current life events.

Several recent volumes have discussed the growing research evidence on these historical influences (7–8,28,81–82). A brief overview of the key findings is presented here.

Cultural Media Forces

As Sarwer and Magee noted in the previous chapter, Western culture's emphasis on beauty and thinness as standards for women permeates all levels of mass me-

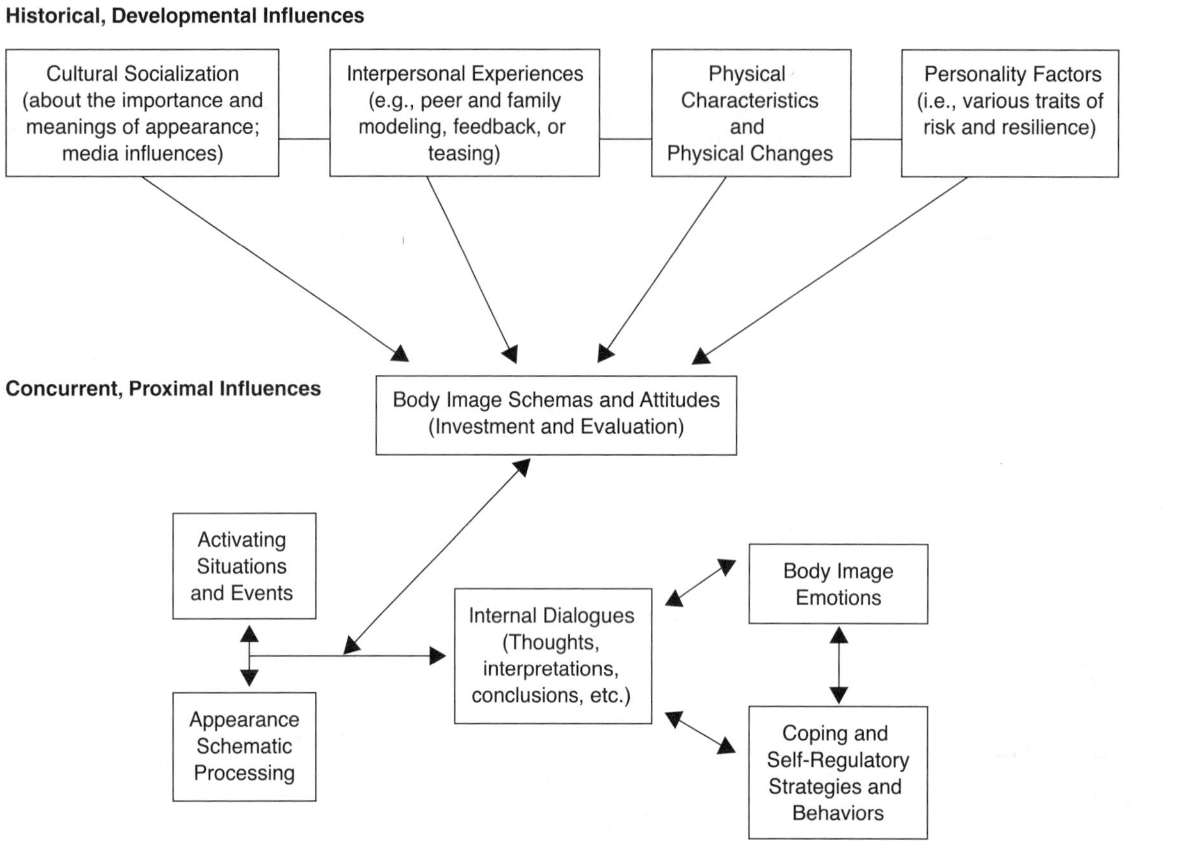

Historical, Developmental Influences

FIGURE 4-1. A cognitive behavioral model of body image development and processes

dia (8,83–84). The widespread dissemination of these cultural expectations fuels the drive for the "ideal female shape" in girls and women. This quest to achieve the societal standard is so common that it has been referred to as a "normative" process (85) even prior to the explosion in cosmetic surgery within the past decade. The internalization of these extreme standards puts females at risk for body image and eating disorders, as well as a host of other psychosocial problems (86–88). The media messages have multiple effects—transmitting the cultural appearance ideal for individual internalization, highlighting the importance of human appearance (the power and necessity of attractiveness), and provoking personal comparisons with these standards in everyday life (potentially inducing recurrent body image dysphoria).

Males do not escape the media's messages about the meaning and ideal of the male body—tall, handsome, lean, broad shouldered, and powerfully muscular. Researchers are beginning to recognize the importance of these cultural images to male body image development (62,65,89). Adoption of these extreme images (such as those seen among professional bodybuilders or wrestlers as well as unrealistically mesomorphic action figure toys) as personal body image ideals may set up the male for body dissatisfaction.

Familial Influences

Expectations, opinions, and verbal or nonverbal messages within the family also influence the formation of body image attitudes (90). Parental modeling conveys the extent to which physical appearance is valued within the family, establishing a yardstick by which the child measures himself or herself. For example, highly appearance-invested mothers who value and engage in dieting behavior or instigate family competition based on physical attractiveness may promote a negative body image in their daughters (91–93). The attractiveness of one's siblings may also affect body image development. Having a more attractive sibling may contribute to a less favorable body image, just as having a less attractive sibling may have the opposite effect (91). Siblings, especially brothers, are frequent perpetrators of appearance-related teasing (91,94). Thus, family members are powerful agents of socialization about the meaning and acceptability of one's physical characteristics.

Peer Influences

As every parent knows, children's peer groups can be very influential on the development of personal values and sense of self. Peers model and reinforce conformity to certain appearance standards, such as what clothing and hairstyles are most desirable. Friendship cliques may also reinforce conformity to group norms about appearance standards and behaviors. For example, research has confirmed greater similarities within such groups of girls on body image concerns and eating/dieting behaviors (95).

Appearance teasing is a common occurrence in childhood and adolescence, and such interpersonal ridicule by peers clearly predisposes body dissatisfaction (96). The child comes to learn that his or her body is an enemy of social acceptance. Correlational evidence confirms a relationship between prior appearance teasing and greater body dissatisfaction in adolescence and adulthood (8,51,91,94,97). Such experiences may play a causal role in faulty body image development (98–99). In addition to teasing, explicit or subtle criticisms about one's appearance may be seen as feedback that one's looks are socially unacceptable (91). A history of appearance-related teasing has differentiated women seeking breast augmentation surgery from similarly small-breasted women not interested in surgery (100).

Romantic Relationships

Physical attractiveness exerts a powerful influence on processes of dating and mating (3–4). However, there has been little research on how body image is affected interpersonally in romantic relationships (96). How one believes one's looks "measure up" to a partner's expectations is an important predictor of one's own body satisfaction (43,101). Of course, sometimes these beliefs about how the partner feels about one's body are merely projections of one's own body image feelings (102). Nevertheless, a more positive body image is associated with having a partner who accepts and compliments one's appearance, and a more negative body image if the partner is critical and demeaning (102).

Childhood Sexual Abuse

In recent years, social and behavioral scientists have made considerable effort to understand the immediate and ultimate impact of childhood sexual abuse (103), including its possible influence on body image development (104–105). Although much of this research has investigated sexual abuse as a risk factor for eating disorders rather than for body image problems per se (106), one plausible hypothesis is that such abuse engenders body contempt, shame, and disgust (105). In Garner's (53) body image survey, 23% of women said sexual abuse was moderately to very important in shaping their body image. While interesting, these data are hardly definitive. The various research reviews provide inconsistent support for the hypothesis (105–106). The aftereffects of sexual abuse are complex and depend on many factors (e.g., timing, duration, and severity of the abuse, relationship with the perpetrator, etc.). Clearly, further prospective research is necessary to clarify the role of childhood sexual abuse in body image development.

Physical Characteristics and Changes

Obesity

Given society's emphasis on thinness and the rampant prejudice and discrimination against fat people, it is not surprising that overweight or obese children, teenagers, and adults often struggle with issues of body image and social acceptance (107–112). The dramatic increases in rates of overweight and obesity in the United States and elsewhere among children and adolescents (113) and adults (114) may place more people at risk for such body image difficulties (82). Obesity affects females' body image attitudes more than it does males' body image (112,115–116). Among obese women, more frequent stigmatizing experiences during childhood, adolescence, and adulthood are associated with poorer body image and psychosocial functioning in adulthood (117). Although weight loss clearly leads to body image improvements (118), a history of obesity may also entail what has been termed "phantom fat," the experience of weight and body image concerns even after weight loss (117,119). This vulnerability may be related to having experienced a weight-related negative body image previously and the realization of the omnipresent potential for weight regain. Following the increasingly popular bariatric surgery for extreme obesity, patients typically report significant improvements in body image (120–121). However, some patients report dissatisfaction with their bodies following the massive weight loss, as a result of loose, sagging skin (122). This dissatisfaction is a likely catalyst to increasing numbers of these individuals who present for a variety of plastic surgical procedures with the hope of reshaping their bodies.

Puberty

The rapid physical change that accompanies puberty can influence body image development. Female puberty often begins about 10 years of age and brings with it adipose weight gain in the hips, abdomen, and breasts. Thus, their body changes in ways contrary to the societal (and perhaps personal) thin ideal, which may provoke self-consciousness, dieting behavior, and concerns about being or becoming fat (123). At about 12 years old, boys enter puberty and experience a broadening of the shoulders, changes in voice, and body growth with increased muscularity. Thus, because boys' physical changes bring them closer to society's standard of "masculinity," they may evaluate their looks more favorably as puberty ensues. Furthermore, some, but not all, research (82) indicates that early pubertal development among girls and late development for boys may exert an adverse impact on body image and self-esteem (124–126).

Pregnancy

Pregnancy is a body-changing experience, but does it affect body image? Davies and Wardle (127) found greater body satisfaction and less weight concern among pregnant than non-pregnant women. However, body image concerns during pregnancy may be especially salient for teenagers (128) and for weight-conscious or eating-disordered women (129). For most women, pregnancy constitutes a period of "suspended reality," in which weight gain is expected and acceptable, trumped by the anticipation of the birth of the baby. The postpartum period, on the other hand, is the "return to reality" that brings concerns about body weight and shape, especially when a woman does not easily return to pre-pregnancy states (127,130).

Personality and Other Individual Difference Factors

A cognitive social learning perspective suggests several factors that may serve as either diatheses or buffers in the development of a negative body image (81). For example, poor self-esteem, social anxiety, and high levels of appearance investment may be predisposing influences. What individual differences, including personality dimensions, operate as protective or resilience characteristics versus vulnerability or risk factors in body image development? This question requires prospective research to provide more definitive answers. Several such longitudinal studies exist, but few include predictors such as self-esteem or specific personality traits, and most examine relatively short-term trajectories of 1 or 2 years during early adolescence. Thus, while it is certainly plausible that positive self-esteem would be protective and negative emotionality would be a risk, the data are simply too limited to reach a conclusion. One factor that emerges as a clearer risk for escalating girls' body image problems is the internalization of the thin-ideal sociocultural standard and beliefs reflecting an investment in one's appearance (82).

One also could hypothesize that traditional gender-role attitudes and values might foster greater appearance investment and body dissatisfaction. Research has pinpointed a link between body image and gender-role attitudes, but only with respect to ideology about male-female social relations (131). Women who endorsed traditional gender attitudes in their social relationships with men were more invested in their appearance, had internalized cultural standards of beauty, and held more maladaptive schemas about their looks. These women also exhibited greater eating disturbance (132). Believing that it is their "feminine duty to be what men want," women not only put their body image in jeopardy, they also are more apt to view other women ambivalently, as their "beauty competitors."

BODY IMAGE: PROXIMAL PROCESSES

Having considered the historical determinants—the cultural, developmental, social, and intrapersonal physical and personality factors—related to acquisition of body image attitudes, it is helpful to consider how such attitudes function within the context of everyday life. Figure 4-1 depicts the cognitive-behavioral model for understanding these influences. Proximal factors refer to current life situations or events and how they are attended to, perceived, processed, and reacted to emotionally and behaviorally (81). These events serve as precipitating or maintaining factors vis-à-vis one's body-image experiences in day-to-day life. As described previously, two attitudinal elements of body image are cognitive-behavioral investment in and affective evaluation of one's appearance.

As discussed above, a core integrative construct of attitudinal body image is the developed *self-schema* as it pertains to one's appearance. Markus (133) defined self-schemas as "cognitive generalizations about the self, derived from past experiences, that organize and guide the processing of self-related information contained in an individual's social experience." The individual who is schematic vis-à-vis a specific self-dimension, such as physical appearance, will likely process information related to that dimension differently than an individual who is not schematic. For example, the appearance-invested cosmetic surgery patient will likely spend considerable mental and behavioral energy thinking about whatever physical characteristic he or she wishes to change.

A situation or event can activate schematic information processing with regard to one's appearance (134). Thus, as Figure 4-1 depicts, contextual cues play an important role in triggering body image experiences at any particular moment. Appearance-schematic persons place more importance on, pay more attention to, and preferentially process information relevant to their appearance. Many events can provoke body image thoughts and emotions. Events such as body exposure, social scrutiny, or wearing certain clothing, among other examples, may trigger automatic thoughts, inferences, interpretations, and conclusions about one's appearance. For appearance-schematic individuals with a negative evaluative body image, these inner dialogues (or "Private Body Talk") are habitual, flawed, and upsetting. They give rise to negative emotions, such as feelings of anxiety or self-consciousness, shame, or anger. Among college women, body image (appearance) schematicity predicted less favorable average body image states (135). It also predicted more variability of body image experiences (e.g., "ups and downs") over time.

People learn a range of strategies to manage or cope with distressing body image thoughts and feelings (81,136). For example, avoidant strategies include behavioral avoidance of certain situations or people or wearing certain body-concealing attire. Appearance-correcting strategies include rituals to alter the perceived "offending" characteristic (e.g., dieting or exercise behavior or perhaps seeking plastic surgery). Seeking social feedback is another approach, whereby individuals solicit reassurance from others to negate or discount their own concerns. Compensatory strategies are attempts to enhance other self-evaluative attributes (physical or otherwise), such as changing a hairstyle to compensate for weight-related concerns. It is important to understand that negative reinforcement processes often govern these habitual, learned efforts, as people seek to escape or avoid bothersome body image experiences. These processes differ from self-regulatory actions motivated by positive self-reinforcement, such as grooming behaviors to enhance thoughts and feelings of body satisfaction or exercise behaviors to promote experiences of physical competence.

There is surprisingly meager research on coping processes in relation to body image functioning. Cash et al. (136) developed the Body Image Coping Strategies Inventory (BICSI) to assess how individuals deal with situations or events that challenge or threaten their body image. Results revealed three body-image coping factors: Coping by *avoidance* entails attempts to avoid the threatening situation or to tune out or ignore the negative emotions associated with the body image threat. Coping by *appearance fixing* involves focusing on and attempting to camouflage or correct one's appearance. Finally, coping by *positive rational acceptance* entails accepting the distress as temporary or illogical and refocusing on personal assets. Although this is a ripe area for research with plastic surgery patients, it is reasonable to expect that they may be very "appearance fixing" in their orientation, yet this and other coping strategies simply do not provide sufficient solace from their body image discomfort. A recent study of college women did confirm that those with more favorable attitudes toward cosmetic surgery were significantly more likely to use appearance-fixing and avoidance coping but neither more nor less likely to cope by positive rational acceptance (50).

In sum, as Figure 4-1 conveys, body image development and functioning entails the complex interaction of multiple determinants and trajectories from the person's social learning history. Understanding these processes requires an appreciation of the fact that body image is "body images"—a pluralistic or multidimensional construct.

BODY IMAGE DISTURBANCES, DISORDERS, AND CONSEQUENCES

Body-image problems may be viewed as falling on a continuum, ranging from mild dissatisfaction to severe psychopathology (7–8,137). For many, negative thoughts and feelings about their appearance are annoying and transient. For others, their chronic preoccupation and distress about their appearance greatly undermine their quality of life. When a negative body image reaches a critical level of severity, it may contribute to several disorders included in the current *Diagnostic and Statistical Manual of Mental Disorders* (DSM-IV-TR) (138). For example, body image disturbances are diagnostic criteria for body dysmorphic disorder (BDD) as well as the eating disorders of anorexia nervosa and bulimia nervosa. As discussed in Chapters 14 and 15, all three disorders may occur with an otherwise higher than expected frequency among cosmetic surgery patients. Furthermore, body image disturbances may also be associated with gender identity disorder (Chapter 13) and certain somatic delusional disorders (138–139).

Body Dysmorphic Disorder

This disorder of "imagined ugliness" entails relentless preoccupation with a perceived defect or minor flaw in one's appearance (140–141). For women and men with BDD, the obsessive worry and compulsive appearance-checking significantly disrupt their functioning, particularly participation in social interactions. BDD involves both perceptual and attitudinal body image disturbances. Individuals with no discernible physical flaw perceive one to exist, and those who exhibit a minor defect perceive it as much more noticeable and "uglier" than objective observers. People with BDD rigidly adhere to distorted thoughts and maladaptive assumptions related to their perceived defect. Although they may recognize the exaggerated nature of their complaints, their self-conscious feelings of unattractiveness are life altering. They frequently feel embarrassed and repulsive to others. They avoid various social events, groom to hide the perceived defect, enact appearance-checking rituals, and make efforts to correct their "defect," including seeking cosmetic surgery, as detailed in Chapter 14.

Eating Disorders and Disturbances

For some people, especially women, being unhappy with one's weight or body shape and being overly invested in one's appearance as a basis for self-evaluation can lead to drastically altered, unhealthy eating behaviors. A multitude of studies have documented both attitudinal and perceptual body image disturbances among eating-disordered patients, as well as those with subclinical eating pathology (8,27,39,142–144). This body of research further suggests that the severity of body image disturbance may determine the severity of eating pathology and that body image problems serve as predisposing, precipitating, and maintaining causes of eating disorders. Chapter 15 includes a discussion of eating disorders among cosmetic surgery patients.

Self-Esteem, Anxiety, Depression, and Sexual Functioning

Most body-dissatisfied people have neither BDD nor a clinical eating disorder. Still, whether cause or consequence, body image is associated with several areas of psychosocial functioning. Body image attitudes and self-esteem are interdependent. Children, adolescents, or adults with negative feelings about their appearance typically report lower self-esteem, especially poorer social self-esteem (58,145–146). Simply stated, if one dislikes one's body, it is difficult to like oneself and vice versa. Body image dissatisfaction and investment also are associated with social anxiety and less secure interpersonal attachment, both in romantic and social relationships (145,147). Furthermore, body image dissatisfaction and investment are related to a greater likelihood of depression (42,148–151).

A reasonable proposition is that body image affects sexual experiences. After all, sexual intimacy entails exposing one's actual unadorned and unconcealed body to another person. Regardless of the causal direction(s) in the relationship, the research literature clearly supports a positive link between body image and the quantity and quality of sexual activity (152–153). One process whereby a poor body image could interfere with sexual pleasure and performance is "spectatoring," an anxious self-focus on one's physical appearance during sex (154–155). Indeed, during sexual activity, persons with generally negative body image attitudes are more likely to attend to those physical attributes they dislike, worry about their partner's perceptions, and try to cover or camouflage those body areas. These immediate body image experiences during sex per se may adversely affect sexual desire, arousal, orgasm, and satisfaction (152–153).

Defining and Measuring Body Image Disturbance

As indicated previously, a good deal of research on body image employs a unidimensional perspective whereby body image is equated with evaluative body image on a continuum of body satisfaction-dissatisfaction. Both Thompson (8,156) and Cash (79,81) have argued for a multidimensional definition of body image disturbance or disorder. Thompson (8) proposed a definition that entails "a persistent report of dissatisfaction, concern, and distress that is related to an aspect of appearance . . . [and] some degree of impairment in social relations, social activities, or occupational functioning." This perspective reflects the contemporary definition of "mental disorder" in the *Diagnostic and Statistical Manual of Mental Disorders* (138).

One attempt to address this problem was the development of an assessment of the impact of body image experiences on individuals' quality of life. The Body Image Quality of Life Inventory (BIQLI) (157–158) measures how persons' body images influence aspects of psychosocial functioning (e.g., self-esteem, moods, social relations, eating behaviors, etc.) known to be related to body image evaluation and investment. The 19 items of the BIQLI are given in Questionnaire 4-2 at the end of this chapter.

A second, recently developed assessment is the Body Image Disturbance Questionnaire (BIDQ) (159), a revised adaptation of the Body Dysmorphic Disorder Questionnaire (140,160) self-report screening tool for BDD. As shown in Questionnaire 4-3, the BIDQ contains seven scaled items that measure (i) concerns about some part(s) of the body felt to be unattractive; (ii) mental preoccupation with these concerns; (iii) experiences of emotional distress over the "defect"; (iv) its production of impairment in social, occupational, or other important areas of functioning; (v) interference with social life; (vi) interference with school, job, or role functioning; and (vii) avoidance of situations due to the "defect." Five of these items also solicit an open-ended clarification of responses that might be helpful in clinical contexts or qualitative research. Initial research is highly supportive of the reliability and validity of the BIDQ. Although this is a promising assessment for plastic surgery patients, it is too new for such data to be available. One study (50) found that college women with more favorable attitudes toward future cosmetic surgery have significantly greater body image disturbance on the BIDQ as well as a poorer body image quality of life on the BIQLI.

PSYCHOSOCIAL APPROACHES TO BODY IMAGE CHANGE

Because a negative body image is a widespread problem that may impair psychosocial functioning and quality of life, professionals have developed a variety of psychotherapeutic treatments for this problem (7). Krueger (161–164) has described a complex and interesting approach to body image problems that derives from developmental and relational psychodynamic theories. Rabinor and Bilich (165) have discussed richly diverse experiential psychotherapeutic approaches to body-image change. Unfortunately, few well-designed studies have been conducted to evaluate the effectiveness of these treatments.

In contrast, a cognitive-behavioral therapy (CBT) approach to body image change has received considerable scientific scrutiny over the past 20 years. This structured, multicomponent derives from the cognitive-behavioral models discussed previously in this chapter and conveyed in Figure 4-1. This treatment (166) actively guides patients in learning new ways to think and behave in order to overcome specific body image problems. As a detailed examination of CBT outcome studies is beyond the scope of this chapter, the reader is referred to recent, comprehensive reviews (167–168). These reviews indicate that body image CBT has emerged as an effective, empirically sound intervention, with efficacy in individual therapy, group therapy, and a self-help format. Outcomes not only reflect body image improvements, but they also confirm positive effects on self-esteem, social functioning, depressive symptoms, eating pathology, and sexual experiences. Although most treatment studies were conducted with extremely body-dissatisfied college women, further evidence confirms the efficacy of body image CBT for obese individuals (169) and BDD patients (170–171). One limitation of these studies is that they have not ascertained the maintenance of these successful outcomes beyond one year.

Cash's CBT program for a negative body image has gone through four generations of development, culminating in *The Body Image Workbook: An 8-Step Program for Learning to Like Your Looks* (77). The elements of this version of the program are summarized as follows:

- **Step 1** involves taking initial self-assessments of various facets of body image. Using interpretations provided for the assessment profile, participants then set specific goals for body image change.
- **Step 2** is a psychoeducational facet of the program, detailing information on the nature of body image and the causes of a negative body image. The self-discovery process also includes mirror-exposure activities and an autobiographical summary of participants' own body-image development. Using a "Body Image Diary," participants learn how to monitor their current body image experiences by attending to and recording the triggers of distress and the effects that these activating events have on their thought processes ("Private Body Talk"), emotions, and subsequent behaviors. This diary is used systematically throughout the program.
- **Step 3** teaches "Body and Mind Relaxation" for managing dysphoric body-image emotions. These skills are applied in desensitization exercises to enable persons to learn how to control and reduce their body-image dysphoria in a variety of troublesome situations.
- **Step 4** identifies 10 problematic "appearance assumptions"—beliefs or schemas about appearance that are the foundation of distressing and disruptive body image experiences. Examples of these assumptions are: "If people knew how I really look, they would like me less." "Physically attractive people have it all." "If I could look just as I wish, my life would be much happier." "The only way I could ever like my looks would be to change them." Participants learn to become cognizant of how these core assumptions operate in daily life and to question and refute them.
- **Step 5** enables participants to identify cognitive errors or distortions in their Private Body Talk and offers strategies for changing them. Such distortions include comparing one's appearance to more attractive persons, thinking of one's looks in dichotomous extremes (e.g., fat or thin, ugly or good-looking), and arbitrarily blaming one's appearance for life's difficulties or disappointments. Participants expand their body image diary to incorporate cognitive restructuring exercises in correcting their distortions and observing the improved consequences.
- **Step 6** details specific behavioral strategies to alter avoidant behaviors related to a poor body image—avoiding certain activities (e.g., exercising, going without make-up, or having sex), situations (e.g., the beach or gym), or people (e.g., attractive women) that might provoke self-consciousness and body-image distress. Participants also target and modify "appearance-preoccupied rituals," such as repeated mirror checking or excessive grooming regimens.
- **Step 7** applies the metaphor of interpersonal relationship satisfaction (e.g., a fulfilling marriage or friendship) to build a proactive, positive relationship with one's

body. Participants engage in prescribed activities for body-image affirmation and enhancement—for instance, "mastery and pleasure" activities for physical fitness and health, sensate pleasure, and grooming for enjoyment instead concealment or repair.

■ **Step 8** concludes the program by having individuals retake the body image tests and receive feedback about their attained changes. Participants then set goals for continued changes. From a perspective of relapse prevention, they learn to identify and prepare for future situations that could place their body image at risk.

The effectiveness of CBT for improving body image is well established (167–168). While body image CBT may be viewed as an alternative to plastic surgery for some body-dissatisfied persons, it may also have value in conjunction with surgery. For example, as an adjunctive, self-help program (77), these patients may benefit by learning more about how their body-image experiences have developed and now influence their lives, as well as how to better manage ongoing threats to their body image and to optimize their psychosocial outcomes from surgery.

THE IMPORTANCE OF BODY IMAGE IN COSMETIC AND RECONSTRUCTIVE SURGERY

The current chapter has maintained that body image is central to both a scientific and clinical understanding of the need for, and effects of, plastic surgery. Patients come to be unhappy, to varying degrees, with some physical characteristic(s), which they seek to alter aesthetically. Their body image experiences and changes are complex, multifaceted, and vary from patient to patient. Some patients will have a focal cosmetic concern that does not greatly impact their overall body image and psychosocial quality of life. At the other extreme are those patients whose body image concerns are more pervasive and psychologically debilitating.

This chapter has offered a framework for understanding how body image difficulties develop as a function of a number of historical determinants. Moreover, it delineated how these experiences unfold and affect day-to-day life. Both preoperatively and postoperatively, a clinical or empirical assessment of body image should pose multiple questions: How does the patient perceive, think, and feel about the physical attribute that she or he wishes to alter? How long has the patient felt this way? How much does this discontent influence the patient's feelings about his or her overall appearance? How invested is the patient in his or her appearance as a criterion of self-worth? How, when, and where does the body image difficulty affect functioning in everyday life (e.g., self-esteem, moods and emotions, social interactions, sexuality, grooming behaviors, eating and exercise behaviors, etc.)? How does the patient attempt to cope with problems engendered by the body image discontent? How realistic are the patient's expectations of the desired surgical changes and psychosocial changes?

Beyond the Hippocratic dictum to do no harm is the wisdom to offer optimal patient care. Physicians and their staff can truly enhance the quality of patient care by understanding body image and applying this knowledge to the individual patient to enhance the quality of embodied life.

Selected Items of the MBSRQ-AS

Instructions: The following are statements about how people might think, feel, or behave. Please indicate the *extent to which each statement pertains to you personally*. Using the scale below, indicate your answer by entering a number from 1 to 5 to the left of the statement. There are no right or wrong answers. Just give the answer that is most accurate for you.

1	2	3	4	5
Definitely Disagree	*Mostly Disagree*	*Neither Agree Nor Disagree*	*Mostly Agree*	*Definitely Agree*

_____ I like my looks just the way they are.

_____ My body is sexually appealing.

_____ Most people would consider me good-looking.

_____ I am physically unattractive.

_____ I like the way I look without my clothes on.

_____ I like the way my clothes fit me.

_____ I dislike my physique.

Use the scale below to indicate how dissatisfied or satisfied you are with each of the following areas or aspects of your body.

1	2	3	4	5
Very Dissatisfied	*Mostly Dissatisfied*	*Neither Satisfied Nor Dissatisfied*	*Mostly Satisfied*	*Very Satisfied*

_____ Face (facial features, complexion)

_____ Hair (color, thickness, texture)

_____ Lower torso (buttocks, hips, thighs, legs)

_____ Mid torso (waist, stomach)

_____ Upper torso (chest or breasts, shoulders, arms)

_____ Muscle tone

_____ Weight

_____ Height

_____ Overall appearance

The Body Image Quality of Life Inventory (BIQLI)

Instructions: Different people have different feelings about their physical appearance. These feelings are called "body image." Some people are generally satisfied with their looks, while others are dissatisfied. At the same time, people differ in terms of how their body-image experiences affect other aspects of their lives. Body image may have positive effects, negative effects, or no effect at all. Listed below are various ways that your own body image may or may not influence your life. For each item, circle how and how much your feelings about your appearance affect that aspect of your life. Before answering each item, think carefully about the answer that is most accurate about how your body image usually affects you.

−3	−2	−1	0	1	2	3
Very Negative Effect	Moderate Negative Effect	Slight Negative Effect	No Effect	Slight Positive Effect	Moderate Positive Effect	Very Positive Effect

1. My basic feelings about myself—feelings of personal adequacy and self-worth   −3 −2 −1 0 +1 +2 +3
2. My feelings about my adequacy as a man or woman— feelings of masculinity or femininity.   −3 −2 −1 0 +1 +2 +3
3. My interactions with people of my own sex.   −3 −2 −1 0 +1 +2 +3
4. My interactions with people of the other sex.   −3 −2 −1 0 +1 +2 +3
5. My experiences when I meet new people.   −3 −2 −1 0 +1 +2 +3
6. My experiences at work or at school.   −3 −2 −1 0 +1 +2 +3
7. My relationships with friends.   −3 −2 −1 0 +1 +2 +3
8. My relationships with family members.   −3 −2 −1 0 +1 +2 +3
9. My day-to-day emotions.   −3 −2 −1 0 +1 +2 +3
10. My satisfaction with my life in general.   −3 −2 −1 0 +1 +2 +3
11. My feelings of acceptability as a sexual partner.   −3 −2 −1 0 +1 +2 +3
12. My enjoyment of my sex life.   −3 −2 −1 0 +1 +2 +3
13. My ability to control what and how much I eat.   −3 −2 −1 0 +1 +2 +3
14. My ability to control my weight.   −3 −2 −1 0 +1 +2 +3
15. My activities for physical exercise.   −3 −2 −1 0 +1 +2 +3
16. My willingness to do things that might call attention to my appearance.   −3 −2 −1 0 +1 +2 +3
17. My daily "grooming" activities (i.e., getting dressed and physically ready for the day).   −3 −2 −1 0 +1 +2 +3
18. How confident I feel in my everyday life.   −3 −2 −1 0 +1 +2 +3
19. How happy I feel in my everyday life.   −3 −2 −1 0 +1 +2 +3

The Body Image Disturbance Questionnaire

Instructions: This questionnaire assesses concerns about physical appearance. Please read each question carefully and circle the answer that best describes your experience. Also write in answers where indicated.

Are you concerned about the appearance of some part(s) of your body which you consider especially unattractive? (Circle the best answer)

1	2	3	4	5
Not at all concerned	**Somewhat concerned**	**Moderately concerned**	**Very concerned**	**Extremely concerned**

What are these concerns? What specifically bothers you about the appearance of these body parts?

_____

_____

_____

If you are at least somewhat concerned, do these concerns preoccupy you? That is, you think about them a lot and they're hard to stop thinking about? (Circle the best answer)

1	2	3	4	5
Not at all preoccupied	**Somewhat preoccupied**	**Moderately preoccupied**	**Very preoccupied**	**Extremely preoccupied**

What effect has your preoccupation with your appearance had on your life? (Please describe):

_____

_____

_____

Has your physical "defect" often caused you a lot of distress, torment, or pain? How much? (Circle the best answer)

1	2	3	4	5
No distress	**Mild, and not too disturbing**	**Moderate and disturbing but still manageable**	**Severe, and very disturbing**	**Extreme, and disabling**

(continued)

QUESTIONNAIRE 4-3 *(continued)*

Has your physical "defect" caused you impairment in social, occupational, or other important areas of functioning? How much? (Circle the best answer)

1	2	3	4	5
No limitation	Mild interference but overall performance not impaired	Moderate, definite interference but still manageable	Severe, causes substantial impairment	Extreme, incapacitating

Has your physical "defect" significantly interfered with your social life? How much? (Circle the best answer)

1	2	3	4	5
Never	Occasionally	Moderately Often	Often	Very often

If so, how?

_____
_____
_____

Has your physical "defect" significantly interfered with your schoolwork, your job, or your ability to function in your role? How much? (Circle the best answer)

1	2	3	4	5
Never	Occasionally	Moderately Often	Often	Very often

If so, how?

_____
_____
_____

Do you ever avoid things because of your physical "defect"? How often? (Circle the best answer)

1	2	3	4	5
Never	Occasionally	Moderately Often	Often	Very often

If so, what do you avoid?

_____
_____
_____

REFERENCES

1. Cash TF. The psychology of physical appearance: aesthetics, attributes, and images. In: Cash TF, Pruzinsky T, eds. *Body Images: Development, Deviance, and Change.* New York: Guilford Press, 1990:51–79.
2. Bull R, Rumsey N. *The Social Psychology of Facial Appearance.* New York: Springer-Verlag, 1988.
3. Etcoff N. *Survival of the Prettiest: The Science of Beauty.* New York: Doubleday, 1999.
4. Jackson LA. *Physical Appearance and Gender: Sociobiological and Sociocultural Perspectives.* Albany, NY: SUNY Press, 1992.
5. Jackson LA. Physical attractiveness: a sociocultural perspective. In: Cash TF, Pruzinsky T, eds. *Body Image: A Handbook of Theory, Research, and Clinical Practice.* New York: Guilford Press, 2002:13–21.
6. Cash TF, Pruzinsky T, eds. *Body Images: Development, Deviance, and Change.* New York: Guilford Press, 1990.
7. Cash TF, Pruzinsky T, eds. *Body Image: A Handbook of Theory, Research, and Clinical Practice.* New York: Guilford Press, 2002.
8. Thompson JK, Heinberg LJ, Altabe M, Tantleff-Dunn S. *Exacting Beauty: Theory, Assessment, and Treatment of Body Image Disturbance.* Washington, DC: American Psychological Association, 1999.
9. Pruzinsky T, Edgerton MT. Body image change in cosmetic plastic surgery. In: Cash TF, Pruzinsky T, eds. *Body Images: Development, Deviance, and Change.* New York: Guilford Press, 1990:217–236.
10. Sarwer DB. Plastic surgery in children and adolescents. In: Thompson JK, Smolak L, eds. *Body Image, Eating Disorders, and Obesity in Youth.* Washington, DC: Amercian Psychological Association, 2001:341–366.
11. Sarwer DB. Cosmetic surgery and changes in body image. In: Cash TF, Pruzinsky T, eds. *Body Image: A Handbook of Theory, Research, and Clinical Practice.* New York: Guilford Press, 2002:422–430.
12. Sarwer DB, Crerand CE. Body image and cosmetic medical treatments. *Body Image: An International Journal of Research* 2004;1:99–111.
13. Sarwer DB, Magee L, Crerand CE. Cosmetic surgery and cosmetic medical treatments. In: Thompson JK, ed. *Handbook of Eating Disorders and Obesity.* Hoboken, NJ: John Wiley and Sons, 2004:718–737.
14. Sarwer DB, Wadden TA, Pertschuk MJ, Whitaker LA. The psychology of cosmetic surgery: a review and reconceptualization. *Clin Psychol Rev* 1998;18:1–22.
15. Sarwer DB, Wadden TA, Whitaker LA. An investigation of changes in body image following cosmetic surgery. *Plast Reconstr Surg* 2002;109:363–369.
16. Pruzinsky T. Body image adaptation to reconstructive surgery for acquired disfigurement. In: Cash TF, Pruzinsky T, eds. *Body Image: A Handbook of Theory, Research, and Clinical Practice.* New York: Guilford Press, 2002:440–449.
17. Rumsey N. Body image and congenital conditions with visible differences. In: Cash TF, Pruzinsky T, eds. *Body Image: A Handbook of Theory, Research, and Clinical Practice.* New York: Guilford Press, 2002:226–235.
18. Rumsey N. Optimizing body image in disfiguring congenital conditions: surgical and psychosocial interventions. In: Cash TF, Pruzinsky T, eds. *Body Image: A Handbook of Theory, Research, and Clinical Practice.* New York: Guilford Press, 2002:431–439.
19. Rumsey N, Harcourt D. Body image and disfigurement: issues and interventions. *Body Image: An International Journal of Research* 2004;1:83–97.
20. Fisher S. The evolution of psychological concepts about the body. In: Cash TF, Pruzinsky T, eds. *Body Images: Development, Deviance, and Change.* New York: Guilford Press, 1990:3–20.
21. Fisher S. *Development and Structure of the Body Image,* Vols. 1, 2. Hillsdale, NJ: Lawrence Erlbaum Associates, 1986.
22. Fisher S. *Body Experience in Fantasy and Behavior.* New York: Appleton-Century-Crofts, 1970.
23. Fisher S, Cleveland SE. *Body Image and Personality,* 2nd rev ed. New York: Dover Publications, 1968.
24. Shontz FC. *Perceptual and Cognitive Aspects of Body Experience.* New York: Macmillan, 1969.
25. Shontz FC. Body image and physical disability. In: Cash TF, Pruzinsky T, eds. *Body Image: A Handbook of Theory, Research, and Clinical Practice.* New York: Guilford Press, 2002:149–169.
26. Thompson JK, ed. *Body Image, Eating Disorders, and Obesity: An Integrative Guide for Assessment and Treatment.* Washington, DC: American Psychological Association, 1996.
27. Thompson JK, ed. *Handbook of Eating Disorders and Obesity.* Hoboken, NJ: John Wiley and Sons, 2004.
28. Thompson JK, Smolak L, eds. *Body Image, Eating Disorders, and Obesity in Youth: Assessment, Prevention, and Treatment.* Washington, DC: American Psychological Association, 2001.
29. Cash TF. Body image: past, present, and future. *Body Image: Int J Res* 2004, 1:1–5.
30. Pruzinsky T, Cash TF. Understanding body images: historical and contemporary perspectives. In: Cash TF, Pruzinsky T, eds. *Body Image: A Handbook of Theory, Research, and Clinical Practice.* New York: Guilford Press, 2002:3–12.
31. Koo JYM, Yeung J. Body image issues in dermatology. In: Cash TF, Pruzinsky T, eds. *Body Image: A Handbook of Theory, Research, and Clinical Practice.* New York: Guilford Press, 2002:333–341.
32. Kiyak HA, Reichmuth M. Body image issues in dental medicine. In: Cash TF, Pruzinsky T, eds. *Body Image: A Handbook of Theory, Research, and Clinical Practice.* New York: Guilford Press, 2002:342–350.
33. Heinberg LJ, Guarda AS. Body image issues in obstetrics and gynecology. In: Cash TF, Pruzinsky T, eds. *Body Image: A Handbook of Theory, Research, and Clinical Practice.* New York: Guilford Press, 2002: 351–360.
34. Tovian SM. Body image and urological disorders. In: Cash TF, Pruzinsky T, eds. *Body Image: A Handbook of Theory, Research, and Clinical Practice.* New York: Guilford Press, 2002:361–369.
35. Gilmour J. Body image issues in endocrinology. In: Cash TF, Pruzinsky T, eds. *Body Image: A Handbook of Theory, Research, and Clinical Practice.* New York: Guilford Press, 2002:370–378.
36. White CA. Body images in oncology. In: Cash TF, Pruzinsky T, eds. *Body Image: A Handbook of Theory, Research, and Clinical Practice.* New York: Guilford Press, 2002:379–386.
37. Rybarczyk BD, Behel JM. Rehabilitation medicine and body image. In: Cash TF, Pruzinsky T, eds. *Body Image: A Handbook of Theory, Research, and Clinical Practice.* New York: Guilford Press, 2002:387–394.

38. Chapman, E. Body image issues among individuals with HIV and AIDS. In: Cash TF, Pruzinsky T, eds. *Body Image: A Handbook of Theory, Research, and Clinical Practice.* New York: Guilford Press, 2002:395–402.
39. Cash TF, Deagle EA. The nature and extent of body-image disturbances in anorexia nervosa and bulimia nervosa: a meta-analysis. *Int J Eat Disord* 1997;22:107–125.
40. Thompson JK, Gardner RM. Measuring perceptual body image among adolescents and adults. In: Cash TF, Pruzinsky T, eds. *Body Image: A Handbook of Theory, Research, and Clinical Practice.* New York: Guilford Press, 2002:135–141.
41. Thompson JK, van den Berg P. Measuring body image attitudes among adolescents and adults. In: Cash TF, Pruzinsky T, eds. *Body Image: A Handbook of Theory, Research, and Clinical Practice.* New York: Guilford Press, 2002:142–154.
42. Cash TF, Szymanski M. Development and validation of the Body-Image Ideals Questionnaire. *J Pers Assess* 1995;64:466–477.
43. Szymanski M, Cash TF. Body-image disturbances and self-discrepancy theory: expansion of the Body-Image Ideals Questionnaire. *J Soc Clin Psychol* 1995;14:134–146.
44. Franzoi SL, Shields SA. The Body Esteem Scale: multidimensional structure and sex differences in a college population. *J Pers Assess* 1984;48:173–179.
45. Brown TA, Cash TF, Mikulka PJ. Attitudinal body-image assessment: factor analysis of the Body-Self Relations Questionnaire. *J Pers Assess* 1990;55:135–144.
46. Cash TF. Body-image assessments: manuals and questionnaires [Author's Web site]. Available at http://www.body-images.com. Accessed May 22, 2005.
47. Cash, TF. *The Multidimensional Body-Self Relations Questionnaire Users' Manual,* 3rd revision. Published by author, Norfolk, VA: Old Dominion University, 2000.
48. Cash TF. The Situational Inventory of Body-Image Dysphoria: psychometric evidence and development of a short form. *Int J Eat Disord* 2002;32:362–366.
49. Cash TF, Melnyk SE, Hrabosky JI. The assessment of body-image investment: an extensive revision of the Appearance Schemas Inventory. *Int J Eat Disord* 2004;35:305–316.
50. Cash TF, Goldenberg R, Grasso K. *Body-image predictors of college women's attitudes toward cosmetic surgery.* Manuscript in preparation, 2005.
51. Cash TF, Winstead BA, Janda LH. The great American shape-up: body image survey report. *Psychol Today* April 1986;20:30–37.
52. Cash TF, Henry PE. Women's body images: The results of a national survey in the U.S.A. *Sex Roles* 1995;33:19–28.
53. Garner DM. The 1997 body image survey results. *Psychol Today* Jan/Feb 1997;30:30–44,75–80,84.
54. Cash TF. A "negative body image": Evaluating epidemiological evidence. In: Cash TF, Pruzinsky T, eds. *Body Image: A Handbook of Theory, Research, and Clinical Practice.* New York: Guilford Press, 2002:269–276.
55. Feingold A, Mazzella R. Gender differences in body image are increasing. *Psychol Sci* 1998;9:190–195.
56. Cash TF, Morrow JA, Hrabosky JI, Perry A. How has body image changed? A cross-sectional investigation of college women and men from 1983 to 2001. *J Consult Clin Psychol* 2004;72:1081–1089.
57. Muth JL, Cash TF. Body-image attitudes: what difference does gender make? *J Applied Soc Psychol* 1997;27:1438–1452.
58. Pliner P, Chaiken S, Flett GL. Gender differences in concern with body weight and physical appearance over the life span. *Pers Soc Psychol Bull* 1990;16:263–273.
59. Sarwer DB, Whitaker LA, Wadden TA, Pertschuk MJ. Body image dissatisfaction in women seeking rhytidectomy and blepharoplasty. *Aesthetic Surg J* 1997;17:230–234.
60. Tiggemann M. Body image across the adult life span: stability and change. *Body Image: An International Journal of Research* 2004;1:29–41.
61. Whitbourne SK, Skultety KM. Body image development: adulthood and aging. In: Cash TF, Pruzinsky T, eds. *Body Image: A Handbook of Theory, Research, and Clinical Practice.* New York: Guilford Press, 2002:83–90.
62. Corson PW, Andersen AE. Body image issues among boys and men. In: Cash TF, Pruzinsky T, eds. *Body Image: A Handbook of Theory, Research, and Clinical Practice.* New York: Guilford Press, 2002:192–199.
63. McCabe MP, Ricciardelli LA. Weight and shape concerns of boys and men. In: Thompson JK, ed. *Handbook of Eating Disorders and Obesity.* Hoboken, NJ: John Wiley and Sons, 2004:606–634.
64. Olivardia R. Body image and muscularity. In: Cash TF, Pruzinsky T, eds. *Body Image: A Handbook of Theory, Research, and Clinical Practice.* New York: Guilford Press, 2002:210–218.
65. Pope HG, Phillips KA, Olivardia R. *The Adonis Complex: The Secret Crisis of Male Body Obsession.* New York: The Free Press, 2000.
66. Pertschuk MJ, Sarwer DB, Wadden TA, et al. Body image dissatisfaction in male cosmetic surgery patients. *Aesthetic Plast Surg* 1998;22:20–24.
67. Celio AA, Zabinski MF, Wilfley DE. African-American body images. In: Cash TF, Pruzinsky T, eds. *Body Image: A Handbook of Theory, Research, and Clinical Practice.* New York: Guilford Press, 2002:234–242.
68. Rucker C, Cash TF. Body images, body-size perceptions, and eating behaviors among African-American and White college women. *Intl J Eat Disord* 1992;12:231–299.
69. Parker S, Nichter M, Vuckovic N, et al. Body image and weight concerns among African-American and white adolescent females: differences that make a difference. *Hum Organ* 1995;54:103–114.
70. Kawamura KY. Asian American body images. In: Cash TF, Pruzinsky T, eds. *Body Image: A Handbook of Theory, Research, and Clinical Practice.* New York: Guilford Press, 2002:243–249.
71. Altabe M, O'Garo KN. Hispanic body images. In: Cash TF, Pruzinsky T, eds. *Body Image: A Handbook of Theory, Research, and Clinical Practice.* New York: Guilford Press, 2002:250–256.
72. Morrison MA, Morrison TG, Sager CL. Does body satisfaction differ between gay men and lesbian women and heterosexual men and women? A meta-analytic review. *Body Image: An International Journal of Research* 2004;1:127–138.
73. Rothblum ED. Gay and lesbian body images. In: Cash TF, Pruzinsky T, eds. *Body Image: A Handbook of Theory, Research, and Clinical Practice.* New York: Guilford Press, 2002:257–265.

74. Gettleman TE, Thompson JK. Actual differences and stereotypical perceptions in body image and eating disturbance: a comparison of male and female heterosexual and homosexual samples. *Sex Roles* 1993;29:545–561.

75. Siever MD. Sexual orientation and gender as factors in socioculturally acquired vulnerability to body dissatisfaction and eating disorders. *J Consult Clin Psychol* 1994;62:252–260.

76. Yelland C, Tiggemann M. Maculinity and the gay ideal: body dissatisfaction and disordered eating in homosexual men. *Eat Behav* 2003;4:107–116.

77. Cash TF. Body image and cosmetic surgery: the psychology of physical appearance. *Amer J Cosmetic Surg* 1996;13:345–351.

78. Cash TF. *The Body Image Workbook: An 8-step Program for Learning to Like Your Looks.* Oakland, CA: New Harbinger, 1997.

79. Cash TF. Women's body images. In: Wingood G, DiClemente D, eds. *Handbook of Women's Sexual and Reproductive Health.* New York: Plenum Publishing, 2002:175–194.

80. Cash TF, Grant JR. Cognitive-behavioral treatment of body-image disturbances. In: Van Hasselt VB, Hersen M, eds. *Sourcebook of Psychological Treatment Manuals for Adult Disorders.* New York: Plenum Publishing, 1995:567–614.

81. Cash TF. Cognitive-behavioral perspectives on body image. In: Cash TF, Pruzinsky T, eds. *Body Image: A Handbook of Theory, Research, and Clinical Practice.* New York: Guilford Press, 2002:38–46.

82. Wertheim EH, Paxton SJ, Blaney S. Risk factors for the development of body image disturbances. In: Thompson JK, ed. *Handbook of Eating Disorders and Obesity.* Hoboken, NJ: John Wiley and Sons, 2004:463–494.

83. Fallon AE. Culture in the mirror: sociocultural determinant of body image. In: Cash TF, Pruzinsky T, eds. *Body Images: Development, Deviance, and Change.* New York: Guilford Press, 1990:80–105.

84. Tiggemann M. Media influences on body image development. In: Cash TF, Pruzinsky T, eds. *Body Image: A Handbook of Theory, Research, and Clinical Practice.* New York: Guilford Press, 2002:91–98.

85. Rodin J, Silberstein L, Striegel-Moore R. Women and weight: A normative discontent. *Nebraska Symposium on Motivation* 1985;32:267–307.

86. Levine MP, Harrison K. Media's role in the perpetuation and prevention of negative body image and disordered eating. In: Thompson JK, ed. *Handbook of Eating Disorders and Obesity.* Hoboken, NJ: John Wiley and Sons, 2004:695–717.

87. Striegel-Moore RH, Franko DL. Body image issues among girls and women. In: Cash TF, Pruzinsky T, eds. *Body Image: A Handbook of Theory, Research, and Clinical Practice.* New York: Guilford Press, 2002: 183–191.

88. Thompson JK, Stice E. Thin-ideal internalization: mounting evidence for a new risk factor for body-image disturbance and eating pathology. *Current Directions in Psychological Science* 2001;10:181–183.

89. Leit RA, Gray JJ, Pope HG. The media's representation of the ideal male body: a cause for muscle dysmorphia? *Int J Eat Disord* 2001;31:334–338.

90. Kearney-Cooke A. Familial influences on body image development. In: Cash TF, Pruzinsky T, eds. *Body Image: A Handbook of Theory, Research, and Clinical Practice.* New York: Guilford Press, 2002:99–107.

91. Rieves L, Cash TF. Social developmental factors and women's body-image attitudes. *J Soc Beh Pers* 1996;11:63–78.

92. Rozin P, Fallon A. Body image, attitudes to weight, and misperceptions of figure preferences of the opposite sex: a comparison of men and women in two generations. *J Abnorm Psychol* 1988;97:342–345.

93. Striegel-Moore RH, Silberstein LR, Rodin J. Toward an understanding of risk factors for bulimia. *Am Psychol* 1986;41:246–263.

94. Cash TF. Developmental teasing about physical appearance: retrospective descriptions and relationships with body image. *Soc Beh Pers* 1995;23:123–130.

95. Paxton SJ, Schutz HK, Wertheim EH, Muir SL. Friendship clique and peer influences on body image concerns, eating restraint, extreme weight-loss behaviors, and binge eating in adolescent girls. *J Abnorm Psychol* 1999;108:255–266.

96. Tantleff-Dunn S, Gokee JL. Interpersonal influences on body image development. In: Cash TF, Pruzinsky T, eds. *Body Image: A Handbook of Theory, Research, and Clinical Practice.* New York: Guilford Press, 2002:108–116.

97. Grilo CM, Wilfley DE, Brownell KD, Rodin J. Teasing, body image, and self-esteem in a clinical sample of obese women. *Addict Behav* 1994;19:443–450.

98. Cattarin JA, Thompson JK. A three-year longitudinal study of body image, eating concerns, and general psychological functioning in adolescent girls. *Eating Disorders* 1994;2:114–125.

99. Thompson JK, Heinberg LJ. Preliminary test of two hypotheses of body image disturbance. *Int J Eat Disord* 1993;14:59–63.

100. Sarwer DB, LaRossa D, Bartlett S, et al. Body image concerns of breast augmentation patients. *Plast Reconstr Surg* 2003;112:83–90.

101. Tantleff-Dunn S, Thompson JK. Romantic partners and body image disturbance: further evidence for the role of perceived-actual disturbances. *Sex Roles* 1995;33:589–605.

102. Cash TF, Grasso K, Rieves L. *Body image and perceived partner attitudes toward one's physical appearance.* Manuscript in preparation for publication, 2005.

103. Kendall-Tackett KA, Meyer-Williams L, Finkelhor D. Impact of sexual abuse on children: a review and synthesis of recent empirical studies. *Psychol Bull* 1993;113:164–180.

104. Fallon P, Ackard DM. Sexual abuse and body image. In: Cash TF, Pruzinsky T, eds. *Body Image: A Handbook of Theory, Research, and Clinical Practice.* New York: Guilford Press, 2002:117–124.

105. Thompson JK, Wonderlich SA. Child sexual abuse and eating disorders. In: Thompson JK, ed. *Handbook of Eating Disorders and Obesity.* Hoboken, NJ: John Wiley and Sons, 2004:679–694.

106. Connors ME. Relationship of sexual abuse to body image and eating problems. In: Thompson JK, Smolak L, eds. *Body Image, Eating Disorders, and Obesity in Youth.* Washington, DC: American Psychological Association, 2001:149–167.

107. Cash TF, Roy RE. Pounds of flesh: weight, gender, and body images. In: Sobal J, Maurer D, eds. *Interpreting Weight: The Social Management of Fatness and Thinness.* Hawthorne, NY: Aldine de Gruyter, 1999: 209–228.

108. Friedman MA, Brownell KD. Psychological correlates of obesity: moving to the next research generation. *Psychol Bull* 1995;117:3–20.

109. Gortmaker SL, Must A, Perrin JM, et al. Social and economic consequences of overweight in adolescence and young adulthood. *N Engl J Med* 1993;329:1008–1012.

110. Sarwer DB, Thompson JK, Cash TF. Obesity and body image in adulthood. *Psych Clin NA* 2005;28:69–87.

111. Schwartz MB, Brownell KD. Obesity and body image. In: Cash TF, Pruzinsky T, eds. *Body Image: A Handbook of Theory, Research, and Clinical Practice.* New York: Guilford Press, 2002:200–209.

112. Schwartz MB, Brownell KD. Obesity and body image. *Body Image: An International Journal of Research* 2004;1:43–56.

113. Ogden CL, Flegal KM, Carroll MD, Johnson CL. Prevalence and trends in overweight among US children and adolescents, 1999–2000. *JAMA* 2002;288:1728–1732.

114. Flegal KM, Carroll MD, Ogden CL, Johnson CL. Prevalence and trends in obesity among US adults, 1999–2000. *JAMA* 2002;288:1723–1727.

115. Cash TF, Hicks KL. Being fat versus thinking fat: relationships with body image, eating behaviors, and well-being. *Cog Ther Res* 1990;14:327–341.

116. Tiggemann M, Rothblum ED. Gender differences in social consequences of perceived overweight in the United States and Australia. *Sex Roles* 1988;18:75–86.

117. Annis NM, Cash TF, Hrabosky JI. Body image and psychosocial differences among stable average weight, currently overweight, and formerly overweight women: The role of stigmatizing experiences. *Body Image: An International Journal of Research* 2004;1:155–167.

118. Foster GD, Matz PE. Weight loss and changes in body image. In: Cash TF, Pruzinsky T, eds. *Body Image: A Handbook of Theory, Research, and Clinical Practice.* New York: Guilford Press, 2002:405–413.

119. Cash TF, Counts B, Huffine CE. Current and vestigial effects of overweight among women: fear of fat, attitudinal body image, and eating behaviors. *J Psychopath Beh Assess* 1990;12:157–167.

120. Dixon JB, Dixon ME, O'Brien PE. Body image: appearance orientation and evaluation in the severely obese. *Obes Surg* 2002;12:65–71.

121. Neven K, Dymek M, leGrange D, et al. The effects of Roux-en-Y gastric bypass surgery on body image. *Obes Surg* 2002;12:265–269.

122. Sarwer DB, Wadden TA, Fabricatore AN. Psychosocial and behavioral aspects of bariatric surgery. *Obes Res* 2005;13:639–648.

123. Attie I, Brooks-Gunn J. Development of eating problems in adolescent girls: a longitudinal study. *Dev Psychol* 1989;25:70–79.

124. Alsaker FD. Pubertal timing, overweight, and psychological adjustment. *J Early Adol* 1992;12:396–419.

125. Brooks-Gunn J, Warren MP. The effects of delayed menarche in different contexts: dance and non-dance students. *J Youth Adol* 1985;14:285–300.

126. Ohring R, Graber JA, Brooks-Gunn J. Girls' recurrent and concurrent body dissatisfaction: correlates and consequences over eight years. *Int J Eat Disord* 2002;31:404–415.

127. Davies K, Wardle J. Body image and dieting in pregnancy. *J Psychosom Res* 1994;38:787–799.

128. Sternberg L, Blinn L. Feelings about self and body image during adolescent pregnancy. *Families in Society* 1993;74:282–290.

129. Fahy TA, O'Donoghue G. Eating disorders in pregnancy. *Psychol Med* 1991;21:577–580.

130. Stein A, Fairburn CG. Eating habits and attitudes in the postpartum period. *Psychosom Med* 1996;58:321–325.

131. Cash TF, Ancis JR, Strachan MD. Gender attitudes, feminist identity, and body images among college women. *Sex Roles* 1997;36:433–447.

132. Cash TF, Shaw KN, Strachan MD, Roy R. The relationship of feminist identity and gender role attitudes to body image. Manuscript in preparation for publication, 2005.

133. Markus H. Self-schemata and processing information about the self. *J Pers Soc Psychol* 1977;35:63–78.

134. Williamson DA, Stewart TM, White MA, York-Crowe E. An information-processing perspective on body image. In: Cash TF, Pruzinsky T, eds. *Body Image: A Handbook of Theory, Research, and Clinical Practice.* New York: Guilford Press, 2002:47–54.

135. Melnyk SE, Cash TF, Janda LH. Body image ups and downs: prediction of intra-individual level and variability of women's daily body image experiences. *Body Image: An International Journal of Research* 2004;1:225–235.

136. Cash TF, Santos ME, Williams, EF. Coping with body-image threats and challenges: validation of the Body Image Coping Strategies Inventory. *J Psychosom Res* 2005;58:191–199.

137. Castle DJ, Phillips KA, eds. *Disorders of Body Image.* Hampshire, England: Wrighton Biomedical Publishing, 2002.

138. American Psychiatric Association. *Diagnostic and Statistical Manual of Mental Disorders.* 4th ed. Washington DC: American Psychiatric Association, 2000.

139. Pruzinsky T. Body image disturbances in psychotic disorders. In: Cash TF, Pruzinsky T, eds. *Body Image: A Handbook of Theory, Research, and Clinical Practice.* New York: Guilford Press, 2002:322–329.

140. Phillips KA. *The Broken Mirror.* New York: Oxford University Press, 1996.

141. Phillips KA. Body image and body dysmorphic disorder. In: Cash TF, Pruzinsky T, eds. *Body Image: A Handbook of Theory, Research, and Clinical Practice.* New York: Guilford Press, 2002:312–321.

142. Garner DM. Body image and anorexia nervosa. In: Cash TF, Pruzinsky T, eds. *Body Image: A Handbook of Theory, Research, and Clinical Practice.* New York: Guilford Press, 2002:295–303.

143. Stice E. Body image and bulimia nervosa. In: Cash TF, Pruzinsky T, eds. *Body Image: A Handbook of Theory, Research, and Clinical Practice.* New York: Guilford Press, 2002:304–311.

144. Stice E. Risk and maintenance factors for eating pathology. *Psychol Bull* 2002;128:825–848.
145. Cash TF, Fleming EC. Body images and social relations. In: Cash TF, Pruzinsky T, eds. *Body Image: A Handbook of Theory, Research, and Clinical Practice*. New York: Guilford Press, 2002:277–286.
146. Powell MR, Hendricks B. Body schema, gender, and other correlates in nonclinical populations. *Genet Soc Gen Psychol Monogr* 1999;125(4):333–412.
147. Cash TF, Theriault J, Annis NM. Body image in an international context: adult attachment, fear of intimacy, and social anxiety. *J Soc Clin Psych* 2004;23:89–103.
148. Cash TF, Labarge AS. Development of the Appearance Schemas Inventory: a new cognitive body-image assessment. *Cog Ther Res* 1996;20:37–50.
149. Marsella AJ, Shizuru L, Brennan J, Kameoka V. Depression and body image satisfaction. *J Cross-Cult Psychol* 1981;12:360–371.
150. Noles SW, Cash TF, Winstead BA. Body image, physical attractiveness, and depression. *J Consult Clin Psychol* 1985;53:88–94.
151. Stice E, Bearman SK. Body image and eating disturbances prospectively predict growth in depressive symptoms in adolescent girls: a growth curve analysis. *Dev Psychol* 2001;37:597–607.
152. Cash TF, Maikkula CL, Yamamiya Y. Baring the body in the bedroom: body image, sexual self-schemas, and sexual functioning among college women and men. *Elect J Human Sex* [serial online]. 2004;vol. 7. Available at http://www.ejhs.org/volume7/bodyimage.html. Accessed June 29, 2004.
153. Wiederman MW. Body image and sexual functioning. In: Cash TF, Pruzinsky T, eds. *Body Image: A Handbook of Theory, Research, and Clinical Practice*. New York: Guilford Press, 2002:287–294.
154. Barlow DH. Causes of sexual dysfunction: the role of anxiety and cognitive interference. *J Consult Clin Psychol* 1986;54:140–148.
155. Masters W, Johnson V. *Human Sexual Inadequacy*. Boston: Little, Brown and Company, 1970.
156. Thompson JK. Body image: extent of disturbance, associated features, theoretical models, assessment methodologies, intervention strategies, and a proposal for a new DSM-IV diagnostic category—body image disorder. In: Hersen M, Eisler RM, Miller PM, eds. *Progress in Behavior Modification*. Sycamore, IL: Sycamore Press, 1992:3–54.
157. Cash TF, Fleming EC. The impact of body-image experiences: development of the Body Image Quality of Life Inventory. *Int J Eat Disord* 2002;31:455–460.
158. Cash TF, Jakatdar TA, Williams EF. The Body Image Quality of Life Inventory: further validation with college men and women. *Body Image: An International Journal of Research* 2004;35:305–316.
159. Cash TF, Phillips KA, Santos MT, Hrabosky JI. Measuring "negative body image": validation of the body image disturbance questionnaire in a non-clinical population. *Body Image: An International Journal of Research* 2004;1:363–372.
160. Dufresne RG, Phillips KA, Vittorio CC, Wilkel CS. A screening questionnaire for body dysmorphic disorder in a cosmetic dermatologic surgery practice. *Dermatol Surg* 2001;27:457–462.
161. Krueger DW. *Body Self and Psychological Self: Developmental and Clinical Integration in Disorders of the Self*. New York: Brunner/Mazel, 1989.
162. Krueger DW. *Creating a New Story: Toward a Psychoanalytic Integration of Body Self and Psychological Self*. New York: Brunner/Routledge, 2002.
163. Krueger DW. Psychodynamic approaches to changing body image. In: Cash TF, Pruzinsky T, eds. *Body Image: A Handbook of Theory, Research, and Clinical Practice*. New York: Guilford Press, 2002:461–468.
164. Krueger DW. Psychodynamic perspectives on body image. In: Cash TF, Pruzinsky T, eds. *Body Image: A Handbook of Theory, Research, and Clinical Practice*. New York: Guilford Press, 2002:30–37.
165. Rabinor JR, Bilich MA. Experiential approaches to changing body image. In: Cash TF, Pruzinsky T, eds. *Body Image: A Handbook of Theory, Research, and Clinical Practice*. New York: Guilford Press, 2002:469–477.
166. Cash TF, Strachan MD. Cognitive behavioral approaches to changing body image. In: Cash TF, Pruzinsky T, eds. *Body Image: A Handbook of Theory, Research, and Clinical Practice*. New York: Guilford Press, 2002:478–486.
167. Cash TF, Hrabosky JI. The treatment of body-image disturbances. In: Thompson JK, ed. *Handbook of Eating Disorders and Obesity*. Hoboken, NJ: John Wiley and Sons, 2004:515–541.
168. Jarry JL, Berardi K. Characteristics and effectiveness of stand-alone body image treatments: a review of the empirical literature. *Body Image: An International Journal of Research* 2004;1:319–333.
169. Rosen JC, Orosan P, Reiter J. Cognitive behavior therapy for negative body image in obese women. *Beh Ther* 1995;26:25–42.
170. Rosen JC. The nature of body dysmorphic disorder and treatment with cognitive behavior therapy. *Cog Beh Practice* 1995;2:143–166.
171. Rosen JC, Reiter J, Orosan P. Cognitive-behavioral body image therapy for body dysmorphic disorder. *J Consult Clin Psychol* 1995;63:263–269.

Psychological Perspectives on Reconstructive Surgery

Chapter 5

Craniofacial Conditions

Kathleen A. Kapp-Simon, PhD

The treatment of individuals with craniofacial conditions of necessity focuses on two aspects of habilitation: (i) functional skills such as speech, mastication, vision, and hearing; and (ii) aesthetic habilitation of the face and cranium. During the early years of a child's life, the necessity of treatment by surgeons and other medical and allied health specialists is seldom questioned by parents, primary care physicians, or insurance companies. Closure of a bilateral cleft lip and palate or release of cranial sutures in the presence of craniosynostosis and significant cranial deformity are considered "medically necessary" procedures. Treatments related to the improvement of speech, such as secondary palatal surgery, are recognized as critical to the child's long-term adjustment and functioning. Similarly, treatment of hearing loss or eye muscle imbalance is readily justified. However, once the initial medical crises have abated, multiple issues emerge in relationship to the necessity and timing of additional treatments. The aspect of treatment which becomes most controversial is the necessity and timing of secondary procedures that have as their primary goal the enhancement of facial appearance.

The habilitation of individuals with congenital craniofacial conditions (CFCs) is a long-term process. Congenital CFCs generally require treatment from a multiplicity of disciplines from birth to at least late adolescence or young adulthood (1). During the early years of treatment, decisions about surgery and other interventions are made by parents in conjunction with the treatment team. At some point during childhood or young adolescence, the child begins to take an active role in these treatment decisions, particularly when they involve elective procedures to improve appearance. At all stages of elective treatment, families and practitioners may find themselves struggling to determine what course of action will lead to the best outcome for the child. This chapter will present an overview of the empirical data that relates to psychological adjustment in individuals with CFCs, identify areas in need of further research that relate to psychosocial adjustment, and discuss the clinical implications of these empirical issues. This material is accompanied by practical information regarding the interrelationships of elective surgery, physical appearance, and psychological adjustment. (See Questionnaires 5-1 and 5-2 at the end of this chapter.)

REVIEW OF EMPIRICAL LITERATURE

Psychological Adjustment

Emotional and behavioral adjustment problems during the childhood years are commonly conceptualized in terms of internalizing and externalizing behavior. Internalizing factors include anxiety, depression, social withdrawal, and somatic complaints, while externalizing factors include aggression, oppositional behaviors, conduct disorders, and attention/hyperactivity disorders (2–3).

Social inhibition is a behavioral characteristic of particular concern for the child with CFC (4–6). In turn, social introversion, withdrawal, loneliness, and problems with social interaction have been associated with dissatisfaction with appearance (7–8). Parents of a child with CFC report peer teasing, exclusion from the peer group, and acting younger or choosing to play with younger peers two to three times more frequently than parents of unaffected children (9–11). Parents frequently attribute those difficulties to facial differences or accommodations of their child to those facial differences. Objective ratings of facial difference have been associated with increased behavioral inhibition (12), which may also be related to quality of social interaction (13). Focus group interviews with adolescents with CFCs provide further information that these teens attribute their perceived lack of welcome by peers to their facial appearance (14). The child who perceives himself to be less welcome by peers may choose to limit their social groups to one or two children with whom they feel safe. Others may choose solitary activities. Either situation serves to decrease anxiety (15–16). A small observational study (13) demonstrated that individuals with CFCs engaged in fewer social interactions than their peers and that those attempts at interaction were more often ineffectual.

Both Spriestersbach (17) and Richman (5) originally focused research attention on behavioral inhibition as a core characteristic of the child with CFC. More recent research has demonstrated that the child who experiences behavior problems frequently experience both externalizing and internalizing problems (9–10,12,18–19). Rogers and Kapp-Simon (18) found that self-reported problems with social interactions and peer popularity were highly associated with parent-reported problems in both internalizing and externalizing psychological adjustment. The behavior problems demonstrated by the child may represent an ineffective attempt to handle the frustration associated with social rejection (20). Robinson et al. (21) have posited that individuals with CFCs who are having social difficulties develop a "negative social interaction style" that results in social shunning. They suggest that initial social rejection may lead individuals with CFCs to act in a manner that is aggressive, defensive, or shy.

Adjustment problems for the child with CFC occur more frequently when he or she must also cope with learning disorders (22). The child with CFC experiences learning disorders at two to three times the rate of nonaffected children (23–25). This combination of findings makes it difficult to disentangle the effects of appearance from those of cognitive functioning. The child with learning problems who does not have a CFC experiences more social and behavioral difficulties than peers without learning problems (26–27). He or she is also more likely to experience specific social skills deficits than a child without such challenges (26–27).

There has been little empirical focus on the adjustment of adults with CFCs. Studies have identified adjustment problems in adults that include less frequent participation in social activities, reports of interpersonal difficulties, and less frequent, and later marriage (28–35). Higher rates of anxiety, depression, and heart palpitations have also been reported in comparison to unaffected individuals (36). Women with CFCs report greater depression than men with similar conditions (35). In addition, greater dissatisfaction with appearance was associated with higher rates of anxiety and depression, fewer friendships, and a belief that appearance affected job choice (35,36). Similarly, Sarwer et al. (37) related negative self-ratings of attractiveness and dissatisfaction with appearance to lower self-esteem, poorer quality of life, and more frequent reports of discrimination.

Facial Appearance

Barden asserts that "facial attractiveness is perhaps one of the most salient and unique characteristic that others may use as a basis for impression formation in any given social context" (38). As reviewed in Chapter 3, there is ample evidence to support the contention that facial configuration and attractiveness influence the reactions and judgments that observers make about an individual, with more attractive individuals receiving positive attributions while less attractive individuals are judged more harshly (39–46). A meta-analysis completed by Langlois et al. (47) concluded that: "Beauty is more than just in the eye of the beholder; people do judge and treat others with whom they interact based on attractiveness; and perhaps most surprisingly, beauty is more than skin deep" (p. 404).

In an effort to relate the broader literature on facial appearance to facial differences in individuals with CFCs, researchers have looked for associations between CFC-related impairment and aspects of psychological adjustment. These empirical investigations have not provided a consistent picture. In part, the inconsistencies are related to differences in research questions and methodologies. However, the complexities of the relationships among the variables in question also thwart simple answers (35).

Ratings of attractiveness have been obtained from treating surgeons, professionals who treat children with CFCs who are not surgeons, parents, naïve observers including other children, and the affected individuals themselves. Using a variety of measurement techniques, this research has found remarkable congruence in judgments of severity or impairment caused by CFCs between parents and other observers (48–52). Studies have also shown that judgments of attractiveness are affected by both severity and type of CFC condition (53–54).

While there may be congruence in ratings of appearance, the relationships between physical appearance and psychological adjustment are more complex. For example, in one study, preschoolers with CFCs reported higher self-concept than a comparison group despite the fact that they were rated as less attractive (55). However, in another study, elementary school children with CFCs demonstrate lower self-concept than comparison children (15,56).

The relationships between appearance ratings and psychological adjustment are even less clear in adolescence, when studies begin to consider self-ratings of appearance and the perceived need for additional surgical treatment. Many of the studies that found congruence between parent and outside raters have found little agreement with self-ratings of appearance (14,48–51,57–58), although a few have found agreement (37,59). When there are discrepancies among raters, adolescents and adults tend to judge their appearance more negatively than others (48–51,57).

Congruent ratings between subjective and outside judges have been associated with better adjustment when the raters are parents or clinicians (7,60). Rogers and Kapp-Simon (18) found that there was considerable congruence between parent and child ratings of social and behavioral concerns in children 9 to 12 years of age; however, self-reported appearance ratings were not predictive of parent-reported psychological adjustment. A more positive rating of appearance than the rating provided by a peer has been associated with a more positive self-concept (61). Yet Topolski et al. (58–59) found that adolescents who were *less* socially isolated had greater dissatisfaction with their appearance and a greater interest in more surgery. Unfortunately, few of the reported studies have evaluated all of the critical variables simultaneously with enough statistical power to provide clarity to these disparate findings.

A common concern of parents of a child with CFC is that their child will experience teasing because of differences in facial appearance. Certainly there is a significant body of literature that supports the concern that individuals with facial differences will be thought of, and possibly treated, less well than their peers (62–63). Children appear to become aware of facial differences at a young age. Children as young as 3 years of age are able to discriminate between attractive and unattractive peers (64). By 6 years of age, children begin to become aware of even minor differences in the facial features of their peers (65). These differences often become the focus of teasing. Therefore, it is not surprising that a sizable percentage of parents reported peer teasing, most often related to facial appearance, to be a problem for their child at 4 to 7 years of age (66). Parents may be able to assist their child in establishing positive relationships by supporting the child's efforts at social interaction and by providing specific social skills training (67–68). Parents also can take comfort from the knowledge that teasing from peers, related to specific aspects of CFC, appears to diminish across the life span for many, but not all, individuals with CFCs (69–70).

Macgregor (69) summarizes the beliefs of many individuals with CFCs: "In all human relationships, it is the face that is the symbol synonymous with the person. . . . Because of its social significance, any condition that distorts it and makes it ugly or unsightly to look at can take precedence over all other personal and social traits and insidiously can become the most important thing about that person" (p. 250). It is this perception among practitioners, families, and patients that focuses treatment upon the amelioration of facial differences.

Summary

The literature has consistently found that individuals with CFCs may demonstrate higher than expected levels of anxiety, acting out behaviors, and difficulty with social interaction leading to social inhibition, isolation, or maladjustment. While these adjustment problems are far from universal, when present, they are often attributed to deviant facial appearance and less frequently to concerns about speech or dentition. Causality is implied, though most research is simply correlational. The broader scholarly literature on attractiveness, discussed in Chapter 3, does support a strong relationship between facial attractiveness and important variables including interpersonal competence, adjustment, social appeal, and academic/developmental competence (47). The specific literature on facial disfigurement demonstrates that the relationship between facial appearance and psychological adjustment is quite complex. Any possible model predicting psychological adjustment for individuals with CFCs is likely multifactorial and will only be elucidated through well-designed, longitudinal, multisite studies. Nevertheless, there is growing evidence that fostering of interpersonal competence can ameliorate some of the negative afteraffects associated with facial disfigurement. Research efforts should continue to investigate the ways in which individuals with facial differences can break down the social barriers that impede total integration into society.

CLINICAL CARE

Team Care for Cleft and Craniofacial Conditions

The American Cleft Palate-Craniofacial Association (ACPA) recommends that clinical care for individuals with CFCs should be delivered within the context of a cleft or craniofacial interdisciplinary team (71). A mental health professional (psychologist, social worker, or psychiatrist) is an integral part of all craniofacial teams and is a recommended member for all cleft teams. It is also expected that team care is based on the "Parameters of Care" developed by ACPA (1). This document urges that teams "weigh all treatment decisions against the expected outcomes and related factors such as facial growth, hearing, speech, dentition, and psychosocial impact on patient and family" (p. 6). In addition, the document advocates that the child should be given age-appropriate information about their craniofacial anomaly, "and should be permitted and encouraged to become active participants in treatment planning. All care providers should be sensitive to how treatment discussions can be perceived by children, and should do everything possible to ensure that the child understands the treatment plan as much as possible. Towards this end, it is helpful for the team to ensure that each child has someone who will listen to his or her fears, concerns, and opinions regarding treatment" (p. 14).

According to the Parameters of Care document, the family, including the child when old enough, is a critical member of the treatment team (1). This mandate raises many issues of clinical importance when treating a child with craniofacial conditions. One issue that occurs frequently is parental confusion due to differing treatment protocols advocated by different treatment teams. Due to increased communication among parents because of Internet access and support organizations, parents quickly realize that there are a variety of approaches to treating a particular problem. For example, one team may advocate use of a presurgical appliance prior to lip surgery for a child with cleft lip and palate, while another team may indicate that the appliance (and associated expense and parental stress) is not necessary. In another scenario, some teams advocate a primary bone graft during the first year of life, while other teams recommend waiting until the age of transition from primary to secondary teeth. In yet another situation, a family may receive a recommendation for midface advancement using a monoblock procedure, while another family whose child has a similar condition may be directed toward an external distraction appliance.

Understandably, parents want to make the best decision for their child and often find themselves with little basis for determining the best course of action. Treatment teams can facilitate parental confidence by helping them to understand that treatment for CFCs is an art as well as a science. Families should be told that there are multiple ways to achieve an excellent outcome for their child and that most teams have adopted a flexible protocol that the individual team members are comfortable implementing. Another team might have a different approach that results in an equally satisfactory outcome for their child.

Surgical Care

Another issue of critical clinical importance relates to the timing and frequency of surgical interventions. Few families have adequate knowledge regarding the various treatments that their child with a CFC will require over his or her lifetime. While they may seek information from other parents, Web sites, and multiple teams, ultimately they place their trust in a selected "team." Families frequently find it difficult to question a recommendation from the team, particularly as it relates to surgical timing and treatment recommendations. Consequently, it is vital that the cleft or craniofacial team educate parents regarding the differences between surgeries that are time-dependent and those that can be scheduled at the discretion of the family.

Some procedures recommended for a child with CFC have greater medical urgency than others. For example, a child should probably have pressure equalizing tubes if they are recommended because of chronic serous otitis media. In contrast, a lip revision or jaw distraction may have a large window of opportunity during which it can be successfully accomplished. Postponement of the procedure even for a year or more may not result in significant harm to the child and may actually benefit him or her. Families can be helped to understand that because a surgery "can be done" or even "should be done" doesn't mean that it "must be done *now*."

In general, the fewer surgeries a child must undergo the better, both for the child and his or her family. Even a minor procedure can be disruptive to the child and family. Often the child is more distressed by blood tests, IVs, anesthetic induction, and postsurgical restrictions than the procedure itself. Scheduling a child for surgery affects the entire family. Parents must get time off from work, siblings must be cared for, and the child undergoing surgery must be supported. Surgery also disrupts a child's social life, including peer relationships, school activities, and athletics. Since few surgeries that are scheduled to treat problems related to CFCs are emergent, it is critical that the treatment team work with the family to determine an appropriate time for scheduling. This often allows for surgical procedures to be combined, cutting down on both the frequency of anesthetics and the individual and family stress involved in a surgery.

There are a variety of factors to be considered when scheduling nonemergency procedures. These include the child's age, temperament, psychological adjustment, motivation, expectations, and family support. Age is an important factor to consider; however, child characteristics such as temperament and psychological adjustment may be even more important. There are developmental, physiological, and temperamental differences among children that affect behavior, activity level, and frustration tolerance. These characteristics likely have a genetic basis that is influenced by environment and behavioral choices (72). There are a number of systems for assessing temperament and adjustment. However, for the purposes of talking about a child's ability to tolerate a surgery Hart et al. (73) provide a useful organizational structure based on three broad personality types that can be fairly easily identified and that have been shown to be related to psychological adjustment. The personality types are defined as (i) the *resilient child* who is socially competent, gets along with both adults and peers, tends to be gregarious, and exhibits positive emotions; (ii) the *overcontrolled child* who typically exhibits extreme shyness, is quite compliant, and highly dependent on others; and (iii) the *undercontrolled child* who is generally uncooperative, has difficulty with social relationships, is noncompliant, and more likely to exhibit negative emotions. A child exhibits these personality traits along a continuum; however, these characteristics do influence how a child thinks, feels, and behaves and consequently can affect his or her response to the surgical experience.

CASE EXAMPLES

Case examples of these different types of temperaments are illustrative and presented below.

Case 1: Resilient Samuel

Samuel is a 17-year-old boy with a repaired bilateral cleft lip and palate. He has undergone multiple surgeries in his life including bilateral lip repair at 2 months, palate repair at 12 months, pharyngeal flap at age 4, columellar lengthening at age 5 and lip revision at age 6. He had bilateral pressure equalizing tubes placed in conjunction with each of his first two surgeries and two additional times during the preschool years. Bilateral maxillary bone grafts were placed at age 8. Nasal tip surgery with a second lip revision took place at age 14. Orthodontic treatment occurred in phases during the preteen and teen years culminating with orthognathic surgery at age 17. Speech therapy was provided between the ages of 3 and 7. He returns for a consultation and a recommendation is made by the surgeon for a minor lip revision and rhinoplasty, likely the last surgery left in his treatment plan.

Samuel has been a model patient in many ways. Even as a young child he had a great sense of humor. He related well to the medical staff and was cooperative for examinations and surgeries. Among his peers his positive attitude and enthusiasm made him a sought-after friend. Between his surgeries he has been active in high school sports and he was recently elected to his school's student council. Although there has been some tension between Samuel and his parents during his high school years, they have generally worked out issues well and there is a positive feeling of mutual respect among them.

Samuel is a great example of the resilient child: cooperative and fun, with a great attitude about the treatment related to his cleft. Consequently, everyone was surprised when he announced that he was not interested in the surgical procedures being recommended at this visit. His parents were upset because these were the "final touches." As they said to him: "You've come so far. How can you quit now?" His surgeon and team all wanted to see him "finish," because they were confident that he would have an excellent result. However, Samuel was quite firm that he was finished with surgeries for now. He was quite pleased with the results of his orthognathic procedure and felt that his lip and nose looked just fine the way they were.

Discussion

It is very disconcerting to parents and sometimes to team members when a teenager decides that he or she is not interested in the treatment recommendations being made. These are complex situations with no easy solutions. Certainly at 17 Samuel has reached a point in his life where his input into the decision making is absolutely necessary and his desires need to be respected. However, his parents have invested a tremendous amount of time and energy, not to mention money, to provide him with the best treatment possible. It is often heartbreaking for these parents to imagine that their child will stop short of what they understand to be the "ideal" outcome.

Kapp-Simon (74) discussed issues related to parent–child disagreement about treatment. She provided a model for helping families to come to an understanding of the differing perspectives of each member. The role of the team members in this situation is to foster communication between the parents and teen. Both may have good reasons for their points of view. Only with honest communication and openness to each others points of view can a resolution to these differing viewpoints be achieved. It must also be understood that the outcome of this communication process will not always be a decision to go forward with surgery.

Case 2: Resilient Rosa

At 5 years of age Rosa presents with a diagnosis of mandibular facial dysostosis (MFD) (Treacher Collins Syndrome) with significant micrognathia and cleft palate. Problems with feeding and breathing were evident from birth. Mandibular distraction successfully alleviated her breathing difficulties and a tracheotomy was not required; however, feeding did not improve. Cleft palate repair occurred after the mandibular distraction allowed adequate access to her mouth. She was fed via an N-G tube for the first two years of life while intensive efforts were directed at facilitating oral feedings. A G-tube was inserted at 2 years of age when it became clear that Rosa was not likely to soon become an oral feeder.

Rosa also was diagnosed with a maximum bilateral conductive hearing loss soon after birth. She was immediately fit with a bone conduction hearing aid, which she has worn continuously since she was 6 weeks of age. Early intervention services were initiated when she was 2 months of age. Speech and language therapy, occupational therapy, and physical therapy were provided as part of a home-based parent–infant program. At 3 years of age, she entered an early childhood preschool program where she continued to receive individual therapies in the context of a classroom setting. Rosa's cognitive development has progressed age appropriately. She uses sign language as her primary means of communication. Oral speech is emerging, although intelligibility has been a persistent issue.

Rosa is a pleasant, happy, and cooperative little girl. She relates well to adults and enjoys the attention she receives during her various therapies. During the current school year she has begun to make noticeable strides in oral communication and, for the first time, is engaging in interactive play with her peers. Her classmates have been accepting of Rosa, although they have been upset by the gagging and retching that accompany Rosa's efforts at oral feeding. In an attempt to minimize the social stigma, Rosa now has lunch, which consists of pureed foods and some liquid, alone with a nurse supervising.

At this point in her development Rosa has a number of treatment needs. A sleep study demonstrated that Rosa has multiple episodes of mild obstructive apnea; however, this problem is successfully treated with nighttime continuous positive airway pressure (CPAP). Videofloroscopy did not reveal aspiration with swallowing but suggests that Rosa's ongoing difficulties with oral feeding may be related to tongue retraction when she initiates the swallow response. To address this concern and also address the mild obstructive apnea, the team has suggested repeat mandibular distraction to increase both the vertical and horizontal dimensions of the mandible. In addition, Rosa is also at an age and stage of development where orbital reconstruction with calvarial bone grafts and correction of the lateral canthal displacement would be appropriate.

Rosa's parents are conflicted about how to proceed at this point. Solving the feeding issue has been a priority for them; however, they were disappointed that the previous distraction procedure did not result in improved oral feeding and are ambivalent about subjecting Rosa to another extended period of distraction. Rosa's appearance has not been an issue to date, yet as she becomes more independent at school these issues related to appearance may become more salient. School staff has raised a concern about the effect of a prolonged distraction process on Rosa's social and speech development. She is just beginning to establish connections with her peers, and they are worried that the extended distraction process would disrupt those relationships. Similarly, they wonder about a decrease in oral speech efforts if Rosa is coping with bilateral distraction appliances.

Discussion

Rosa is characterized as a resilient child due to her positive emotional presentation, ability to cooperate with adult demands during therapy, and her tolerance of complex medical interventions. She displays positive social relatedness with adults and can be quite endearing to her teachers and therapists. Peer relationships have been more of a struggle. Many of the natural occasions when peer interactions develop have not been available to Rosa due to her therapies and feeding needs. Rosa's communication difficulties also have limited her ability to relate in an inclusion classroom where most children do not use sign language.

There is no real disagreement about Rosa's ability to cooperate with a distraction procedure; the issue is whether it is in her best interests to have this procedure at this time. Her teachers and therapists are advocating against having the procedure because they see her making strides in speech and social relatedness and fear that she will not maintain this growth if she is also coping with distraction appliances. The surgical team maintains that the potential gains in terms of improved oral feeding and nasal airway should take precedence. Her parents feel trapped, wanting both improved speech and social relatedness and improved feeding and breathing.

The ideal way to resolve these issues would be to schedule a team conference where school representatives, such as the speech therapist, classroom teacher, and feeding therapist, are invited. Including school staff in the team meeting would facilitate decision making. Ultimately, Rosa's parents have to make the decision about which treatment should receive highest priority. They would benefit by having a professional skilled in communication, such as a mental health professional, participate in the conference. That person can help parents understand the potential benefit/risk ratios for each course of action and support them as they make a decision.

Case 3: Overcontrolled Bryan

Bryan is an 11-year-old boy with a unilateral cleft lip and palate. He has undergone three cleft-related surgeries: lip closure at 10 weeks, palate closure at 9 months, and maxillary bone graft placement at age 8. He has had 5 sets of pressure equalizing tubes and currently has a set of T tubes in place due to repeated episodes of otitis media. Bryan has been enrolled in speech therapy since age 3 and continues to receive services on a weekly basis.

Bryan has struggled in school due to a developmental reading disorder. Although early evidence of the reading disorder was present in first and second grade, no formal intervention was offered by the school until third grade. The psychoeducational evaluation completed when Bryan was 8 confirmed a diagnosis of learning disabilities (LD). Consistent with that LD diagnosis, Bryan displayed normal intelligence with above average Performance IQ and low normal Verbal IQ. Reading and spelling skills were at a beginning first grade level. Inclusion special education services have been provided to address Bryan's learning problems; however, he continues to lag behind his classmates in achievement.

On his first clinic visit to a new treatment team, he presents with a well-healed lip scar with mild mismatch of the vermillion border, some fullness of the lip with incorrect muscle placement, and some nasal asymmetry. Dentally, he presents with a crossbite, crowding, and multiple rotations.

At age 11, Bryan is a shy, somewhat inhibited young boy. At times he appears sullen or angry. He is reluctant to answer direct questions during the clinic exam. His parents report that Bryan has been experiencing significant peer difficulties in school. He does not have any good friends and is seldom invited to parties or other activities by his classmates. He does not participate in school sports and has no other interests that would enable him to have social interaction with his peers outside of school. According to his parents, his classmates call him "fat lip" and "smashed face." They report that he used to try to ignore them and walk away when the taunting started, but recently he has become aggressive and fights back. He has been suspended from school one time during the past school year because of fighting. Bryan has told his parents that he would like them to make his cleft "go away." The family is requesting a lip and nose revision so that Bryan receives less teasing at school.

Clinical examination reveals that the ideal treatment plan for Bryan would include (i) additional maxillary expansion combined with second stage orthodontic treatment to bring teeth in better alignment; (ii) probable repeat bone grafting due to limited bone in the area of the cleft to occur following the maxillary expansion; and (iii) lip and nasal tip revision 6 months to a year after bone graft with definitive rhinoplasty deferred until later teen years.

Discussion

Bryan displays a personality that is consistent with what has been called the "over-controlled child." During his early childhood and elementary school years he was extremely shy, withdrawn, and compliant. Teachers seeing his facial differences may have assumed that he was a "little slow." However, since he was such a well-behaved boy who brought little attention to himself, the possibility of treatable learning disabilities was initially overlooked. Bryan's lack of assertiveness and inhibition impaired his ability to establish friendships with his peers. This same lack of assertiveness along with his facial differences made him a likely scapegoat for peer taunting. Although Bryan may be an internalizer by personality, with enough provocation he and other children with this personality style will explode with an aggressive response when pushed beyond their endurance.

Often children and parents in this situation imagine that removing the facial stigmata of clefting would also remove the social isolation and peer stigmatization that they experience. In reality, the issues are far more complex. Surgeries for congenital birth defects like cleft lip and cleft palate seldom erase all of the stigmata related to the birth defect. Although an individual surgery may occasionally result in dramatic improvement, small improvements that enhance appearance, but do not eliminate the scars, are typical. Even when the surgical results are ideal, the boost in self-esteem lasts only if the child has good social support from his family, coupled with the behavioral control and social skills to establish or maintain steadfast peer relationships. Consequently, the intervention plan developed by the treatment team must take into account the emotional and social needs of the child. For Bryan, this will likely mean a referral for psychological treatment with a specific focus on the development of social skills. The psychological treatment should run parallel to the medical treatment and, if the therapist is not a member of the team, the therapist must be in contact with the team so that he or she develops an understanding of the treatment goals and realistic expectations for outcome.

The family must also be educated about the stages of treatment. At 11, Bryan can understand that maxillary expansion, tooth alignment, and bone grafting may change the orientation of his lip and nose and, therefore, should be done prior to a lip revision. However, he will probably be upset and disappointed by this information. It is important that the members of the team acknowledge and accept that disappointment while continuing to educate Bryan and his family about the goals of treatment.

Case 4: Undercontrolled Jayne

Jayne is a 4-year-old girl with a significant hemifacial microsomia and left microtia. Her left facial asymmetry is striking and her parents are invested in achieving correction as soon as possible. They report that Jayne stares at her face in the mirror and they worry about the effect of her facial difference on her self-esteem. They also fear that she will be subjected to teasing in school and, thus far, have kept her out of preschool to protect her.

Observation of Jayne in the clinic setting shows her to be a very active girl. In the waiting room she climbs on the chairs, pulls books from the book shelf, and interferes with the play of other children. In the exam room she twirls on the chair, pulls open drawers, and dumps a box of tongue blades on the floor. Her parents' efforts to contain her are ineffectual; however, they excuse her behavior by stating that she is hungry and tired.

Despite their defense of her clinic behavior, they also complain that they have a hard time getting Jayne to sleep at night, that she doesn't listen to them, that she can't sit still at home, and that she fights with her brother a great deal.

The clinical exam, accomplished with great effort and some tantruming on the part of Jayne, reveals that she would be a candidate for a distraction appliance to lengthen her mandible, if her behavior were under better control. Parents are eager to pursue the treatment. The treatment team members are concerned about Jayne's ability to cooperate with the medical staff and her parents to allow for cleaning of the surgical sites, the screw turning, and other aspects of care related the distraction appliance.

Discussion

Jayne displays many of the characteristics of an undercontrolled child. She has difficulty managing her impulses, is not particularly cooperative, doesn't get along well with her brother or other children, and frequently displays negative emotions. The procedure recommended to address her facial asymmetry (distraction osteogenesis) requires considerable cooperation from the child. She needs to be compliant with medical staff and her parents need to be able to manage hygiene and screw turning at home. Despite the eagerness of her parents for treatment, Jayne is probably not a good candidate at this point in time. Children who display similar characteristics to Jayne have been known to develop infection due to poor hygiene in the area of the appliance, to loosen the distraction appliance because of their activity level and lack of care, and to experience extreme upset around the times of screw turning, which has been very difficult for the parents to endure.

What is the best way for the treatment team to proceed? Direct communication with the parents about the risks of proceeding with surgery at this point in time is recommended. Parents should be told that deferring surgery now does not mean that it will not be offered as Jayne matures. They can be offered information regarding parent education programs that would enable them to understand their child's behavior and perhaps develop better strategies for helping her to manage over-stimulating situations. Parents also can be educated about the social and behavioral factors that are most important for helping Jayne cope socially with her peers, an important aspect of her development at this age. While her appearance may draw attention to her in unwanted ways, her behavior is likely to compound that negative attention. Helping Jayne to develop more appropriate behavior will make a big difference in her social acceptance.

In addition, if the team can help Jayne's parents find positive ways to talk about her appearance, her parents, in turn, will be able to provide Jayne with a model of appropriate responses to questions or comments. Parental modeling takes many forms. For example, when a parent is asked about Jayne's face in an appropriate way by an adult in her hearing, they can reply: "One side of Jayne's face didn't develop completely before she was born, so it's a bit smaller, but she's a great kid. She loves to dance and she's learning to swim like a fish (*or some other appropriate talent*)." Often parents are faced with another child coming to them with the question, "What's wrong with her face?" Parents can be coached to answer that question directly at a level appropriate to the questioner's age. Similar to the response given to the adult, a parent might say: "When Jayne was born one side of her face was smaller than the other. It doesn't hurt her at all, even though it does look different than your face. But you know what? I bet she likes to do some of the same things you like to do." As Jayne's parents become comfortable talking about her condition, Jayne herself will begin to develop confidence about her ability to talk directly about her facial differences and this will also help her to interact more appropriately with her peers as she begins school.

FOSTERING SOCIAL SKILLS

The child with facial differences who has developed positive social interaction skills experiences peer acceptance, demonstrates social competence, and is far less likely to exhibit significant adjustment problems than a child who does not have these skills (18,55,75–76). One goal of team treatment for a child with CFC should be to help families develop strategies to foster skills that will enhance their child's social confidence (77). Strauss (78) urged members of cleft and craniofacial teams to provide families with information on individuals who have successfully coped with the challenges of living with facial disfigurement. The idea is to encourage families to establish an optimistic outlook about their child's future. To this end, a number of Web-based support groups provide a mechanism for families to share their child's treatment progress and antidotes about their successes (e.g., www.aboutfaceusa.org; www.cleftadvocate.org). A similar optimistic attitude should be communicated by members of the cleft or craniofacial team. While parents may feel distressed, worried, sad, or sometimes even angry that their child has a CFC, the team members can help them work through these feelings by both acknowledging them and encouraging them to focus on active ways to support their child (77).

There are many ways that parents can help their child develop social competence. One of the first is to develop their own parenting skills so that they are able to provide their child with emotional support, positive discipline, and ultimately promote social interaction. The skills outlined by Gottman (79) on emotion coaching provide an excellent foundation for parents who want to improve their sensitivity to their children. Emotion coaching encourages parents to become aware of their child's emotions and to recognize that times of emotional upset are also moments of potential intimacy with their child. Emotion coaching advocates that parents respond with empathy to their child's distress. This empathic response can help the child find labels for their strong emotions so that together parent and child can find an appropriate way to respond to a difficult situation. There are a number of other parenting programs that teach similar skills (80–82). Children have a better chance of learning to use these skills when interacting with peers if the skills are consistently modeled by their parents.

Learning appropriate social skills is a lifelong process. The types of skills needed will vary based on the age of the child. The goal for parents is to provide their child with a variety of tools for establishing friendly encounters with peers. Thus, even a preschool child can learn to respond to a question about their facial asymmetry in a friendly and effective manner if parents have provided the child with a simple, age-appropriate vocabulary to describe the condition and have modeled the responses in similar situations. Clinical experience has demonstrated that a major part of the training comes from talking about the facial difference with the same level of emotional intensity that they talk about the color of their child's hair or eyes.

Older children may need more specific training in social skills (68,83). Specific attention should be given to pragmatic communication skills such as eye contact, tone of voice, and social distance, as well as specific skills for entering and maintaining conversations. Some children may need help with anxiety management or responding to peer teasing. All children should be taught to be friendly and empathic toward their peers.

CONCLUSIONS

A child with CFC faces many challenges. Most undergo multiple surgical procedures during childhood, which involve hospitalizations of various lengths, loss of time from school and other social activities, and incorporation of a new appearance into their identity. Despite the surgeries, residual disfigurement and scaring typically remain. Consequently, this child also must possess social skills that enable him or her to negotiate childhood peer relationships with the added stress of a facial difference.

Being the parent of a child with a CFC requires learning a new vocabulary and becoming intimately familiar with numerous medical specialties, treatments, and procedures. Parents are asked to participate in medical decision making because they are their child's primary advocate. Parents are most familiar with their child's temperament, needs, and abilities. Nonetheless, they often feel anxious as they try to make treatment decisions for their child. These stressors are best minimized when care for these conditions is delivered within the context of a multidisciplinary cleft or craniofacial team that includes the support of a mental health professional.

Cleft/Craniofacial Surgery Questionnaire   Ages 4–12

Parent/guardian: Please complete the following questions so that we might better understand your child's needs.

1. How concerned are **you and/or your child** about his/her facial appearance?

	Not at All	A Little	Moderately	A Lot	Extremely
Lips	(0)	(1)	(2)	(3)	(4)
Nose	(0)	(1)	(2)	(3)	(4)
Ear(s)	(0)	(1)	(2)	(3)	(4)
Eye(s)	(0)	(1)	(2)	(3)	(4)
Teeth/jaws	(0)	(1)	(2)	(3)	(4)
Other _____	(0)	(1)	(2)	(3)	(4)

2. How worried does your child become when surgery is planned?

	Not at All	A Little	Moderately	Lot	Extremely
General anxiety/fear	(0)	(1)	(2)	(3)	(4)
Preoperative blood work/anesthesia	(0)	(1)	(2)	(3)	(4)
Postoperative pain	(0)	(1)	(2)	(3)	(4)
Missing school	(0)	(1)	(2)	(3)	(4)
Possible disappointment with outcome	(0)	(1)	(2)	(3)	(4)

3. In what ways do **you** believe that your child's cleft or craniofacial condition affects him/her?

	Not at All	A Little	Moderately	Lot	Extremely
Facial appearance differences	(0)	(1)	(2)	(3)	(4)
Teasing from peers	(0)	(1)	(2)	(3)	(4)
Speech problems	(0)	(1)	(2)	(3)	(4)
Hearing problems	(0)	(1)	(2)	(3)	(4)
Vision problems	(0)	(1)	(2)	(3)	(4)
Learning problems	(0)	(1)	(2)	(3)	(4)
Unhappiness with life in general	(0)	(1)	(2)	(3)	(4)
Negative self-esteem	(0)	(1)	(2)	(3)	(4)
Social problems	(0)	(1)	(2)	(3)	(4)
Self-consciousness	(0)	(1)	(2)	(3)	(4)

(continued)

4. Do you expect surgery to make a difference for your child in any of these areas?

	No Change	A Little Better	Moderately Better	A Lot Better	Totally Better
Speech	⓪	①	②	③	④
Teasing by peers	⓪	①	②	③	④
Appearance	⓪	①	②	③	④
Social activities/involvement	⓪	①	②	③	④
Satisfaction with life in general	⓪	①	②	③	④
Self-esteem	⓪	①	②	③	④
Self-consciousness	⓪	①	②	③	④

5. To what degree does the appearance of your child's face concern **you and/or your child**?

   Not at all ____   **A little** ____   **Moderately** ____   **A lot** ____   **Extremely** ____

6. How interested are you in surgery for your child at this time in his/her life?

   Not at all ____   **A little** ____   **Moderately** ____   **A lot** ____   **Extremely** ____

Cleft/Craniofacial Surgery Questionnaire   Ages 13–18

Please complete the following questions so that we might better understand your needs.

1. How concerned are you about these areas of your face?

	Not at All	A Little	Moderately	A Lot	Extremely
Lips	⓪	①	②	③	④
Nose	⓪	①	②	③	④
Ear(s)	⓪	①	②	③	④
Eye(s)	⓪	①	②	③	④
Teeth/jaws	⓪	①	②	③	④
Other_____	⓪	①	②	③	④

2. In what ways do you believe that the appearance of your face affects you?

	Not at All	A Little	Moderately	A Lot	Extremely
More determined	⓪	①	②	③	④
Improved social skills	⓪	①	②	③	④
Social isolation	⓪	①	②	③	④
Self-consciousness	⓪	①	②	③	④
Staring by others	⓪	①	②	③	④
Teasing by peers	⓪	①	②	③	④
Limitation in social activities/ involvement	⓪	①	②	③	④
Problems with dating	⓪	①	②	③	④
Unhappiness with life in general	⓪	①	②	③	④
Negative self-esteem	⓪	①	②	③	④
More accepting of others	⓪	①	②	③	④

(continued)

3. Which of these areas do you expect to change following surgery?

	No Change	A Little Better	Moderately Better	A Lot Better	Totally Better
Appearance	⓪	①	②	③	④
Peer Acceptance	⓪	①	②	③	④
Speech	⓪	①	②	③	④
Social activities/involvement	⓪	①	②	③	④
Determination	⓪	①	②	③	④
Satisfaction with life in general	⓪	①	②	③	④
Improved self-esteem	⓪	①	②	③	④
Compassion for others	⓪	①	②	③	④
Increased social involvement	⓪	①	②	③	④
Self-consciousness	⓪	①	②	③	④
Dating	⓪	①	②	③	④

4. To what degree does the appearance of your face concern you?

Not at all _____ **A little** _____ **Moderately** _____ **A lot** _____ **Extremely** _____

5. How interested are you in having surgery for your face at this time in your life?

Not at all _____ **A little** _____ **Moderately** _____ **A lot** _____ **Extremely** _____

6. Do you have other goals for this surgery not mentioned above?

No ___ **Yes** ___ **If yes, please explain**

_____

_____

_____

REFERENCES

1. ACPA. Parameters for the evaluation and treatment of patients with cleft lip/palate and other craniofacial anomalies. *Cleft Palate Craniofac J* [serial online]. 1993, volume 30 (supplement 1). Available at http://http://www.cleftpalate-craniofacial.org/teamcare. Accessed February 15, 2005.
2. Achenbach TM, Rescorla LA. *Manual for the ASEBA Preschool Forms & Profiles.* Burlington, VT: University of Vermont, Dept of Psychiatry, 2000.
3. Achenbach TM, Rescorla LA. *Manual for the ASEBA School Age Forms & Profiles.* Burlington, VT: University of Vermont, Dept of Psychiatry, 2001.
4. Rumsey N, Harcourt D. Body image and disfigurement: issues and interventions. *Body Image: An International Journal of Research* 2004;1:83–97.
5. Richman LC. Behavior and achievement of cleft palate children. *Cleft Palate J* 1976;13:4–10.
6. Richman LC, Harper DC. School adjustment of children with observable disabilities. *J Abnorm Child Psychol* 1978;6:11–18.
7. Richman LC. Self-reported social, speech, and facial concerns and personality adjustment of adolescents with cleft lip and palate. *Cleft Palate J* 1983;20:108–112.
8. Pope AW, Ward J. Self-perceived facial appearance and psychosocial adjustment in preadolescents with craniofacial anomalies. *Cleft Palate Craniofac J* 1997;34:396–401.
9. Kapp-Simon KA, Dawson P. Behavior adjustment and competence of children with craniofacial conditions. Paper presented at American Cleft Palate-Craniofacial Association Meeting; April 20–25, 1998; Baltimore, MD.
10. Long BC, Kapp-Simon KA. Psychological adjustment and self-perception in children with nonsyndromic cleft lip and palate. Paper presented at American Cleft Palate-Craniofacial Meeting; March 19, 2004; Chicago.
11. Pillemer FG, Cook KV. The psychosocial adjustment of pediatric craniofacial patients after surgery. *Cleft Palate J* 1989;26:201–208.
12. Richman LC, Millard TL. Cleft lip and palate: longitudinal behavior and relationships of cleft conditions to behavior and achievement. *J Pediatr Psychol* 1997;22:487–494.
13. Kapp-Simon KA, McGuire DE. Observed social interaction patterns in adolescents with and without craniofacial conditions. *Cleft Palate Craniofac J* 1997;34:380–384.
14. Edwards TC, Topolski TD. Conceptual foundations and studies of quality of life in persons with craniofacial conditions. Paper presented at American Cleft Palate-Craniofacial Association Meeting; April 10, 2003; Asheville, NC.
15. Kapp-Simon KA. Self-concept of primary school-age children with cleft lip, cleft palate or both. *Cleft Palate J* 1986;23:24–27.
16. Richman LC. Fearful shyness versus solitary passivity in socially inhibited children with cleft. Paper presented at American Cleft Palate Craniofacial Association Meeting; April 20–25, 1998; Baltimore, MD.
17. Spriesterbach DC. *Psychological Aspects of the Cleft Palate Problem.* Iowa City, IA: University of Iowa Press, 1973.
18. Rogers J, Kapp-Simon KA. A comparison of parent and child ratings of psychological adjustment and social functioning. Paper presented at American Cleft Palate-Craniofacial Association Meeting; March 19, 2004; Chicago.
19. Speltz ML, Morton K, Goodell EW, Clarren SK. Psychological functioning of children with craniofacial anomalies and their mothers: follow-up from late infancy to school entry. *Cleft Palate Craniofac J* 1993;30:482–489.
20. Endriga MC, Kapp-Simon KA. Psychological issues in craniofacial care: state of the art. *Cleft Palate Craniofac J* 1999;36(1):3–11.
21. Robinson E, Rumsey N, Patridge J. An evaluation of the impact of social interaction skills training for facially disfigured people. *Br J Plast Surg* 1986;49:281–289.
22. Dawson P, Kapp-Simon KA. Risk and resistance factors on behavior and adjustment in children with craniofacial conditions. Paper presented at American Cleft Palate-Craniofacial Association Meeting; May 4, 2002; Seattle, WA.
23. Broder H, Richman LC, Matheson PB. Learning disabilities, school achievement, and grade retention among children with cleft: a two-center study. *Cleft Palate Craniofac J* 1988;37:127–131.
24. McWilliams BJ, Matthews HP. A comparison of intelligence and social maturity in children with unilateral complete clefts and those with isolated cleft palates. *Cleft Palate J* 1979;16:363–372.
25. Kapp-Simon KA, Figueroa A, Jocher CA, Schafer M. Longitudinal assessment of mental development in infants with nonsyndromic craniosynostosis with and without cranial release and reconstruction. *Plast Reconstr Surg* 1993;92(5):831–840.
26. Prior M, Smart D, Sanson A, Oberklaid F. Relationships between learning difficulties and psychological problems in preadolescents from a longitudinal sample. *J Am Acad Child Adolesc Psychiatry* 1999; 38(4):429–436.
27. Wiener J, Schneider B. A multisource exploration of the friendship patterns of children with and without learning disabilities. *J Abnorm Child Psychol* 2002;30(2):127–141.
28. Bjornsson A, Agustsdottir S. A psychosocial study of Icelandic individuals with cleft lip or cleft lip and palate. *Cleft Palate J* 1987;24:152–157.
29. Clifford E, Crocker E, Pope B. Psychological findings in adulthood of 98 cleft lip-palate children. *Plast Reconstr Surg* 1972;50:234–236.
30. Heller A, Tidmarsh W, Pless IB. The psychological functioning of young adults born with cleft lip or palate. *Clin Pediatr* 1981;20:459–465.
31. McWilliams BJ, Paradise LP. Educational, occupational, and marital status of cleft palate adults. *Cleft Palate J* 1979;10:223–229.
32. Peter JP, Chinsky RR. Sociological aspects of cleft palate adults: education. *Cleft Palate J* 1974;11:443–449.

33. Peter JP, Chinsky RR. Sociological aspects of cleft palate adults, I: marriage. *Cleft Palate J* 1974;11:295–301.
34. Peter JP, Chinsky RR, Fisher MJ. Sociological aspects of cleft palate adults, IV: social integration. *Cleft Palate J* 1975;12:304–310.
35. Rumsey N, Clarke A, White P, Wyn-Williams M, Garlick W. Altered body image: appearance-related concerns of people with visible disfigurement. *J Adv Nurs* 2004;48(5):1–11.
36. Ramstad T, Ottem E, Shaw WC. Psychosocial adjustment in Norwegian adults who had undergone standardized treatment of complete cleft lip and palate. II Self-reported problems and concerns with appearance. *Scand J of Plast Reconstr Surg Hand Surg* 1995;29(4):329–336.
37. Sarwer DB, Bartlett SP, Whitaker LA, Paige KT, Pertschuk MJ, Wadden TA. Adult psychological functioning of individuals born with craniofacial anomalies. *Plast Reconstr Surg* 1999;103(2):412–418.
38. Barden RC. The effects of craniofacial deformity, chronic illness, and physical handicaps on patient and familial adjustment. In: Laheyt B, Kazdin A, eds. *Advances in Child Clinical Psychology*. New York: Plenum Publishing, 1990:343–375.
39. Miller AG. Role of physical attractiveness in impression formation. *Psychomic Science* 1970;19:241–243.
40. Dion KK, Berscheid E, Walster E. What is beautiful is good. *J Pers Soc Psychol* 1972;24:285–290.
41. Adams GR. Physical attractiveness, personality and social reactions to peer pressure. *J Psychol* 1977;96:287–296.
42. Adams GR. Physical attractiveness research: toward a developmental social psychology of beauty. *Hum Dev* 1977;20:217–239.
43. Langlois J, Stephan C. Beauty and the beast: the role physical attractiveness in the development of peer relations and social behavior. In: Brehm SS, Kassin SM, Gibbons FX, eds. *Developmental Social Psychology: Theory and Research*. New York: Oxford University Press, 1981:152–168.
44. Unger R, Hilderbrand M, Madar T. Physical attractiveness and assumptions about social deviance: some sex by sex comparisons. *Personality and Social Psychology* 1982;107:23–28.
45. Kenealy P, Frude N, Shaw WC. Influence of children's physical attractiveness on teacher expectations. *J Soc Psychol* 1987;128:373–383.
46. Maner JK, Kenrick DT, Becker DV, et al. Sexually selective cognition: beauty captures the mind of the beholder. *J PersSoc Psychol* 2003;85(6):1107–1120.
47. Langlois JH, Kalakanis L, Rubenstein AJ, et al. Maxims or myths of beauty? A meta-analytic and theoretical review. *Psychol Bull* 2000;126(3):390–423.
48. Lefebvre A, Barclay S. Psychosocial impact of craniofacial deformities before and after reconstructive surgery. *C J Psychiatry* 1982;27(7):579–587.
49. Lefebvre A, Munro IR. Psychological adjustment of patients with craniofacial deformities before and after surgery. In: Herman P, Zannna MP, Torry Higgins E, eds. *The Ontario Symposium*. Hillsdale, NJ: Lawrence Earlbaum Associates, 1986:53–62.
50. Sinko K, Jagsch R, Prechtl V, et al. Evaluation of esthetical, functional, and quality of life outcome in adult cleft lip and palate patients. Paper presented at American Cleft Palate-Craniofacial Association Annual Meeting; April 9–13, 2003; Asheville, NC.
51. Tobiasen JM, Hiebert JM. Facial impairment scales for clefts. *Plast Reconstr Surg* 1994;93(1):31–41.
52. Strauss RP, Broder H, Helms RW. Perceptions of appearance and speech by adolescent patients with cleft lip and palate and by their parents. *Cleft Palate J* 1988;25(4):335–342.
53. Reed J, Robathan M, Hockenhull A, et al. Children's attitudes toward interacting with peers with different craniofacial anomalies. *Cleft Palate Craniofac J* 1999;36(5):441–447.
54. Okkerse JME, Beemer FA, Cordia-De Haan M, et al. Facial attractiveness and facial impairment ratings in children with craniofacial malformations. *Cleft Palate Craniofac J* 2001;38(4):386–392.
55. Krueckeberg S, Kapp-Simon KA, Ribordy SC. Social skills of preschoolers with and without craniofacial anomalies. *Cleft Palate Craniofac J* 1993;30:475–481.
56. Broder H, Strauss RP. Self-concept of early primary school age children with visible or invisible defects. *Cleft Palate J* 1989;26(2):114–117.
57. Turner SR, Thomas WN, Dowell T, et al. Psychological outcomes amongst cleft patients and their families. *Br J Plastc Surg* 1997;50:1–9.
58. Topolski TD, Edwards TC, Patrick D. Understanding quality of life among adolescents with craniofacial differences. Paper presented at American Cleft Palate-Craniofacial Annual Meeting; March 17, 2004; Chicago.
59. Thomas PT, Turner SR, Rumsey N, et al. Satisfaction with facial appearance among subjects affected by a cleft. *Cleft Palate Craniofac J* 1997;34(3):226–231.
60. Slifer KJ, Beck M, Amari A, et al. Self-concept and satisfaction with physical appearance in youth with and without oral clefts. *Child Health Care* 2003;32(2):81–101.
61. Tobiasen JM, Hiebert JM. Combined effects of severity of facial impairment and facial attractiveness of social perception: an experimental study. *Cleft Palate Craniofac J* 1993;30:82–86.
62. Schneiderman CR, Harding JB. Social ratings of children with cleft lip by school peers. *Cleft Palate J* 1984;21:219–223.
63. Rankin M, Borah G. Perceived functional impact of abnormal facial appearance. *Plast Reconstr Surg* 2003;111(7):2140–2146.
64. Langlois JH, Styczynski L. The effects of physical attractiveness on behavioral attributions and peer preferences of acquainted children. *Int J Behav Dev* 1979;2:325–341.
65. Chang PP, Levine SC, Benson PJ. Children's recognition of caricature. *Dev Psychol* 2003;38(6):1038–1051.
66. Reid AC, Vig K, Lidral A, Johnston W. Perceptions of treatment satisfaction: a questionnaire survey of parents whose children attend a cleft palate-craniofacial team. Paper presented at American Cleft Palate-Craniofacial Association Annual Meeting; April 2001; Minneapolis, MN.
67. Pope AW, Ward J. Factors associated with peer social competence in preadolescents with craniofacial anomalies. *Pediatrics* 1997;22:455–469.
68. Kapp-Simon KA, McGuire DE, Long BC, Simon DJ. Addressing quality of life issues in adolescent: social skills interventions. *Cleft Palate Craniofac J*. In Press.

69. MacGregor FC. Facial disfigurement: problems and management of social interaction and implications for mental health. *Aethetic Plast Surg* 1990;14:249–257.
70. Nash P. *Living with Disfigurement: Psychosocial Implications of Being Born with Cleft Lip and Palate.* Brookfield, VA: Avebury, 1995.
71. ACPA Team Standards Committee. The cleft and craniofacial team. ACPA Web site. Available at: http://www.acpa-cpf.org/teamcare/ccteam.htm. Accessed June 1, 2005.
72. Kagan J. Biology, context, and developmental inquiry. *Annu Rev Psychol* 2003;54:1–23.
73. Hart D, Atkins R, Fegley S. *Personality and Development in Childhood: A Person-Centered Approach.* Boston: Blackwell, 2003.
74. Kapp-Simon KA. Psychological interventions for the adolescent with cleft lip and palate. *Cleft Palate Craniofac J* 1995;32:104–108.
75. Kapp-Simon KA, Simon DJ, Kristovich S. Self-perception, social skills, adjustment, and inhibition in young adolescents with craniofacial anomalies. *Cleft Palate Craniofac J* 1992;29:352–356.
76. Krueckeberg S, Kapp-Simon KA. Longitudinal follow-up of social skills in children with and without craniofacial anomalies. Paper presented at American Cleft Palate-Craniofacial Association Annual Meeting; April 7–12, 1997; New Orleans, LA.
77. Kapp-Simon KA. Psychological care of children with cleft lip and palate in the family. In: Wyszynski DF, ed. *Cleft Lip and Palate: From Origin to Treatment.* New York: Oxford University Press, 2002:412–423.
78. Strauss RP. "Only skin deep": Health resilience and craniofacial care. *Cleft Palate Craniofac J* 2001;38:226–230.
79. Gottman J. *Raising an Emotionally Intelligent Child.* New York: Fireside, 1997.
80. Gordon T. *P.E.T. Parent Effectiveness Training.* New York: Peter H. Wyden, 1970.
81. Nelsen J. *Positive Discipline.* Rev 2nd ed. New York: Ballantine, 1996.
82. Faber A, Mazlish E. *Siblings Without Rivalry.* New York: Avon, 1998.
83. Kapp-Simon KA, Simon DJ. *Meeting the Challenge: A Social Skills Program for Adolescents with Special Needs.* Chicago: Kapp-Simon & Simon, 1991.

Pediatric Burn Injury

Mary Rose, PsyD, and Patricia Blakeney, PhD

No injury is more painful than a severe burn; no image more horrifying than that of a child transformed by burns. Burns destroy ears and noses, fingers and toes; vision and hearing fade. Burn injuries induce immense pain as do the treatments to combat infections and burn-scar contractures. Many survivors must learn to walk without legs, to write without fingers, and to dance without toes. Exercise to regain strength necessitates more pain in a body already fatigued by healing, hormone depletion, and chemical imbalance.

Yet, it is the nonphysical child who suffers the most enduring pain—the psychological "spirit" of the child, who must constantly be on guard, prepared to defend against stares and taunts of others who fail to understand the journey behind burn scars. Ordinary outings to a grocery store or movie present emotionally charged and exceptionally difficult interpersonal challenges. A burned child constantly monitors his or her behavior for any action that is likely to attract attention, while simultaneously mustering the courage to tolerate and cope with potential responses that attention may invoke (1). It is impossible for the burn-scarred child not to attract attention. An "appearance impaired" child rarely has an opportunity to remain anonymous, to be respectfully ignored, or to blend into the crowd (2).

PURPOSE OF THIS CHAPTER

Consequent to scientific advances in treating acute burns, the number of children in the United States who survive massive burns has increased significantly (3–4). Whereas 25 years ago only half of the children with greater than 50% Total Body Surface Area burns (TBSA) survived, now half of those who have 85% TBSA burns and essentially all those with smaller burns routinely survive (5). As the number of children living with burns has increased, so too has concern for psychosocial outcomes and interest in interventions to enhance quality of life for burned children. The quality and quantity of published articles in this field improves each year, reinforcing that psychological and social interventions must be integral to burn treatment throughout care, from acute injury through the years of rehabilitation and reconstruction.

This chapter is written for health care professionals who engage in the difficult, but rewarding endeavor of helping children and their families recover from massive burns. First is a summary of what is known about long-term outcomes, psychosocial adaptation, and quality of life for pediatric burn survivors en route to adulthood.

Acknowledgments: We would like to thank the National Institutes of Disability and Rehabilitation Research Grant #H133A70019 and the Shriner Multicenter Outcomes Research Grant #9115 for their funding support.

Knowing the possibilities of remarkable success as well as the common pitfalls during recovery can encourage both professional and patient through these times. Findings based on these studies can be used to guide patients and their families through what may seem like a massive obstacle course. We describe psychological issues and their importance as they evolve in a typical pattern of recovery through time. Regardless of when one first becomes involved in the care of a burned child, it is helpful to have a perspective of the typical process of rehabilitation. Although the patient may be focused on the present moment, the helper who has awareness of both the child's history and future possibilities is better able to assist the patient in moving through the moment adaptively. We suggest interview questions, therapeutic tasks, and interventions to assist burned children, their families, and the professionals who care for them as they all move through the process of healing and growing together.

LONG-TERM PSYCHOSOCIAL OUTCOMES OF PEDIATRIC BURN INJURIES

Contrary to expectations, empirical data indicate that most burn survivors, even those with the most extensive and disfiguring injuries, demonstrate long-term adjustment comparable to normative values of standard psychometric measures. Only 20% to 30% of pediatric burn survivors demonstrate moderate to severe behavioral problems (6–9). This lack of observable psychopathology does not equate to a happy or easy adjustment (10,11). When competence (comprised largely of socialization skills) is evaluated, another 20% to 30% show mild to moderate diminished competence. When both behavioral problems and competence are assessed, approximately 50% of each sample indicates at least mild deficits in competence and/or elevated behavioral problem scores (12). The difficulties of most pediatric burn survivors are not obvious. In a recent study examining psychological adjustment of 50 adolescents identified as "troubled" on a standardized screening instrument, 52% of the sample assessed 10 years postburn had developed symptoms meeting criteria for psychiatric diagnoses. Of those who did, the most frequently occurring diagnoses (36%) were anxiety disorders, especially social phobia and separation anxiety, which often go unnoticed by others or are known only to the individual's closest confidantes. These and other data (10) suggest that while most burn survivors appear to be doing well, they may be suffering internally. They develop the public persona of a person doing well much of the time, especially in familiar situations. They may also feel a sense of well-being. However, like all people, they also have a private persona, a part of themselves that is shared selectively with people they trust. The private persona of a burned child is sensitized to looking "different" and is anxious about being rejected, teased, or ridiculed. These private feelings vary in their saliency and are situation-specific. For example, a child may feel comfortable and confident in a group of other burned children, but feel terrified at the prospect of walking into a classroom of unfamiliar, unburned children.

Factors Associated with Positive Adjustment

Postburn adjustment has neither been predicted by characteristics of the burn itself, nor is there clear evidence that burn size or location is related to quality of adjustment (13), although some have reported visible disfigurement to be associated with poorer adjustment (14–15). The most significant determining factor of psychosocial adjustment for pediatric burn survivors appears to be family support (9,16–17). For the older child or adolescent, support received from peers is also important (14). Two personality characteristics, extraversion and social risk taking, are important influences on long-term outcomes (15). In one study, high extraversion and social risk taking, together with the family characteristics of high cohesion and low conflict, accounted for 80% of the variance between well-adjusted and poorly adjusted adolescent survivors of pediatric burns (17).

LONG-TERM DIFFICULTIES FOLLOWING PEDIATRIC BURNS—SURVIVORS AS YOUNG ADULTS

The ultimate goal of pediatric burn care, beyond survival and functional restoration, is to restore the quality of life and the potential for productive adult lives. We recently examined the success of 101 survivors of childhood burns between the ages of 18 and 28. Their mean burn size was 54% TBSA, averaging 14 years postinjury. By several objective criteria (e.g., educational achievement and employment) these young adults were doing well. Examination by a physical therapist found them to be without significant impairment, capable of self-care and independent living. Overtly, the burn survivors appeared to be functioning satisfactorily in their lives. However, they differed significantly from the nonclinical reference groups in several psychological and emotional areas. Burned males reported significantly more somatic complaints; burned females reported not only significant elevations in somatic complaints, but also greater withdrawal, more thought problems, and more aggressive and angry behavior (18–19), supporting findings that appearance impairment is a greater source of distress and has stronger impact for females than for males (20–22).

Burn survivors appeared to feel adequate self-worth within the context of family and friends. Outside those arenas, they expressed lowered self-esteem manifested through anxiety and withdrawal as well as intrusive thoughts and difficulty with concentration. Burned males and females indicated that they were acutely aware of their bodies and felt that they make poor first impressions when interacting with others.

A high percentage (46%) of young adult survivors had significant personality disorders, a finding not found in our studies of younger children and adolescents. Individually administered standardized interviews revealed a high (44%) incidence of current psychiatric diagnoses among this sample of adult survivors. As with the adolescent sample, anxiety disorders were the most common diagnoses for the young adults.

These results indicate that a significant number of young adults who survived severe burn injuries as children suffer major mental illness likely complicated by their injuries and resultant scars. Moreover, many others without major mental illness are distressed in social and interpersonal situations, hampered by keen awareness of their disfigurement (23). The "illness" or distress may be managed in a way that makes it invisible to all but those individuals closest to them; and the commonly reported withdrawal behaviors of burn survivors limit the numbers of people in that category. Their behaviors also impede the opportunity to have positive, corrective experiences without external therapeutic assistance. Notably, most survivors in the study sample were not involved in psychological or psychiatric treatment, and most would have gone unnoticed as needing help except by professionals who were sensitized to their experiences.

Long-Term Sequelae for Burned Children

The most significant limitations on the long-term quality of life for the pediatric burn survivor seems not to be functional impairment (24), but rather anxiety and social impairment in relating to others. The gestalt of disfigurement, unhappiness with appearance, stigmatization, social anxiety, maladaptive coping, and social discomfort is more likely to result in significant long-term impairment than the physical results of severe burn injuries (25). Physical impediments of burn scar contractures, amputations, diminished hearing and/or eyesight do not prevent burn survivors from performing activities required for self-care (8). But coping with isolation related to disfigurement requires skills and confidence many survivors never achieve. For these individuals, social and emotional challenges during childhood and adolescence lead to long-lasting anxieties, fear of new social settings, and decreased self-esteem.

Survivors' inhibitions in taking interpersonal initiative are reinforced by rejecting or demeaning attitudes of others. This cycle of appearance distinction, anxiety, and withdrawal to avoid rejection creates barriers to the success of many burn survivors. Researchers are increasingly focused on stigmatization, dissatisfaction with appearance, social anxiety, and development of interventions to assist survivors in coping with these social obstacles (26–27).

Body Image Dissatisfaction

Body image is multidimensional, including self-perceptions and expectations of how others evaluate appearance. Beliefs about one's strength, physical sensations, sexuality, movement, facial features, and physical boundaries are integral (28). Burn survivors may experience alterations in all of these areas. Survivors rate their unusual appearance and others' responses as most salient to how they adjust (1). Developmental stage impacts body image throughout childhood and, thus is assumed to be the same for burned children (29). Whether gender contributes differentially to the effect of burn on body image is unclear (1,30).

Most of the literature on body image of the burned child is based on clinical observation with scant empirical data. The paucity of studies in this area reflects the difficulty in assessing relevant aspects of body image in burned children. Lawrence et al. have developed the Satisfaction With Appearance Scale (SWAP), which examines the degree to which appearance affects interpersonal relations and satisfaction with specific areas of the body (31). Validated for older adolescents (16 and over) and adults, it appears to be appropriate for preteens as well, and plans are underway at our institution to develop a version for young children.

Stigmatization

According to Goffman (32), the original Greek word *stigma* referred to bodily signs designed to expose something unusual and bad about the moral status of the individual who bore the signs. Stigmatization has retained a similar purpose of separating some individuals from larger society. Burn survivors often relate experiences in which they feel discredited by others because of their scars. The stigmatizing behaviors may be obvious such as staring, teasing, or bullying; or they may be subtle such as avoiding eye contact, ignoring, or expressing pity (33).

Bull and Rumsey hypothesized that experiencing stigmatization has three specific effects on people with appearance distinctions: poor body-esteem, a sense of social isolation, and a violation of privacy effect (34). This refers to the inability of the person to be anonymous, without undue attention. The burned child can rarely be anonymous; even the act of ignoring is a form of recognition and rejection. Sometimes the extraordinary attention is meant to be positive, but is nonetheless intrusive and dehumanizing. One young woman, whose survival and accomplishments had received a great deal of public praise, described her experience when she attended her first class at a large university in a city near her home. Several people greeted her, calling her by name; but she had no idea who they were. She fled, dropping out of school for the semester. She explained that she felt she had been performing to live up to her reputation as a "wonder" for years; and that, even in a setting where she knew no one, she already felt pressured to be an example to the world.

Social Anxiety

Social anxiety is an important factor in social impairment and emotional functioning among nonclinical populations of children and adolescence. Children who are rejected or neglected by their peers report substantially more social anxiety than their accepted classmates (35). Those with high social anxiety perceive themselves as less socially accepted and report lower levels of global self-esteem compared with less socially anxious peers (62). Among middle-school students, high levels of social anxiety at the beginning of the school year have also been found to predict low levels of companionship and intimacy in friendships during the school year (36). Not all children with social anxiety develop psychopathology; levels of social anxiety appear to be important risk markers and may help to differentiate clinically anxious children with and without impairments in their social functioning (37). As yet, there are no published studies of social anxiety in the adaptation of burned children. However, given the findings related to adolescent and young adult burn survivors, such investigation is imperative for early identification of risk for developing more serious psychopathology.

Social Learning

Social learning theory suggests that diminished social competence, increased behavioral problems, and anxiety may be related to maladaptive coping techniques that the burned child has utilized to deal with disfigurement. Social learning theory emphasizes that the individual forms a vision of "self" and "reality" through reciprocal interaction (i.e., the impact of the individual upon his environment and vice versa) and feedback (38). People's behavior determines aspects of their environment to which they are exposed and to which they attend; and their behavior is, in turn, modified by that environment. Based on learned preferences and competencies, humans select with whom they interact and in which activities they participate. Thus, the individual's behavior determines which of many potential environmental influences come into play.

Humans evoke reactions from the social environment as a result of physical characteristics, such as age, race, sex, and physical appearance. One's interpretations of the reactions of the social environment feed into concepts of "self" and expectations of the future. The individual develops "cognitions," for example, beliefs, values, expectations, through interactions with the social environment. These cognitions guide behavior. Cognitions change as a function of maturation and experience, but without corrective experience, ideas do not change. Beliefs or expectations that served the person well historically may, over time and in new situations, become maladaptive unless the person learns to adapt their beliefs and behaviors to match new experiences.

Clinical Example

In order to understand how these theoretical constructs apply to burned children, it is helpful to imagine a hypothetical burned boy who leaves the hospital in bandages and splints. He returns to school, in spite of his parents' anxieties, feeling timid and anxious because he knows his body looks and functions differently than in the past and differently from others' bodies. His parents' anxieties affirm his own fears. In the school cafeteria, he notices that some of the children stare at him, but look away when he looks at them. He interprets that behavior as indicating that he looks like a "freak." When he walks by those children, one of the boys says "Hey, Freddy" referring to a burned villain in a horror movie. The burned child perceives that response as further evidence that he looks like a monster. The child begins to incorporate this feedback into his self-image. With recurrent similar experiences, the child is likely to misinterpret all looks from others as related to his appearance without considering other possible explanations (such as his own perceptible misery). Because he cannot change his appearance and does not know how to decrease the discomfort of others (which he interprets as evidence of his own worthlessness), he may well decide that he should not approach people whom he expects to be uncomfortable with him. He becomes fearful of approaching any-one except his most trusted friends and family. His mother, wanting to protect him, asks for a homebound teacher so he will not have to interact with others. This affirms his beliefs that others will hurt and reject him. The more he avoids others, the more his dysfunctional beliefs are unchallenged; the more he refuses to inter-act with others, the more others exclude him.

The child may decide to stay away from other people whenever possible; he may decide to avoid situations in which he is likely to call attention to himself; or he may decide to attack others before they can hurt him. This hypothetical child will develop strategies to maintain, to the degree possible, his own comfort. These strategies may facilitate successful interactions with others, but they are just as likely to work against his adjustment. The more strategies the child develops and the more helpful feedback he receives, the more likely he is to identify strategies that are effective in social interactions. Without helpful feedback and/or a variety of coping techniques, the child develops a feedback loop of social anxiety that may become disabling. If the burned child chooses a strategy of striking out at others to protect himself, he would be called a "behavior problem"; as that role became integral to his self-concept, he would feel angrier and increasingly negative about himself. Thus, he would strike out more, eventually perhaps meeting criteria for the psychiatric diagnosis of conduct disorder.

THE FAMILY'S INVOLVEMENT

Burn injury and its treatment are family affairs from the beginning, particularly for pediatric patients. The family unit is disrupted and traumatized. The premorbid characteristics of the family are important in predicting the course of recovery. At the time of injury, family members face not only the life-threatening event to the child but other losses as well. They are conflicted by desire to provide love and sup-port while mourning the loss of their imagined perfect child. In many instances, the fire has taken the home, loved ones, pets, and/or property. Families may be facing the loss of a wage earner and/or financial ruin while caring for the patient. Even at hospitals where medical care is free of charge to the families, attendant costs of lost wages, travel expenses, and special arrangements to care for the patient postdis-charge can be devastating.

Family members play a critical role in long-term care and rehabilitation of the burned child and are often extended members of the treatment team. Family mem-bers can be extremely helpful in supporting the best interests of the child during the difficult months or years ahead. But even well-adapted and healthy families have dif-ficulties, and a serious injury exacerbates pre-existing problems (70). Identification of psychosocial strengths and vulnerabilities of family members, including those that contributed to the burn injury, help the team to develop a treatment plan that will facilitate adjustment of the child and the entire family unit.

THE PSYCHOLOGIST'S INVOLVEMENT

Burn care is improved by a comprehensive multidisciplinary program in which men-tal health professionals are integral. A psychotherapists should be involved in the treatment of the burned child throughout recovery (39–41). However, all caregivers, including the patient's family, are instruments of therapeutic intervention (42). An essential role of the psychotherapist is to consult with and guide other burn care professionals and patients' families about psychosocial issues and to collaborate in cross-disciplinary therapeutic interventions (69).

PSYCHOLOGICAL CONCERNS DURING BURN RECONSTRUCTION AND REHABILITATION

Adaptation to burn injury is a complex process occurring throughout several months or years following injury. Psychological healing occurs across time commensurate with physical healing in a pattern that is relatively predictable and consistent, although mediated by individual dynamics (43–45). Awareness of this pattern allows caregivers to anticipate emergence of psychosocial issues and to prepare patients for coping with those issues. Predicting problematic issues for patients normalizes reactions and avoids patients/families perceiving themselves as psychologically disturbed. Recognizing that recovery is a lengthy process, we have, for convenience, arbitrarily designated a pre-injury phase and four phases of recovery: *critical care, recuperation, reintegration, and rehabilitation.* Psychosocial issues to be addressed during acute treatment are addressed elsewhere (42); in this chapter we focus on preburn issues and on issues arising later during reintegration and rehabilitation.

Pre-burn Psychological Concerns

Because problematic issues in the life of the child prior to the burn are exacerbated by the additional difficulties of living with burn scars and disfigurement, it is important to be aware of historical concerns that may complicate or facilitate recovery, reconstructive, and rehabilitation success. Demographics provide important information for rehabilitation of young survivors. Many parents of burned children have few financial resources (46–47), and limited education. Additionally, the family of the burned child is likely to have at least one parent who is seriously dysfunctional, for example, chronic substance abuser, incarcerated, or mentally ill (48). Restricted time, distraction, limited knowledge about child development, and unrealistic expectations of children puts parents at risk for providing inadequate supervision of their children despite their positive attachment to them. Because the child recovering from serious burns and reconstructive procedures requires even more time and attention from a caretaker than prior to injury, the burn team must assist the family by teaching the caretaker what a child needs as well as providing emotional support to the caretaker, helping to obtain resources, and monitoring the child's care.

Sometimes parental inadequacy involves more sinister neglect and/or abuse of a child. Perhaps as many as 30% of U.S. pediatric burn injuries are incurred through either abuse or neglect serious enough to warrant involvement of child welfare services (18,49). The abused child has complications throughout recovery related to family and care provider dysfunctions, making identification of risk factors critical (18,49–50). Abuse and neglect cases demand professional demeanor and diplomatic skills. The burn team must find ways to work effectively with the family of the abused child over the long term, sometimes including the abuser, as the child often returns to the family. At times it may be necessary for the team to report suspicious injuries or negligent behavior while simultaneously maintaining rapport with the family. Care providers can be honest with families about reports that are mandated by law and will be made while projecting a nonjudgmental attitude (49).

A child's characteristics may be important in the etiology of burns as well as major factors in recovery. Pre-existing psychiatric disorders are common in histories of older burned patients, and frequently have contributed to the etiology of the injury (51–52). This is probably true for the young child as well, although the young child is less likely to have been given a psychological diagnosis, limiting availability of data to substantiate such a hypothesis (53). ADD and ADHD are predisposing conditions for burns (54), especially during periods of "drug holiday" (55). Serious burn injuries from purposeful self-immolation are extremely rare among pediatric patients; but they do occur, usually preceded by a major depression with psychotic features, including suicidal ideation (56). Substance abuse often plays a causal role in burn injuries of the older child. Those abusing flammable inhalants are at particular risk for burn injury (57–58). Obviously, adequate management of such conditions is necessary for successful reconstruction and rehabilitation.

Reconstructive Surgery and Rehabilitation

Reconstructive procedures for a child may begin during the first year postinjury, and continue for many years. Throughout those years, psychosocial processes challenge the well-being of the child. Early after discharge from acute treatment, wound breakdown, dressing changes, exercises, splints, and pressure garments force the child to confront anew the losses and possibly to experience a delayed grief reaction. After leaving the protective hospital environment, symptoms of traumatic stress that had remitted in the hospital may recur. Social encounters are critical experiences for the burned child during these early months.

Massive burns do not follow a steady trajectory toward health and well-being where progress can be tracked by visible improvement. Following many traumatic injuries, patients undergo a relatively steady progression toward recovery with occasional setbacks. The burn-injured child, however, may appear more "normal" at acute discharge than at a year postburn when the child is actually healthier. Initially following debridement of dead tissue, a child's skin is discolored but retains its shape; missing ears, nose, or lips may be obscured by dressings. Scars, as well, are covered by dressings, splints, and pressure garments. As the child heals, the patchwork of grafted skin becomes more apparent, and disfigurement may become more pronounced with contractures, keloid or hypertrophic scarring, and distorted appearance and function in digits, joints, and posture.

A burned face is much like a masked one. Even with undamaged muscle tissue, it is sometimes difficult for a child to project the former level of facial animation. Normal skin reveals much about the individual's emotional state through blushing, blanching, sweating, or bristling of hair (59); burns change all of this. Nuances in facial expression may be gone, requiring one to "read" emotional expression in the child's eyes (60). Burn associated growth delays may have negative effects on psychological functioning as has been found for people with other growth hormone–related deficiencies (61–62). These distinctive characteristics of appearance seem to be at the heart of stigmatization and social obstacles with which the child must cope.

Early in the rehabilitation phase, focus is primarily on functional physical recovery. Often ignored are the changes in body image, self-esteem, and social identity consequent to disfigurement. While children are wearing pressure garments or splints, they tend to think of their bodies as *temporarily* different, and they hope that, at the end of treatment, their old bodies will magically reappear. When the devices are discontinued, a new phase of body image adaptation begins. Children are confronted with the permanence of their scars. Disfigured children must find ways of developing positive self-esteem despite reactions from others that communicate that the very sight of them brings horror, shock, sadness, or pity (63). Burned children typically pass through a period of dysphoric self-worth lasting several months before recovering their feelings of value by adopting a strategy of rationalization, denying importance of those things that they cannot change and turning their attention and energy to areas where they can succeed (64–65). Unlike nonburned children, burned children rate personal appearance, athletic competence, and social acceptance as less important to self-esteem than scholastic competence, job competence, and romantic appeal (65).

Families also continue the stressful process of adaptation. Feelings related to the traumatic incident resurface frequently and must be resolved. Parents must cope with ordinary pressures of life while also grieving. Care for an injured child requires a great deal of time and energy, which may compete with the care available for the uninjured family members. The early adaptation period (about 1 year) of this phase is tumultuous and gradually calms down. By about 2 years postinjury, most families are able to focus more on ordinary tasks of life and less on recovery from burns. During this time they begin to realize fully the long-term implications of the irrevocable changes created by the injury.

Psychotherapeutic Tasks of the Reconstructive and Rehabilitative Phase

- Help children cope with social anxiety and stigmatization. Rehearse use of diverse coping skills and practice empathetic perceptions of others. Provide assistance as needed with integration in community and school.
- Promote development of positive self-image. It is helpful to remind children of the courage and strength required to have survived the injury and to have accomplished the difficult work of rehabilitation, that is, to promote a "heroic" identity. This gives children a positive frame through which to view their burn scars as visible signs of what they have achieved. Be aware, however, that over time this image should evolve into a self-concept that includes more realistic aspects. The ultimate goal is for the children to think of themselves as persons who were burned and have many interests and strengths as well as vulnerabilities and difficulties to overcome.
- Assist in developing an overall plan for reconstruction and rehabilitation.
- At each opportunity, assess the patient's and/or family's desires and expectations for reconstruction and assist them to communicate clearly with the burn team.

RECONSTRUCTIVE INTERVENTIONS FOR LONG-TERM BENEFIT

Though burned children celebrate cessation of acute treatment and rehabilitation, they may yet have years of reconstructive procedures ahead of them, each followed by new rehabilitation routines, that offers hope for eventual salvation from the constant tension of being physically distinct. Although children in the United States grow up hearing truisms such as "Beauty is only skin deep," for burned children this carries special meaning. First impressions are appearance-based, and often dictate availability of future interactions. For disfigured children, the first impression is quite likely to interfere with willingness of others to continue investing interpersonally. In pursuit of physical normalcy, burned children and their parents cling to the hope that plastic surgery will actualize access to social options.

Children with large burns and/or contractures over joints must live with delayed gratification while their burn scars mature. Problems emerge when the surgeon's priorities appear to be quite different from those of the child and/or parent. Surgeons prioritize surgeries to first prevent deformity, second to reconstruct active function, and finally to restore passive function (66). Factored into surgical plans must be potential viable donor sites and how to accomplish the best long-term outcome. Multiple surgeries are often extended over years, subsequent to which new splints and pressure garments are worn, and passive and active range of motion is essential. In the eyes of the child, the surgeon's order of priorities may represent a long and painful delay in addressing the child's own priorities. As early as possible after acute healing, a reconstruction and rehabilitation plan should be developed with the child and participation of the family. Child, family, and surgeon must agree on common goals, and the child and family must understand how each step of the plan is necessary to achieve the end goal. Active family cooperation with recommended aftercare is pivotal to the success of postsurgical recovery. If the child and family understand the plan and trust that the surgeon and burn team are assisting them in achieving their goals, they have a far greater likelihood to adhere to the plan (67).

As children mature, their concern with their appearance intensifies, as does their independence, that is, their ability *not* to cooperate. When their wishes clash with surgical priorities, the surgeon must find a way to give something to the children to validate their needs. For example, a hand must be made functional before addressing a facial scar; but it might be possible to resurface an area during the same operation in which a contracture is released. Alternatively, scheduling a time when the facial scar will be surgically addressed may support the child's hope, and show collaboration and respect for the child's priorities. When issues of appearance cannot be quickly addressed or when the child's fantasies of how appearance will be changed by surgery are unrealistically high, a "cosmetic" nonsurgical intervention can be prescribed as an interim solution. Skin camouflage techniques or particular styles of dressing to de-emphasize disfigurement can be helpful in supporting children through periods of desensitization to their scars. This gives them an active and alternative approach to improving their appearance, as well as time to adapt to the realistic prognosis that their skin will never look completely "normal."

Scheduling sequential surgeries for a child must promote, to the degree possible, normal socialization and developmental goals of children. Some children have been unable to attend burn camp or play on a Little League team for years because reconstructive surgeries were scheduled at times that prohibited participation. Although the visual drama of disfigurement invites the assumption that surgical correction must be top priority in the child's life, sometimes psychosocial needs may outweigh need for an operation.

Motivation for surgery is often taken for granted. As most plastic surgeons have learned, it is a mistake to guess a patient's reason for consult based upon how they appear. A desire to forego certain surgeries may represent an earnest comfort with one's physical appearance and disfigurement. One may have awareness of disfigurement, but nevertheless have high self-regard in other ways and be truly disinterested in surgery to improve aesthetics. A developing child sometimes desires, more than an improved appearance, an opportunity to break from the role of being constantly readmitted to a hospital. Returning for surgery is not only a continuous reminder of being burned and being different. As one survivor of 95% TBSA burns states, "The reconstruction just isn't worth the pain and bother. . . . I'm tired of it." One frustration in working with a child is the child's reluctance to proceed with surgeries that the adults (surgeons, parents, etc.) think are in his best interest. Improved management of pain has likely removed some posttraumatic blocks to children's willingness to undergo reconstructive surgeries. Despite advances in pain management, myths regarding analgesics causing drug addiction, and our hasty failure to use topical analgesics for minor procedures and needle placement, painful previous treatments have a profound effect on our patients' decision not to pursue reconstructive surgery. The memories of pain from an earlier experience may fade and lay dormant, but be rekindled when the child is readmitted to a hospital. Additionally, the suffering of pain is sometimes believed to be deserved. Particularly when one pursues elective "aesthetic" surgery, society is quick to lose empathy. This social stigma is not only inflicted upon the patient, but is integrated into the patients' self-perceptions; he or she may view disfigurement as a part of themselves that he or she must endure as a deserved "punishment" for some imagined behavior.

Over time, poor families and the uninsured may have financial trouble accessing follow-up care. Insurance benefits may terminate, and reconstructive procedures may be denied as "unnecessary." Cost is critical not only with reconstructive procedures, but also in applying prostheses for amputated limbs. Prostheses must be replaced as a child grows, and even after growth has stopped, sockets need replacement every 2 to 3 years (68). Lack of access to these parts essentially means that the burn victims again lose their limbs.

Unlike an adult, a child's developmental issues may hinder participation in reconstructive surgery. Teens may decline or desire reconstructions that are incompatible, unbeknownst to them, with their future identities as adults (attested by the success of laser tattoo removal). Reconstructive surgery for the burned child may also serve purposes not immediately obvious to adults. For example, one teen with >95% full thickness burn set as a major reconstruction goal to have ear lobes so that she might wear earrings.

In general, strategies that combine a sense of collegiality, guidance, and empathy work best for children and families. Interventions by child life, music therapists, psychologists, psychiatrists, and carefully selected experienced burn survivors have been instrumental at our institution in creating trust and in conveying issues that interfere with a child or family in making decisions.

PSYCHOSOCIAL INTERVENTIONS TO ADDRESS LONG-TERM CONCERNS

Many burn centers provide psychosocial care for burn survivors during acute hospitalization and in conjunction with reconstructive and rehabilitation procedures. However, limited funding for mental health services means that only those with the most disruptive psychiatric disorders can access such attention; most burn survivors do not meet those criteria. The care they receive as children from the burn teams acutely may be the only opportunity to receive professional attention for their distress. Fortunately, the intensity of the relationship between the burn team with burned children and their families can facilitate psychosocial interventions provided in the brief time that children usually receive their reconstruction and rehabilitative treatments. The strength of those relationships also ensure success of referrals for continued treatment when necessary and available. Our therapeutic strategy is designed to break maladaptive connections between cognition, emotion, and behavior, and to replace them with more adaptive thought and behavioral patterns through cognitive behavioral therapy (CBT), family systems therapy, psycho-education, and psychopharmacology (33). Early recognition of distress, well-directed interventions, psycho-education, and supportive therapy in the context of a strong therapeutic relationship may prevent much of the paralyzing anxiety previously noted, thus limiting the need for more in-depth and long-term treatment.

Summer camps are designed to provide activities to promote self-esteem and self-efficacy in a setting where burned children can relax their usual hyperawareness of their burns. Studies have reported decreased behavioral problems, especially decreased aggressive behaviors, (69) improved self-esteem, and enhanced psychological well-being (70) following burn camp experience.

Another promising intervention is social skills training in a group setting with a curriculum aimed at specific concerns of burned children. The goal is to help children develop ways to manage and control their social interactions (71). *Changing Faces*, a nonprofit organization, has reported this psycho-educational program to be effective with adults with facial disfigurement (72–73), and we have been pleased with outcomes thus far in our work with adolescents.

CASE EXAMPLES

The following cases illustrate some issues important in the psychosocial treatment of burned children and the importance of these issues for outcome. Two 19-year-old men, both seriously burned as children with resulting visible scars including face and hands, were seen for assessments. Both had been followed by our staff since their acute burns as children years earlier. There are other similarities; both boys have two siblings, and both live in working class families. Both receive their basic financial support from their parents. And both may be said to be functioning satisfactorily with no psychiatric diagnoses. However, the outcomes are strikingly different.

Case 1: A.C.

At the age of 8, A.C. received burns over 58% of his body, following the malfunction of a household appliance. His father and younger sister were also burned in the accident. The two children, accompanied by their mother, were flown to our hospital while their father received treatment in a burn center local to their home. Although extremely stressful for the family, the acute hospitalization was uneventful; the family was reunited within weeks and began reintegrating into the community. The children were homeschooled by their mother, as they had been prior to the accident. Their social activities centered on church where their parents were actively involved. During the first year A.C. demonstrated more distress, usually manifested as anger, than did his sister, who was the more compliant of the two. He and his family entered counseling together to address not only A.C.'s anger, but the many stressors the accident had precipitated, for example, rebuilding a home, father's lengthy physical disability, and mother's burdens in caring for the burned family members as well as a healthy infant. The family received a great deal of help and support from relatives and friends. During the second year postinjury, the family life became more normal; the home was built and father returned to work. Return trips to the hospital for the children diminished to one time a year with usually one reconstructive procedure per child occurring during those trips. Often the whole family traveled together to the city where the children received their treatment. Reconstruction went smoothly at each occasion, and the children adhered to their recommended postoperative care. In the summers, the children attended a camp for burned children, a church camp, or both. A.C. began attendance in public school as he entered middle school; he made good grades and excelled at sports. After the first year postinjury, he accepted his scars and they never appeared to impede his activities. At 19, he is attending a college on a scholarship, majoring in biology, and working during the summers teaching basketball.

Case 2: C.J.

C.J. was 13 when he received full thickness burns over 76% of his body also resulting from an appliance malfunction. Both of his parents traveled the short distance to be with him in the hospital; however, their relationship was fraught with tension. They had been divorced for 2 years. Now, with their middle son struggling to survive his burns, they decided to resume living together as a family in order to care for him; however, they made it clear that they would not live together as man and wife. The father was primarily focused on his busy life coaching a Little League baseball team. C.J.'s older brother played on the team and apparently showed athletic promise, whereas C.J. showed neither interest nor talent and was not involved in Little League. The mother worked outside the home in a government service position with good benefits that would allow her to assume a primary role in caring for C.J. during the early months postdischarge. The father stayed near the hospital until his son was medically stable and then returned to his job and activities. Though his father returned to visit on weekends, C.J.'s brother never visited C.J. at the hospital. It became clear that C.J. and his mother shared a closeness that the boy did not have with the other members of the family. In fact, C.J. seemed distant from everyone. He had stopped going to school, with his parents' permission, a few weeks prior to the accident. He felt rejected by peers at school and placed the blame on the fact that he was mildly overweight. School personnel had recognized his unhappiness and tried to convince his parents that he needed special attention. However, the parents, believing that the school unjustly wanted C.J. in special education, declined assistance, thereafter allowing him to remain out of school. The boy had poor socialization beyond his family. Neither parent seemed concerned that C.J. was not attending school and was without friends. The one positive thing with which both parents agreed was that he enjoyed playing guitar and possessed some talent for that.

As C.J. was discharged from acute hospitalization, he allowed members of the burn team to conduct a school visit and educational program to assist his re-entry into school. However, his school attendance, predictably, lasted less than one week. The family physician, at the father's request, wrote a letter recommending homebound study. Our team also submitted referrals for C.J. to receive outpatient therapy for physical as well as psychiatric care. The parents refused counseling for themselves and/or the other boys, but agreed reluctantly to C.J.'s participation in a program that included physical therapy, psychotherapy, and academic work in a day program. However, they could not arrange their schedules to get him to his appointments regularly. Finally, a case manager threatened to file "medical neglect" charges, leading the parents to relent and arrange for physical therapy. Psychotherapy in the community was terminated and a homebound teacher resumed teaching him one hour a day, 4 days per week.

Over the next 2 years, there were no significant changes in C.J.'s life. He returned on schedule for surgeries and assessments. During each hospitalization, C.J.'s demands for pain medicine frustrated the staff and consumed much of the time the staff had available to work with him. The only consistent attention from mental health professionals the boy received was from the psychologist and psychiatrist at the burn center. These professionals treated the boy (with CBT and psychopharmacology) and his mother (with CBT and supportive therapy) whenever they came to the hospital. Slowly, the boy began socializing with others his age and developed friendships. He eventually returned to public school and graduated from high school at age 19. He currently is working as a car washer. He expresses anger with his father, but continues to live at home with both parents, who continue to live separate lives within the same household. C.J. can verbalize no specific ambitions or goals except to play his guitar and hang out with friends. No one in the family receives any mental health treatment except for the sporadic visits the boy makes to the hospital, visits that have become fewer and fewer over the years and will cease when he is 21.

Discussion

Both boys might be said to be doing fine after a superficial interview. However, A.C. began his ordeal from the resilient position of being a treasured son in a cohesive family with parents who supported each other and who encouraged age-appropriate independence in their children. His family also had good social support. And they were, as a family, open to facing the emotional ordeal of adjustment, accepting, and seeking help from appropriate sources. Together, they dealt with the stares and questions, stigmatization and anxieties so that A.C. could learn quickly how to cope with social situations. C.J., on the other hand, prior to his burn injury was well into the cycle of rejection, body image dissatisfaction, and social anxiety; his burn injury and scars exacerbated his anxiety and intensified his withdrawal. His parents, focused on their own goals, were unable to provide time and attention to their son. Their own insecurities prohibited them from acknowledging that the boy needed professional help. The burn care team failed to mobilize the mother to take a more active role in decision making for her son and failed to establish the relationship with the boy's father that would have been necessary to help the boy cope more effectively at an earlier age. In some way, the fact that C.J. did finish high school and has a circle of friends may be marks of success; but like many other burn survivors, C.J. is just "getting by". . . not excelling, not failing, and trying not to be noticed.

SPECIAL NOTES TO THE RECONSTRUCTIVE SURGEON AND TEAM

Perhaps the most difficult point in treatment for a surgeon is the moment when a surgeon informs the patient that further reconstruction is unlikely to provide additional aesthetic or functional benefit. The surgeon, trained with focus on more refined procedures that should result in significant aesthetic improvement, may feel disappointed and inadequate when viewing completed work with patients who remain seriously disfigured. Discomfort on the part of both the patient and the surgeon may create a synergistic dissatisfaction. Surgeons working with burn survivors must set expectations based not on social norms of aesthetics, but rather upon the gains from pretreatment conditions.

There are several strategies we recommend for those working with pediatric burn reconstruction patients to facilitate trust as well as to understand and manage potential compliance difficulties and unrealistic expectations. Questionnaires 6-1 and 6-2 at the end of the chapter have been designed to obtain, quickly and efficiently, basic information as an initial step to assisting the patient, family, and surgical team through the reconstructive process.

1. Be familiar with the circumstance of the original burn. Burns that are the result of fire play, antisocial activity, parental depression resulting in neglect, or parental abuse represent different etiologies that will likely continue to play a role in future compliance and surgical outcomes. Such burn related issues may complicate postsurgical recovery, dissatisfaction, and pain management.
2. Psychosocial staff should be involved in the team when possible. Such personnel should be familiar with the procedures used. A basic understanding of procedures and the risks and contraindications allows the psychosocial staff to converse with the patient more comfortably and to evaluate expectations.
3. Use touch. Nonthreatening physical touch has been shown to significantly facilitate doctor–patient communication (74). For the reconstruction patient, touch may be a subtle way to dispel the patient's fears that disfigurement is dirty or repulsive to the physician. Children's boundaries are such that physical bonding at different stages may be crucial to building trust, particularly in nonverbal children. Contrarily, one must be conscientious of how the child sets such boundaries.
4. Introduction of oneself and greetings first to the child, then the parent, is well received by both. This pleases children of verbal age as adults rarely introduce themselves, and almost never first, to the child. It reminds the child and family that the child is first in the equation and allows the doctor to initiate a physical bond with a handshake or touch. It also impels the child to be participatory during the visit.
5. Children and adolescents may have inaccurate beliefs about how a surgery will affect function or appearance. Reassure parents and children about time issues related to multistep procedures. Families are sometimes eager to cram surgeries into spring breaks or summer vacations. They may feel that perceived delays in reconstructive surgery are solely scheduling issues. Families need to be reassured about issues such as the importance of matured scarring in successful outcomes.
6. Trust your instinct regarding suspicions of neglect or abuse. Even with families for whom protective services has closed or dismissed the case, staff often have

continued serious concerns regarding the family and worry about the possibility of repeat injury (75). Concerns regarding abuse can often be partially evaluated by long bone scans and involvement of psychological services. Defensiveness, aggressive behavior, and a reticent child who the caregiver will not permit to speak with staff alone, are significant red flags for maladaptive home environments that warrant further investigation.

7. Do not underplay disfigurement with statements you truly cannot defend such as "looks don't really matter." In her young adult novel, Teena Booth writes: "If there is one thing worse than being an ugly duckling in a house of swans, it's having the swans pretend there's no difference" (76, p. 17).

8. An expectation that appearance is more important to girls than to boys may create anxiety for boys who wish to discuss aesthetic and reconstructive desires. Open the discussion for them and offer reassurance of normalcy.

9. Ask "why" when patient motivations or rationale for treatment seem unclear.

10. Statements such as "many of our patients tell us . . ." and "if you were my child. . . ." help establish normalcy, connection, and investment in the child's situation.

11. Create at least the guise of modesty for patients. Children at specific developmental stages experience greater modesty issues. We have encountered many children whose growing affection for their surgeon complicates their embarrassment during surgeries and examinations. We generally allow children to wear underwear into the operating room as it can easily be removed and replaced when needed without the child ever being faced with the modesty issue.

12. Take delight and celebrate the achievement of each survivor. Accept the patient's moments of sadness and anger as normal human responses that are to be expected as part of life.

CONCLUSIONS

There are many reasons to believe that survivors of serious burn injuries, even those who appear well-adjusted as children, will be impaired in their abilities to develop into well-adjusted adults. Even after years of work in rehabilitation, disfigurement is the norm for individuals with massive burns. The years of special treatment impose major disruptions to the family and interfere with the child's normal development and social integration. Yet many can serve as models of resilience; they survive and they succeed in spite of dramatic mitigating circumstances (77). Today, improvement in burn survival has greatly surpassed our ability to improve the aftermath of burn injuries aesthetically and psychosocially. As more children survive, research focuses on more holistic aspects of outcome and ultimately on improving quality of life.

Surgery General Information Questionnaire | Ages 6–12

Parent/guardian: Please complete the following questions so that we might better understand your child's needs.

1. How worried is your *child* about having reconstructive surgery?

	Not at All	A Little	Moderately	A Lot	Extremely
Missing school	⓪	①	②	③	④
Possible postoperative pain	⓪	①	②	③	④
General anxiety/fear	⓪	①	②	③	④
POSSIBLE DISAPPOINTMENT WITH OUTCOME	⓪	①	②	③	④

2. How concerned are *you* about surgery for your child?

	Not at All	A Little	Moderately	A Lot	Extremely
Cost of surgery	⓪	①	②	③	④
POSSIBLE POSTOPERATIVE PAIN	⓪	①	②	③	④
Possible disappointment with outcome	⓪	①	②	③	④
Lost time from school	⓪	①	②	③	④
My (parent's) time from work	⓪	①	②	③	④

3. In what ways do *you* believe that aspects of your child's burned skin affect him or her?

	Not at All	A Little	Moderately	A Lot	Extremely
Lack of symmetry (balance on both sides)	⓪	①	②	③	④
Discoloration of burned areas	⓪	①	②	③	④
Teasing from peers	⓪	①	②	③	④
Pain	⓪	①	②	③	④
Limitation in social activities/involvement	⓪	①	②	③	④
Dependence upon others physically	⓪	①	②	③	④
Unhappiness with life in general	⓪	①	②	③	④
Negative self-esteem	⓪	①	②	③	④
Poor sports participation and skill	⓪	①	②	③	④
Self-consciousness	⓪	①	②	③	④

(continued)

4. In what ways do *you* anticipate surgery to affect your child in the following areas?

	No Change	A Little Better	Moderately Better	A Lot Better	Totally Better
Improved symmetry (balance on both sides)	⓪	①	②	③	④
Decreased teasing by peers	⓪	①	②	③	④
Decrease pain/discomfort	⓪	①	②	③	④
Improved social activities/involvement	⓪	①	②	③	④
Decreased dependence on others physically	⓪	①	②	③	④
Satisfaction with life in general	⓪	①	②	③	④
Improved self-esteem	⓪	①	②	③	④
Increased/better sports participation/skill	⓪	①	②	③	④
Increased social involvement	⓪	①	②	③	④
Self-consciousness	⓪	①	②	③	④

5. To what degree do burned area(s) of your child's body concern *you and/or your child*?

Not at all _____   A little _____   Moderately _____   A lot _____   Extremely _____

6. Was anyone else injured when the child was burned?

No _____   Yes, who? _____

Surgery General Information Questionnaire Ages 13–18

Please complete the following questions so that we might better understand your needs.

1. How worried are *you* about having reconstructive surgery?

	Not at All	A Little	Moderately	A Lot	Extremely
Missing school	⓪	①	②	③	④
Possible postoperative pain	⓪	①	②	③	④
General anxiety/fear	⓪	①	②	③	④
POSSIBLE DISAPPOINTMENT WITH OUTCOME	⓪	①	②	③	④
Cost of surgery	⓪	①	②	③	④

2. In what ways do you believe that aspects of your burned skin affect *you*?

	Not at All	A Little	Moderately	A Lot	Extremely
Lack of symmetry (balance on both sides)	⓪	①	②	③	④
Discoloration of burned areas	⓪	①	②	③	④
Isolation/rejection by peers	⓪	①	②	③	④
Pain	⓪	①	②	③	④
Limitation in social activities/involvement	⓪	①	②	③	④
Dependence upon others physically	⓪	①	②	③	④
Unhappiness with life in general	⓪	①	②	③	④
Negative self-esteem	⓪	①	②	③	④
Poor sports participation and skill	⓪	①	②	③	④
Self-consciousness	⓪	①	②	③	④
Negatively affect dating/intimacy	⓪	①	②	③	④

3. In what ways do you anticipate surgery to affect *you* in the following areas?

	No Change	A Little Better	Moderately Better	A Lot Better	Totally Better
Improved symmetry (balance on both sides)	⓪	①	②	③	④
Isolation/rejection by peers	⓪	①	②	③	④
Decrease pain/discomfort	⓪	①	②	③	④
Improved social activities/involvement	⓪	①	②	③	④
Decreased physical dependence on others	⓪	①	②	③	④
Satisfaction with life in general	⓪	①	②	③	④
Improved self-esteem	⓪	①	②	③	④
Increased/better sports participation/skill	⓪	①	②	③	④
Increased social involvement	⓪	①	②	③	④
Self-consciousness	⓪	①	②	③	④
Improved dating/intimacy	⓪	①	②	③	④

(continued)

4. **To what degree do burned area(s) of your body concern *you*?**
   Not at all ____   **A little** ____   **Moderately** _____   **A lot** ____   **Extremely** _____

5. **Was any one else injured when you were burned?**
   No ___   **Yes, who?** _____

6. **Do you have other goals for this surgery not mentioned above?**
   No ___   **Yes** ___   **If yes, please explain**

   _____
   _____
   _____
   _____
   _____
   _____

REFERENCES

1. Knudson-Cooper MS. Adjustment to visible stigma: the case of the severely burned. *Soc Sci Med* 1981;15B(1):31–44.
2. Hill-Beuf A, Porter JD. Children coping with impaired appearance: social and psychologic influences. *Gen Hosp Psychiatry* 1984;6(4):294–301.
3. Wolf SE, Rose JK, Desai MH, et al. Mortality determinants in massive pediatric burns—an analysis of 103 children with >=80% TBSA burns (>=70% full-thickness). *Ann Surg* 1997;225(5):554–565.
4. Sheridan RL, Remensnyder JP, Schnitzer JJ, et al. Current expectations for survival in pediatric burns. *Arch Pediatr Adolesc Med* 2000;154(3):245–249.
5. Rashid A, Khanna A, Gowar JP, et al. Revised estimates of mortality from burns in the last 20 years at the Birmingham Burns Centre. *Burns* 2001;27(7):723–730.
6. Blakeney P, Portman S, Rutan R. Familial values as factors influencing long-term psychological adjustment of children after severe burn injury. *J Burn Care Rehabil* 1990;11(5):472–475.
7. Moore P, Moore M, Blakeney P, et al. Competence and physical impairment of pediatric survivors of burns of more than 80% total body surface area. *J Burn Care Rehabil* 1996;17(6Pt1):547–551.
8. Meyers P, Blakeney P, Robert R, et al. Physical and psychological rehabilitation outcomes for pediatric patients who suffer 80% or more TBSA, 70% or more third degree burns. *J Burn Care Rehabil* 2000; 21(1Pt1):43–49.
9. LeDoux J, Meyer WJ III, Blakeney PE, et al. Relationship between parental emotional states, family environment and the behavioural adjustment of pediatric burn survivors. *Burns* 1998;24(5):425–432.
10. Holaday M, Blakeney P. A comparison of psychologic functioning in children and adolescents with severe burns on the Rorschach and the Child Behavior Checklist. *J Burn Care Rehabil* 1994;15(5):412–415.
11. Holaday M, Terrell D. Resiliency characteristics and Rorschach variables in children and adolescents with severe burns. *J Burn Care Rehabil* 1994;15(5):455–460.
12. Meyer WJ, Blakeney PE, Holzer CE, et al. Inconsistencies in psychosocial assessment of children after severe burns. *J Burn Care Rehabil* 1995;16(5):559–568.
13. Lawrence JW, Fauerbach JA, Heinberg LJ, et al. Visible versus hidden scars and their relation to body esteem. *J Burn Care Rehabil* 2004;25(1):25–32.
14. Love B, Byrne C, Roberts J, et al. Adult psychosocial adjustment following childhood injury: the effect of disfigurement. *J Burn Care Rehabil* 1987;8(4):280–285.
15. Abdullah A, Blakeney P, Hunt R, et al. Visible scars and self-esteem in pediatric patients with burns. *J Burn Care Rehabil* 1994;15(2):164–168.
16. Blakeney P, Herndon DN, Desai MH, et al. Long-term psychosocial adjustment following burn injury. *J Burn Care Rehabil* 1988;9(6):661–665.
17. Blakeney P, Portman S, Rutan R. Familial values as factors influencing long-term psychological adjustment of children after severe burn injury. *J Burn Care Rehabil* 1990;11(5):472–475.
18. Weimer CL, Goldfarb IW, Slater H. Multidisciplinary approach to working with burn victims of child abuse. *J Burn Care Rehabil* 1988;9(1):79–82.
19. Meyer WJ, Blakeney P, Russell W, et al. Psychological problems reported by young adults who were burned as children. *J Burn Care Rehabil* 2004;25(1):98–106.
20. Ramsey JL, Langlois JH. Effects of the "beauty is good" stereotype on children's information processing. *J Exper Child Psychol* 2002;81(3):320–340.
21. Leonard BJ, Brust JD, Abrahams G, et al. Self-concept of children and adolescents with cleft lip and/or palate. *Cleft Palate Craniofac J* 1991;28(4):347–353.
22. Van Loey NE, Van Son MJ. Psychopathology and psychological problems in patients with burn scars: epidemiology and management. *Am J Clin Dermatol* 2003;4(4):245–272.
23. Robert R, Berniger F, Thomas C, et al. *Suicide Probability in Young Adult Survivors of Pediatric Burn Injury*. Seattle, WA: International Society of Burn Injuries, 2002.
24. Saigh PA, Green BL, Korol M. The history and prevalence of posttraumatic stress disorder with special reference to children and adolescents. *J Sch Psychol* 1996;34(2):107–131.
25. Meyer W III, Thomas C, Holzer C, et al. Incidence of major psychiatric illness in young adults who were burned as children. Proceedings of the American Burn Association 35th annual meeting, Miami: 2003.
26. Fauerbach JA, Heinberg LJ, Lawrence JW, et al. Effect of early body image dissatisfaction on subsequent psychological and physical adjustment after disfiguring injury. *Psychosom Med* 2000;62(4):576–582.
27. Fauerbach JA, Heinberg LJ, Lawrence JW, et al. Coping with body image changes following a disfiguring burn injury. *Health Psychol* 2002;21(2):115–121.
28. Cash T, Pruzinsky T, eds. *Body Images: Development, Deviance and Change.* New York: Guilford Press, 1990.
29. Stoddard FJ. Body image development in the burned child. *J Am Acad Child Adolesc Psychiatry* 1982; 21(5):502–507.
30. Jessee PO, Strickland MP, Leeper JD, et al. Perception of body image in children with burns, five years after burn injury. *J Burn Care Rehabil* 1992;13:33–38.
31. Lawrence JW, Heinberg LJ, Roca R, et al. Development and validation of the Satisfaction With Appearance Scale: assessing body image among burn-injured patients. *Psychol Assess* 1998;10(1):64–70.
32. Goffman E. *Stigma.* Englewood Cliffs, NJ: Prentice-Hall, 1963.
33. Pruzinsky T, Doctor ME. Body images and pediatric burn injury. In: Tarnowski K, ed. *Behavioral Aspects of Pediatric Burns.* New York: Plenum Publishing, 1994:169–191.
34. Bull RHC, Rumseg N. *The Social Psychology of Facial Appearance.* New York: Springer-Verlag, 1988.
35. La Greca AM, Dandes SK, Wick P, et al. The Social Anxiety Scale for Children-Revised: factor structure and concurrent validity. *J Clin Child Psychol* 1993;22:17–27.
36. Vernberg EM, Abwender DA, Ewell KK, et al. Social anxiety and peer relationships in early adolescence—a prospective analysis. *J Clin Child Psychol* 1992;21(2):189–196.
37. Ginsburg GS, La Greca AM, Silverman WK. Social anxiety in children with anxiety disorders: relation with social and emotional functioning. *J Abnorm Child Psychol* 1998;26(3):175–185.

38. Blank K, Perry S. Relationship of psychological processes during delirium to outcome. *Am J Psychiatry* 1984;141(7):843–847.
39. Morris J, Mcfadd A. mental-health team on a burn unit—multidisciplinary approach. *J Trauma* 1978;18(9):658–664.
40. Blakeney P, Meyer WJ. Psychological aspects of burn care. *Trauma Quarterly* 1994;11(2):166–179.
41. VanderPlate C. An adaptive coping model of intervention with the severely burn-injured. *Intl J Psychiatr Med* 1984;14(4):331–341.
42. Blakeney P, Fauerbach J, Meyer W III, Thomas C. Psychosocial recovery and reintegration of patients with burn injuries. In: Herndon DN, ed. *Total Burn Care.* London, England: WB Saunders, 2002:783–797.
43. Blakeney P, Robert R, Meyer WJ. Psychological and social recovery of children disfigured by physical trauma: elements of treatment supported by empirical data. *Int Rev Psychiatry* 1998; 10:196–200.
44. Watkins PN, Cook EL, May SR, et al. Psychological stages in adaptation following burn injury: a method for facilitating psychological recovery of burn victims. *J Burn Care Rehabil* 1988;9(4):376–384.
45. Knudson-Cooper MS. Emotional care of the hospitalized burned child. *J Burn Care Rehabil* 1982;3:109–116.
46. Tarnowski KJ, Rasnake LK, Linscheid TR, et al. Ecobehavioral characteristics of a pediatric burn injury unit. *J App Beh Anal* 1989;22(1):101–109.
47. Pruitt BA, Goodwin CW, Mason AD. Epidemiological, demographic, and outcome characteristics of burn injury. In: Herndon DN, ed. *Total Burn Care.* London, England: WB Saunders, 2002:16–30.
48. Kendall-Grove KJ, Ehde DM, Patterson DR, et al. Rates of dysfunction in parents of pediatric patients with burns. *J Burn Care Rehabil* 1998;19(4):312–316.
49. Robert R, Blakeney P, Herndon D. Abuse, neglect, and fire setting: when burn injury involves reporting to a safety officer. In: Herndon DH, ed. *Total Burn Care.* London, England: WB Saunders, 2002:774–782.
50. Hammond J, Perez-Stable A, Ward CG. Predictive value of historical and physical characteristics for the diagnosis of child abuse. *South Med J* 1991;84(2):166–168.
51. Fauerbach JA, Lawrence J, Haythornthwaite J, et al. Preinjury psychiatric illness and postinjury adjustment in adult burn survivors. *Psychosomatics* 1996;37(6):547–555.
52. Fauerbach JA, Lawrence J, Haythornthwaite J, et al. Preburn psychiatric history affects posttrauma morbidity. *Psychosomatics* 1997;38(4):374–385.
53. Tarnowski KJ, Rasnake LK, Gavaghanjones MP, et al. Psychosocial sequelae of pediatric burn injuries—a review. *Clin Psychol Rev* 1991;11(4):371–398.
54. Mangus RS, Bergman D, Zieger M, et al. Burn injuries in children with attention-deficit/hyperactivity disorder. *Burns* 2004;30(2):148–150.
55. Thomas C, Ayoub M, Rosenberg L, et al. Attention deficit hyperactivity disorder and pediatric burn injury: a preliminary retrospective study. *Burns* 2004;30(3):221–223.
56. Stoddard FJ, Pahlavan K, Cahners SS. Suicide attempted by self-immolation during adolescence. I. Literature review, case reports, and personality precursors. *Adolesc Psychiatry* 1985;12:251–265.
57. Sheridan RL. Burns with inhalation injury and petrol aspiration in adolescents seeking euphoria through hydrocarbon inhalation. *Burns* 1996;22(7):566–567.
58. Cole M, Herndon HN, Desai MH, et al. Gasoline explosions, gasoline sniffing: an epidemic in young adolescents. *J Burn Care Rehabil* 1986;7(6):532–534.
59. Kligman AM. Medical aspects of the skin and its appearance. In: Graham JA, Kligman AM, eds. *The Psychology of Cosmetic Treatments.* New York: Praeger, 1985:3–25.
60. Partridge J. *Changing Faces.* 2nd ed. London, England: Changing Faces, 1994.
61. Riva G, Molinari E. Body-image and social attitude in growth-hormone-deficient adults. *Percept Mot Skills* 1995;80(3):1083–1088.
62. Erling A, Wiklund I, Albertssonwikland K. Prepubertal children with short stature have a different perception of their well-being and stature than their parents. *Qual Life Res* 1994;3(6):425–429.
63. Bernstein NR. Objective bodily damage: disfigurement and disability. In: Cash TF, Pruzinsky T, eds. *Body Images: Development, Deviance and Change.* New York: Guilford Press, 1990:131–148.
64. LeDoux JM, Meyer WJ, Blakeney P, et al. Positive self-regard as a coping mechanism for pediatric burn survivors. *J Burn Care Rehabil* 1996;17(5):472–476.
65. Robert R, Bishop B, Rosenberg L, et al. The impact of time and facial disfigurement on children's self-perception post-burn injury. *Current Concepts in Pediatric Burn Care* 1999:101–106.
66. Robson MC. Overview of burn reconstruction. In: Herndon DH, ed. *Total Burn Care.* London, England: WB Saunders, 2002: 620–627.
67. Bjarnason D, Phillips LG, McCoy B, et al. Reconstructive goals for children with burns: are our goals the same? *J Burn Care Rehabil* 1992;13(3):389–390.
68. Serghiou MA. 2004. Personal communication.
69. Doctor M, Meyer W III, McShan S, et al. Burn camp: Impact of psychosocial adjustment. Proceedings of the American Burn Association 29th annual meeting, New York: 1997.
70. Gaskell SL. The impact of a burn camp on children's psychological well-being: a quantitative evaluation. Lyon, France: European Burns Association 79; 2001.
71. Blakeney P, Thomas C, Holzer C, et al. Efficacy of a short-term social skills training program for burned adolescents. *J Burn Care Rehabil* 2002;23:S99.
72. Robinson E, Rumsey N, Partridge J. An evaluation of the impact of social interaction skills training for facially disfigured people. *Br J Plast Surg* 1996;49(5):281–289.
73. Clarke A, Cooper C, Partridge J, et al. *Reach Out! Developing the Tools for Successful Social Interaction After Burns: A 2, 3 or 4 Day Program.* London, England: Changing Faces, 1997.
74. Bruhn JG. The doctor's touch: tactile communication in the doctor-patient relationship. *South Med J* 1978;71(12):1469–1473.
75. Andronicus M, Oates RK, Peat J, et al. Non-accidental burns in children. *Burns* 1998;24(6):552–558.
76. Booth T. *Falling from Fire.* New York: Wendy Lamb Books, 2002.
77. Luthar SS, Zigler E. Vulnerability and competence: a review of research on resilience in childhood. *Am J Orthopsychiatry* 1991;61(1):6–22.

Chapter 7

Adult Burn Injury

James A. Fauerbach, PhD, Robert J. Spence, MD, and David R. Patterson, PhD

Understanding the person who presents for reconstructive surgery after a major burn is often contingent on understanding the nature and course of their lives before, during, and after the injury. Major burn injury has been defined by the American Burn Association (1) as meeting one of the following criteria:

■ Deep second and third degree burns greater than 10% Total Body Surface Area (TBSA) in patients under 10 or over 50 years old,
■ Deep second and third degree burns greater than 20% TBSA in other age groups,
■ Deep second and third degree burns with serious threat of functional or cosmetic threat that involve face, hands, feet, genitalia, perineum, and major joints,
■ Third degree burns greater than 5% TBSA in any age group,
■ Deep electrical burns including lightning injury; inhalation injury with burn injury, or
■ Circumferential burns of an extremity or chest.

Individuals who sustain these burns experience substantial biological, psychological, and social stressors (2–4). Burns may result in traumatic stress, pain, shock, sepsis, and altered functioning of the hypothalamic–pituitary–adreno-cortical system or the immune system. These can eventuate from the burn event and injury, as well as subsequent treatment components such as medication regimens, daily aversive dressing changes, physiotherapy, and surgical debridement or wound closure.

A major burn injury can substantially impair skin integrity and sensation and may lead to hypertrophic scarring. In addition to changes in appearance and function brought about by scarring, deeper burns may result in damage to, or complete loss of, functionally or cosmetically important body parts. Furthermore, many forms of psychological disturbance have been noted beyond generic distress, including body image dissatisfaction, depression, and posttraumatic distress. The physical and psychological consequences of major burn injury can interfere significantly with social and occupational role performance, which may be either minimized or exacerbated by environmental barriers or social support. The psychological well-being of patients seen in the burn reconstruction clinic becomes an important consideration not only because of the recent disfigurement, functional losses, and trauma, but also because even total compliance with preventive measures (e.g., to treat hypertrophic scarring via pressure garments) yield a demoralizing result.

The goals of this chapter are to review the growing scientific literature on the psychological, social, and physical health functioning of adult burn survivors,

Preparation of this chapter was supported by funds from the National Institute on Disability and Rehabilitation Research in the Office of Special Education and Rehabilitative Services in the U.S. Department of Education (Grant #H133A020101).

including examining the role of personality variables, the size of a burn injury, stigmatization, and body image. Particular attention is given to recent research on patient experience of posttraumatic stress disorder (PTSD). The final section of the chapter reviews specific methods by which members of the plastic surgery treatment team can help burn survivors learn to cope with the effects of their injuries and to identify those patients who are in particular need of more intensive forms of psychological intervention. In many cases, because of the scarcity of work done specifically with patients presenting for burn reconstruction, it is necessary to extrapolate from the acute injury literature.

SOCIAL, PSYCHOLOGICAL, AND PHYSCIAL ADJUSTMENT FOLLOWING MAJOR BURN INJURY: A REVIEW OF THE EMPIRICAL LITERATURE

Quality of Life and Burn Injury

Quality of life is composed of many facets including disease symptoms, functional capacity, impairment, role performance, perceived well-being, and satisfaction (5). A significant measure of the degree of recovery from major burn injury is health-related quality of life (HRQL) (6). HRQL has been defined as a multifactorial construct that involves an individual's degree of satisfaction and level of functioning in several core domains, including physical–behavioral function, psychological well-being, social and work role performance, and personal perception of health (7).

A recent literature review presents a profile of the patient at risk for lower quality of life following a major burn injury (8). The profile includes pre-injury factors (e.g., premorbid psychiatric disorder, personality structure), peritraumatic factors (e.g., TBSA, pain, and coping behavior) and postburn factors (e.g., social support). Re-establishing pre-injury quality of life seems problematic for some survivors, especially for those with history of preburn psychiatric disorder (9) as well as those who develop symptoms of depression (10), body image dissatisfaction (11), or posttraumatic distress (12) following the injury. Each of these is addressed in detail below.

Pre-injury Personality Variables and Postburn Adjustment

Individuals who sustain a burn are more likely to have pre-existing psychosocial needs that are important determinants of postburn psychosocial adjustment. The process of psychological coping involves any thought or behavior that a person uses with the intention of reducing negative affect. Poorer postburn adjustment appears to be a function of a combined approach and avoidant personality coping style (10,13–14) and exhibit personality traits such as high neuroticism and low extraversion (15–16). Patients who use approach-avoidant coping will typically alternate between ruminative thinking about the stressor (e.g., disfiguring scar) and blocking out awareness of the stressor or denying its impact. Additionally, a patient who is high in the personality trait "neuroticism" will experience more frequent, prolonged, and intense episodes of negative affect (e.g., anxiety, depression, irritability). A patient with low trait "extraversion" will experience less energy and positive affect, as well as increased social withdrawal.

The patients' pre-injury quality of life also has been shown to influence postburn status. For example, one study has shown that the pre-injury psychosocial adjustment of burn patients, relative to published norms, was typified by greater psychological distress, anxiety, depression, and loss of behavioral and emotional control (17). Marital status, mental health treatment, and length of intensive care stay predicted satisfaction with life at discharge and at 6-month follow-up, and satisfaction at both assessments was significantly lower than norms (4). Thus, patient coping style, personality variables (neuroticism-extraversion), and pre-injury psychological adjustment all can affect how a person adapts to a burn injury.

Extent of Burn Injury and Psychological Outcome

Despite repeated evidence to the contrary, many anecdotal and intuitive suggestions have been made over the years that psychosocial adjustment to burn scar disfigurement is related to the size and visibility of the scars. For example, the psychosocial adjustment of adults was related to current unemployment, reduced job status, avoidance coping, and restricted recreational activity; however, the severity of the burn and time since the burn were not related to psychosocial adjustment (18).

Some studies are beginning to use burn-specific measures of quality of life, such as the Burn-Specific Health Scale (19). For example, Finnish investigators, observed reduced self-reported general health among older survivors, those with larger TBSA or larger full thickness burns (TBSA-FT), and those with longer length of hospitalization. Interestingly, larger burns and hand burns were associated with greater physical impairment, and both body image and sexual functioning were associated with TBSA-FT but not the presence of hand or facial injuries (20).

Recently, investigations with adults and children have documented a fairly optimistic outlook for long-term quality of life outcome following major burn injuries. A study of survivors of massive burns in childhood, approximately 15 years after injury, found that adjustment was generally similar to published normative data (21). However, roughly 20% of the burn survivors reported substantially impaired physical functioning and had significant role interference from these impairments. Better functional status of the family predicted less role performance limitations due to physical problems, and early reintegration with preburn activities predicted better physical functioning and fewer role limitations from physical problems. A study of adult burn survivors evaluated roughly 5 years postburn, relative to a matched unburned control group, found similar level of quality of life (22). However, 25% of burn patients report clinically significant psychological disturbances compared to 12% of controls. Importantly, burn survivors with abnormal sensations in their healed wounds, relative to burn patients with normal sensation, report more somatizing and obsessive-compulsive behaviors.

Another study of burn survivors roughly 5 years after trauma found that functional impairment, regardless of its extent, was related to severe depression (23). This is of particular concern, given the chronicity of depressive symptoms among burn survivors. For example, 43% of burn survivors reported moderate to severe symptoms of depression 2 years postburn (24). Furthermore, even mild symptoms of depression are associated with an increased likelihood of becoming disabled and a decreased chance of recovery (25). Thus, even under the best of circumstances, roughly 20% to 25% of those who survive major burn injury can be expected to evidence significant physical (21) or psychological (23) impairment even years after the injury.

We recently reported a prospective, longitudinal study examining the influence of baseline physical and psychological burden on HRQL among adults with major burns from three regional burn centers (26). Physical Burden groups were defined by TBSA <10%, 10% to 30%, or >30%. Psychological Burden groups were defined by in-hospital distress on the Brief Symptom Inventory Global Severity Index (27–28). The SF-36 Health Survey (7) was used to assess HRQL during the preburn month, at the time of discharge from acute hospitalization, and at 6 and 12 months postburn. Greater in-hospital psychological distress (i.e., high Psychological Burden) was associated with greater impairment and role disruption in both physical and psychosocial domains at least as far as 6 and 12 months after injury, as well as a slower rate of recovery in both physical and psychosocial health and function. To the contrary, larger burn size (i.e., high Physical Burden) was only associated with more physical impairment and role disruption and a slower rate of physical recovery at 6 and 12 months postburn.

The differential effect of high and low distress (i.e., Psychological Burden) on quality of life was clearly demonstrated. At discharge, and at one-year postburn, the high distress group, relative to the low distress group, demonstrated significantly worse health and function in both physical and psychosocial domains. Furthermore, both Psychological Burden levels, relative to published U.S. population norms, experienced dramatic and statistically significant deficits in all areas of function at discharge. Importantly, at one year postinjury, the high distress group was still functioning at significantly lower physical and psychosocial levels relative to norms. Interestingly, the low distress individuals, although not differing from normative data in mental health or physical functioning domains, remained impaired in their ability to perform work and social roles requiring physical health and emotional stability. This underscores the need to evaluate psychological function at the time of the clinic visit as well as prompting early intervention when indicated.

Findings indicate that the larger the Physical Burden of injury, the longer the recovery of physical functioning. However, Physical Burden was not differentially related to the degree of loss or recovery of psychosocial function. Furthermore, relative to norms for the population of community dwelling adults (7), each of the Physical Burden groups evidenced significant deficits at baseline in all physical and psychosocial domains of function. Interestingly, by one year postburn, only the physical composite score and the Physical Functioning subscale scores differed significantly across the three Physical Burden groups. Thus, the size of the burn does not appear to be the most important determinant of health and function. Individual differences appear to play a more central role.

This point, regarding the lack of a clear relationship between the extent of an injury and the nature of psychosocial adjustment, cannot be emphasized strongly enough. It is a theme that recurs in the scientific and clinical literature reviewed in multiple chapters throughout this volume.

Social Perception, Stigmatization, and Body Image

The study of the social perception and body image of burn survivors, while still in its infancy (29–30) is central to understanding the lives of adult burn survivors. In fact, it is a common thread that links together each of the chapters in this section of this volume.

Social Perception and Stigmatization

Stigmatization is a social process that characterizes individuals as deviant and subjects them to a variety of dehumanizing behaviors that may be overt (i.e., staring, startled reaction, double takes, whispering, teasing, bullying) or subtle (i.e., avoiding eye contact, ignoring, walking faster when approaching, ambivalence about engaging in an interaction, pity) (30–32). Teasing and negative verbal commentary are stigmatizing acts that have been shown to negatively affect body image and self-esteem for prolonged periods (33). Bull and Rumsey (34) hypothesized that when individuals with physical distinctions experience stigmatizing behavior, they may develop poor body esteem, a sense of social isolation, and a violation of their privacy. The frequency and severity of such discrimination among burn survivors is unknown (29–30). However, a number of studies have found that positive social support is associated with better adjustment for burn survivors (35–36). The consistency of these findings support the urgency of putting in place programs of psychosocial assessment and interventions geared towards assisting survivors accept scars, reduce depression, cope with social stigmatization, and build a strong support system.

Body Image

We recently examined the relationship among burn scar severity and visibility, and body esteem (37). Scar visibility was significantly related to reduced satisfaction with one's appearance, increased perception of others' negative reactions to one's appearance, and perceived stigmatization. Social adjustment and depression accounted for substantial variance in body esteem. In contrast, scar severity and visibility accounted for very little variance in body esteem, or social and emotional adjustment. Finally, outpatients with visible distinctions reported experiencing significant anxiety, depression, social anxiety, social avoidance, and poor quality of life. Severity of disfigurement was not strongly related to distress or adjustment (38).

The impact of in-hospital body image dissatisfaction on subsequent quality of life after severe burn injury has only recently been studied (11,39). Most prior studies lacked a measure of body image satisfaction, and many did not control for other determinants of outcome including injury location, other forms of psychological distress, and preburn quality of life. Quality of life measured 2 months after discharge of groups with, and without, body image dissatisfaction during hospitalization was studied, controlling for the effect of preburn quality of life. Among those with greater in-hospital body image dissatisfaction, significantly lower psychosocial and physical quality of life was reported at 2 month follow-up. Further analyses indicated that symptoms of depression and posttraumatic distress moderated the impact of body image dissatisfaction on physical but not psychosocial health. Finally, postburn physical adjustment was poorer among all burn survivors relative to published norms, while psychosocial adjustment was poorer only for those with body image dissatisfaction. Although body image is a clinically recognized determinant of adjustment in other populations, these findings empirically demonstrated the significant negative impact of poor body image on quality of life in a representative sample of burn survivors. Typically, and perhaps not surprisingly, the body image of patients presenting for burn reconstruction is substantially worse than that observed at earlier stages of recovery.

The impact of body image dissatisfaction on psychosocial quality of life suggests the importance of early identification of populations at risk. A number of cognitive-behavioral treatments have been developed with demonstrated efficacy in treating (40) or preventing (41–42) body image dissatisfaction. Unfortunately, no controlled studies have been completed involving individuals with burn injuries. Nevertheless, these treatment models potentially hold great promise in the treatment of body image concerns of burn survivors.

Summary

Amid the complexity of empirical findings regarding the psychosocial adjustment of burn survivors a few critical themes emerge. One is that pre-existing personality variables (e.g., coping style) can significantly affect long-term outcome. A second theme is that there is no necessary correlation between the extent of the injury and the long-term psychological affects of the injury; individual psychological differences appear to play a more influential role. And finally, a great deal of empirical and clinical attention needs to be given to the social and body image experiences of burn survivors.

POSTTRAUMATIC DISTRESS

When evaluating any burn survivor, health care providers must be sensitive to the patients' possible experience with Post Traumatic Stress Disorder (PTSD). PTSD is characterized by three symptom clusters: (i) re-experiencing—intrusive, distressing thoughts, dreams, or images of the traumatic event; (ii) avoidance—avoidance of trauma-related thoughts, feelings, and situations; and (iii) hyperarousal—persistent sleep disturbance, easy startle, increased tension and irritability (43). Between 25%

and 38% of burn survivors meet criteria for PTSD in the first postburn year, and almost 50% of survivors meet criteria for at least one of the symptom clusters. PTSD among burn survivors has not been found to be related to the severity of the injury (46–48). On the other hand, posttrauma distress is positively related to more intense pain among hospitalized burn patients (49–50).

We have studied the impact of mild to moderate symptoms of in-hospital posttrauma distress following severe burn injury on quality of life at 2 month follow-up (12). After adjusting for preburn psychosocial adjustment, greater in-hospital posttraumatic distress was associated with poorer psychosocial functioning at follow-up. This effect remained after covarying preburn physical domain quality of life. However, the most robust finding was that posttraumatic distress influences psychosocial but not physical adjustment over and above the influence of personality characteristics such as neuroticism.

As Patterson et al. have noted, symptoms of distress "tend to dissipate by the time of hospital discharge" for the greatest number of burn patients (29, p. 374). Similarly to the posttraumatic distress findings just described, baseline trait negative affectivity was inversely correlated and baseline trait positive affectivity was associated with better psychological and psychosomatic functioning 12 months after discharge from an acute hospitalization for burn injury (9). The results of these two studies suggest that personality traits may be important latent variables contributing to symptom report (e.g., posttraumatic distress) and level of postburn adjustment.

The Relationship of Personality Structure and Coping Style with Psychological Distress

In this vein, we recently examined how personality traits relate to the emergence of PTSD in persons with recent, major burns. Overall, relative to published norms, the sample of burn survivors scored significantly higher on neuroticism and extraversion and lower on openness, agreeableness, and conscientiousness (15). The low conscientiousness suggests that it is prudent to incorporate compliance enhancement procedures when the reconstruction patient is responsible for complex rehabilitation or wound care. Individuals who are high in neuroticism are predisposed to frequent bouts of strong negative affect (e.g., anxiety, depression) of greater intensity and duration, and those with low extraversion typically have very little counterbalancing energy or interest in people (51). These personality traits are also associated with ineffective coping styles (e.g., avoidance). We have found it helpful to provide these people with a specific contact person in our office who is available for presurgery and follow-up phone calls for support and information.

A recent meta-analytic review assessed the relations between causal attributions, coping, and psychological adjustment in medical patients (52). Overall, individuals who achieve better psychosocial adjustment do so by thinking more flexibly about ways to improve their situation and blaming themselves less. In addition, individuals who experience poor psychosocial outcome are more likely to feel they have no control over their coping behavior or their situation. These results suggest the central importance of coping thoughts and behaviors within the context of illness.

We have examined the influence of emotion-focused coping on symptoms of PTSD, body image dissatisfaction, and depression. Coping by emotion-approach and emotion-avoidance was assessed during acute hospitalization for burn injury and the symptoms were assessed in-hospital, and at 1 week and 2 months following discharge. The group of individuals who employed a combination of both emotion-approach and emotion-avoidance (i.e., ambivalent coping), compared with those who used only one of these coping methods, reported significantly greater body image dissatisfaction and negative social impact of disfigurement at the 2 month follow-up (13) and higher levels of posttraumatic stress disorder symptoms even when controlling for baseline symptoms (14). Symptoms of depression also persisted at higher levels even when controlling baseline depression (10).

Thus, when a person copes by combining emotion-avoidance and emotion-approach, they are at tremendous risk of greater psychological distress and poor psychosocial quality of life. We have proposed that the desire to enhance control motivates one to cope by using emotion-avoidance (10). For example, by avoiding stressful situations (looking at scars in mirror; going to novel social situations) one attempts to control the emotional distress related to body image dissatisfaction. Conversely, we have suggested that the desire to increase predictability motivates one to cope by using emotion-approach. For example, by ruminating over adverse social interactions one tries to make unpleasant interactions more predictable. Similar to classic descriptions of approach-avoidance conflict, we suggest that ambivalence between the motive to enhance controllability and the motive to increase predictability of distressing thoughts, images, and feelings leads to worsened distress.

Limitations of Current Empirical Research and Suggestions for Future Research Progress

Many of the studies reported in this review of the empirical literature have not as yet been replicated during periods following scar maturation. Nor have they been replicated in patients presenting to reconstruction clinics. It remains to be seen whether the effects documented thus far persist, resolve, or are exacerbated over longer periods of time. As physical changes stabilize and permanent disfigurements are more evident, body image dissatisfaction may emerge among those who had initially been relatively well adjusted in the acute period given that appearance and functional outcomes were more ambiguous. Additionally, many of the studies cited employed designs that are correlational, and, therefore, causal inferences are not warranted. The burn reconstruction clinic is a prime setting for "natural experiments" using pretest and posttest designs. Careful attention to design and measurement of studies with this population may usefully elucidate cognitive and behavioral processes that augment or interfere with body image, emotional adjustment, social integration and role performance, and overall quality of life.

Thus far, key limitations exist in most of the studies, such as excessive reliance on cross-sectional or retrospective designs, self-report measures, and simplistic data analytic strategies. On the other hand, recent studies indicate an increased use of prospective, longitudinal designs assessing pre-injury status on dependent measures and employing sophistic analytic strategies such as latent growth curve models.

HELPING BURN SURVIVORS COPE WITH DISTRESS

Clearly, severe burn is one of the most disruptive and disturbing events for a person to experience. In the next two sections we provide practical guidelines for facilitating adaptive coping and for identifying those patients in greatest need of help while undergoing reconstruction and rehabilitation.

Assisting patients in coping is not solely the domain of a mental health professional; arguably surgeons and burn therapists have a greater role in managing distress than social workers or psychologists. Virtually any patient hospitalized for burn care will show distress, and there are many choices that the burn team can make that will have a great effect on distress levels. For example, the empirical and clinical literature is clear about the observation that the amount of pain reported by patients has a greater impact on their long-term psychological well being than does the size of the burn injury or length of hospitalization (53). Therefore, at all stages of patient care, it is essential to closely monitor and effectively treat the patient's pain symptoms.

When intervening to help reduce patient distress, it is essential to tailor approaches to stress reduction according to where the patient is in their burn care. Burn reconstructive surgery usually occurs on an outpatient basis, but it also can take place during early care and hospitalization. In general, burn care can be thought of as three stages: intensive, acute, and outpatient (rehabilitation) care. We note, however, that the distinction between these stages can be quite arbitrary. For example, physical and occupational rehabilitation usually begins during intensive care.

Intensive Care

During the intensive care phase, patients are often critically ill, intubated, and fighting for survival. At this stage, patients are likely sedated and minimally responsive, and their coping resources may be exhausted, leading to high levels of anxiety. When patients are in intensive care or are critically ill, it is important that interventions focus on the patient's basic needs. Such patients are focused on survival or controlling their pain during their next surgery or dressing change. Consequently, coping interventions might include family visits, physical touch and reassurance, and encouraging the patient to accept and let go of things that cannot be controlled. Issues such as long-term adjustment, grieving losses, and adapting to disfigurement are not typically of greatest concern to patients at this time.

Acute Care

During this stage patients are less critically ill, more awake, and better able to realize the magnitude of their injury, and the patient often has a greater capacity to understand fluctuations in pain control and sources of their distress. With greater cognitive capacity, patients may be more concerned about disfigurement, loss of loved ones or possessions in the fire, and vocational issues. Facilitating coping can now involve more elaborate discussion with the burn team (e.g., what will be the long-term consequences of this injury?). Patients can receive education and interventions for problems such as acute stress disorder or PTSD, preparation for school return, and community reintegration.

Rehabilitation

The third stage of care is rehabilitation. Care is typically provided on an outpatient basis and initial reconstruction evaluations will often occur at this phase. Pain associated with open wounds and anxiety about survival becomes less of an issue. However, patients are faced with new issues that might include itching, poor sleep, and integration into the community, including a return to work. Depression and PTSD often become more solidified at this time. Relationship issues and problems with sexual functioning may come to the forefront. It is at this phase that long-term psychotherapy with a mental health professional may become particularly important. Sleep is often a neglected topic, and teaching patients sleep hygiene may be of use (e.g., eliminating day time naps, waking at the same time every morning). Limited use of mixed agonist benzodiazepines (e.g., zolpidem, zaleplon) can be warranted. Trazodone can be useful for patients that do not respond to the mixed benzodiazepine agonists, avoid sleep because of nightmares or hypervigilance, or who have a history of depression (54).

Almost every burn patient will experience suffering that can be reduced by timely attention from the burn treatment team. An important role of the burn team is to recognize when distress reaches the level where the patient meets the criteria for a DSM-IV-TR psychiatric diagnosis and the need for psychological or psychiatric assessment. Early in care, the more common diagnoses to be aware of include adjustment disorders, acute stress disorder, and PTSD. Labels of depression are often prematurely applied when the patient is in the early stages of burn care. It is important to remember that one or more "down days" do not constitute major depressive disorder; patients must show a constellation of symptoms persisting 2 weeks, causing significant distress, and interfering with function. In turn, the use of anti-anxiety agents such as benzodiazepines (e.g., lorazepam, diazepam) is often neglected in favor of anti-depressants. However, when a patient develops PTSD or a major depressive disorder, then SSRI antidepressant agents are often warranted either alone or in combination with cognitive-behavioral therapy.

Coping with Disfigurement

As described above, it is difficult to determine which patients will experience body-image dissatisfaction after a burn injury. For example, the size or location of a burn injury does not necessarily tell us how disturbed a patient will be about scarring. Additionally, it is not possible to determine at what point in their recovery a patient may experience body-image dissatisfaction. A patient may voice no concerns at hospital discharge, only to become unhappy with appearance over time. It can be a mistake to assume a patient will be disturbed over their appearance, and interactions based on this assumption may lead to creation or exacerbation of body image distress. Asking patients about how satisfied they are with their appearance or what reactions they have experienced from other people can be awkward topics. For this reason, it can be useful to routinely use patient self-report measures (e.g., Satisfaction with Appearance Scale) (39). Such tools can be valuable, not only to obtain an accurate gauge of patient concerns, but to do so in a manner that is minimally intrusive for the patient.

Plastic surgery is a source of tremendous hope and comfort for patients. The notion that the patients have options that can improve their appearance may provide some of the strongest coping assistance imaginable. The point at which patients become satisfied with their appearance and no longer desire surgical interventions is highly subjective. Clinicians have to be careful not to assume that their opinion of a patient's scar will match either the patient's self-perception or desire for additional procedures.

A practical approach to facilitate burn survivors' adaptation to disfigurement has been described by James Partridge, a burn survivor in Great Britain. With Dr. Nichola Rumsey, a clinical psychologist, Partridge has developed Changing Faces, a series of programs for improving the quality of life of people with disfigurement. This group has developed a cognitive-behavioral approach to treating disfigurement that relies heavily on social skills training.

The Changing Faces approach essentially involves two components, which will be briefly reviewed here (55). The first involves the use of a variety of techniques to help people understand their emotional, cognitive, and behavioral reactions when they encounter others in public. For example, a burn survivor may feel self-conscious, conspicuous, anxious, embarrassed, or different when he or she encounters another in public. These thoughts and feelings can lead to shyness, fearfulness, aggressiveness, retreating, evasiveness, or defensive behaviors. The first component of the model enables the burn survivor to understand the thoughts, feelings, and behaviors of others when they encounter them. For example, the people the burn survivor encounters in public may feel shocked, confused, anxious, or any other number of thoughts and feelings. This may lead them to behave clumsily, awkwardly, rudely, or evasively. By taking into account the most common social responses of others to their appearance the model enables burn survivors to develop new cognitive and social skills that can enhance confidence during challenging social interactions (4).

The second component of the model provides a set of skills and strategies for burn survivors to address the problems in social interactions. The acronym for this set of strategies is REACH OUT, with each letter indicating a strategy that, if practiced, can increase one's confidence in handling social challenges:

R–Reassurance
E–Energy/Effort
A–Assertiveness
C–Courage
H–Humor
O–Over there!
U–Understanding
T–Tenacity

The skills and strategies are taught in various formats, including face-to-face sessions, group activities, workshops and weekends, self-help guidelines and social skills videos. At the Galveston Shriner's Burn Center, Drs. Rose and Blakeney (the authors of Chapter 6 on pediatric burn injury) and their colleagues have successfully pilot tested this program to facilitate socialization of adolescents with severe burn injuries (56). This program is particularly appealing because it is based on cognitive-behavioral principles, is simple to teach and learn, and does not rely on long-term forms of psychotherapy.

In coping with both distress and disfigurement, peer support from other burn survivors also can be of immeasurable value. Some burn centers have active programs that encourage peer support visits. Others use professionally run support groups. Additionally, there are a number of burn camps available to children nationwide. The Phoenix Society (57) provides a means for burn survivors to get in touch with other survivors and available programs. This well-known organization has recently released a very informative book, video, and CD set related to image enhancement for burn survivors (58).

It is also important to emphasize that specific psychologically based treatment programs with empirically demonstrated efficacy for adults have been described to treat PTSD (59–60) and acute stress disorder (46). Good self-help materials have been developed including social skills training for coping with disfigurement (55) and anxiety management and self-paced in vivo exposure therapy for anxiety problems (61). In addition, a number of cognitive-behavioral treatments have been developed and demonstrated to be efficacious for treating, or preventing, body image dissatisfaction in other populations (40–41) and a recent book contributes to understanding how disfigurement impacts both the individual with the visible distinction and those who are among the observers of these individuals (62). All of these interventions can be used, alone or in combination, to enhance the quality of life and reduce the suffering of burn survivors.

IDENTIFYING PATIENTS IN GREATEST NEED OF PSYCHOLOGICAL SERVICES

At the heart of providing the most comprehensive and effective psychosocial rehabilitation services possible is the ability to identify those patients and families in the greatest need of such services. Therefore, we next describe cognitive-behavioral assessment of individuals coming for burn reconstruction evaluation.

Psychological Assessment

The first step in comprehensive assessment ideally includes using standardized measures of personality, coping, psychological distress, and health-related quality of life. However, in many cases and for a variety of reasons, this often is not practical. For this reason, we present an abbreviated screening tool in Questionnaire

7-1 at the end of this chapter. This brief screening tool can help to identify those patients who are in need of more comprehensive psychological assessment and intervention.

Our assessment model proposes that personality structure (i.e., enduring patterns of thoughts, feelings, behaviors, and motivations) works to influence appraisal of and coping with perceived stressors (e.g., traumatization, social stigmatization). Appraisal and coping methods influence the degree of distress one experiences in various contexts (e.g., body image dissatisfaction when looking in mirror or engaged in sexually intimate behavior). The degree of distress one experiences then contributes to social and occupational functioning, well-being, and quality of life. In situations where a more formal evaluation is possible, we recommend use of the following psychometrically sound assessment instruments, both at baseline and during the course of rehabilitation.

1. To assess relevant personality and psychological coping characteristics it is helpful to use *The Revised NEO Personality Inventory (NEO PI-R)* or *The NEO Five Factor Inventory (NEO-FFI)* (51) in addition to the *The COPE* (63).

2. An excellent measure of health status and function is the *SF-36 Health Survey* which is currently the most widely used measure of general health-related quality of life in medical settings (7).

3. Particularly useful measures of psychosocial distress, include the *Beck Depression Inventory* (BDI) (64–65), a frequently used measure in medical populations, and the *Davidson Trauma Scale* (66), which evaluates the frequency and severity of all the posttraumatic stress symptoms contained within the *Diagnostic and Statistical Manual of Mental Disorders IV TR* (43). The measure has proven to be a reliable and valid measure of PTSD symptoms among burn survivors (67).

4. Assessment of patient distress related to changes in appearance is accomplished effectively with the *Perceived Stigmatization Questionnaire* (PSQ) (68), which was developed to assess appearance-related perceived stigmatizing behavior. The PSQ is not a burn-specific measure, but rather, a general measure of stigmatizing behaviors applicable to any population with appearance concerns. Also very useful is the *Satisfaction With Appearance Scale* (SWAP) (39), which assess patient satisfaction with facial and nonfacial aspects of appearance, as well as the amount of social discomfort one experiences, and one's perception of the negative social impact of burn scars.

Clinical Interview

Behavioral treatment planning is also based on continual clinical assessment of how particular thoughts that occur in specific social and environmental contexts become associated with adaptive or maladaptive behavior (69). The framework for comprehensively understanding the patient's current adaptation and psychosocial rehabilitation is provided by the measures described above. This can be further refined to understand how specific undesirable behaviors are maintained and other more desirable ones are avoided. This enables the cognitive behavioral therapist to evaluate how (i) specific situations affect thoughts; (ii) thoughts affect feelings; and (iii) thoughts and feelings affect behavior. As mentioned earlier, Questionnaire 7-1 at the end of this chapter may supplement this clinical interview when a more complete assessment is not practical.

CASE EXAMPLES

The following two cases illustrate the psychosocial assessment and treatment of adult burn survivors.

Case 1: Kyle

Kyle is a 21-year-old male with a well-healed, 25% TBSA flame burns. One year ago, Kyle was injured while emulating a popular TV show. He stood in the middle of his front yard, poured a circle of gasoline around himself on the ground, and ignited it. The explosion and flames were much higher and hotter than he expected. He panicked and leapt through the flames, resulting in his injury. During his 4-week inpatient stay, Kyle required split thickness skin grafts to his leg and arm, while the rest of the burns closed with routine debridement and wound care. He underwent inpatient and outpatient physical and occupational therapy that included scar massage, range of motion, conditioning, and pressure therapy.

Kyle has been a model patient in many ways. Even shortly after his injury, he was able to laugh about his mistaken judgment and accept the changes in his appearance. Kyle made friends easily; he was always quite outgoing and energetic, and had a good sense of how to help people accept the changes in his appearance. However, Kyle has recently started a job as a local delivery man and has become more aware of initial reactions that customers have when first viewing his scars. He remains quite comfortable with his appearance, but wants to limit the awkwardness that others feel when first interacting with him.

Approximately half of the burns were deep partial and full thickness burns to his left foot and calf, left hand and forearm, and left cheek, lip, and ear. He has a red, raised plaque of hypertrophic scar occupying the lower three quarters of the left cheek and his earlobe as well as marked asymmetry of the lip. The forearm has a well-healed split-thickness skin graft that occupies the distal third of the extensor forearm and extends across the dorsal wrist onto the hand. His left hand is grafted over the entire dorsum distally to the proximal phalanges. There is tightness of the graft over the entire dorsum with inability to completely make a fist due to this tightness, particularly when he flexes. A hypertrophic scar contracture runs along the ulnar aspect of his forearm, wrist, and hand into the ulnar aspect of the little finger, thereby preventing complete adduction of the little finger and interfering with finger posture and wrist range of motion. There are webspace contractures of the thumb preventing full abduction of the thumb. His left leg and foot also have residual scarring but are of minor concern to the patient at this time.

Kyle returns to the Center for Burn Reconstruction (CBR) for a team consultation including reconstructive surgery, physical and occupational therapy, psychosocial evaluation, and case management. As a result of his compression and silicone gel sheeting therapy, the red, raised plaque of hypertrophic scar occupying the lower third of his left cheek and extending into his lower lip and chin is now flatter, softer, and is much more the color of normal skin. However, it still differs noticeably from normal skin. The scar of the lower lip continues to pull the lower lip inferiorly causing a distinct asymmetry of the lower portion of Kyle's mouth. His left earlobe also continues to be contracted to the skin at the angle of his jaw and neck.

A secondary concern regards the use of his left wrist and hand. Over the last several months, function has improved tremendously secondary to hand therapy. His ability to make a fist has improved with continued stretch exercises. The hypertrophic burn scar contracture along the ulnar aspect of his forearm, wrist, and hand still restricts the radial deviation of his wrist and hand, thereby preventing his little finger from completely adducting his fingers and he has difficulty making a fist. He would also like to improve his ability to spread his thumb, which is limited by a contracture of his thumb webspace. He also does not like the appearance of the webspace contractures between his fingers.

The surgeon discusses all of these problems with Kyle in detail. This discussion is used as an opportunity to try to establish realistic expectations regarding the results of reconstructive surgery as well as to detail the procedures themselves. The relative benefits and disadvantages of each treatment are reviewed. Kyle and the surgeon agreed to resurfacing the left cheek, lower lip, and chin.

Kyle's personality is characterized by high energy. He is outgoing and optimistic. He is quite unorthodox (e.g., identifying with a "rebel skateboarder" persona) and not very conscientious. He generally copes by avoiding stressful situations and through the use of humor. Despite these characteristics, he has a supportive social network. Interestingly, his personality and coping style also relates well to his body image issues and reason for the CBR consult: although comfortable with his own appearance, he is most concerned with the way his scars interfere with some people being spontaneous and "real" with him. Kyle's combination of energy, optimism, and agreeableness makes other people more tolerant of his lack of conformity and irregular performance. However, his lack of conscientiousness and his avoidance of unpleasantness put him at high risk for noncompliance with self-care. Kyle's parents, with whom he is living, are quite supportive; however, they are not likely to provide the structure required to help Kyle follow the necessary self-care recommendations.

Discussion

In many ways, Kyle's personality style, his social support network, as well as the presence of scars that are quite amenable to reconstruction, make him a very good candidate for surgery. The greatest concerns are that Kyle's lack of conscientiousness and avoidance coping may impair his ability to perform important self-care tasks; and, that his impulsivity, high energy, and active lifestyle may put him at risk for complications (e.g., suture tears, infections). It is often necessary to assist people like Kyle in following through with treatment recommendations. Since the social network is not able to provide sufficient structure for Kyle, the CBR team provides a clinic coordinator who works closely with him to coordinate his care.

The therapists trained Kyle to competence in performing specific self-care behaviors, and demonstrated how certain movements can tear the skin around sutures. The surgeon and case manager helped Kyle to delineate his goals for the surgery and draw clear connections between these goals and his compliance with prescribed self-care behavior and activity limitations. At one point, it became clear that Kyle had engaged in work-related activities likely to put his surgical outcome at risk. At the weekly meeting, the necessity of Kyle's compliance was reiterated. A problem-solving approach to compliance was inaugurated that emphasized Kyle's responsibility for his own behavior and, ultimately, for the success or failure of the surgery. With this approach, Kyle was able to identify other ways of doing things that would not put the outcome at risk.

Case 2: Rebecca

Rebecca is a 36-year-old woman who was injured as a 4-year-old girl at her parents' home. She was dancing in the kitchen, bumped into the stove, and spilled the scalding hot contents of a large cooking pot onto herself. She does not recall the accident or her recovery except "unending pain" and "really missing my mother a lot." The burn involved 25% TBSA deep partial and full thickness scald burns to her face, chest, and bilateral upper extremities. Her facial burn scars consisted of hypertrophic scars of the posterior half of her cheeks and forehead. Her hands and forearms clearly had been burned, but her mature burn scars in these areas were apparently acceptable to her. She had severe truncal burn scarring with contractures of the inferior aspects of her breasts. Rebecca selectively focused on the deformities of her face and breasts and gave no indication of concern about the generalized scarring of her abdomen and back.

Rebecca reported that she first became aware of her different appearance when noticing the stares and the awkwardness of adults she encountered as a child. As she got older she became the object of cruel comments from her peers. Although naturally social and likable, she became hesitant to approach new people and developed a reticent style of interaction, marked by poor eye contact, tense body posture, and avoidance of conversation. She has struggled with episodes of major depression throughout her adult life, although she has never been psychotic or suicidal. These episodes have either spontaneously remitted or been successfully treated with antidepressants. Her few friends are clearly of great benefit to her; they provide emotional support, engage her in interesting cultural activities, and provide assistance when requested. However, she remains quite uncomfortable with her appearance. Interestingly, she is just as distressed about the deformities of her face as she is with the deformities of her breasts. Rebecca is hopeful that surgical reconstruction will boost her confidence sufficiently that she will feel more comfortable in novel social situations and in making new friends.

Rebecca presented to the CBR for a team consultation including reconstructive surgery, physical and occupational therapy, psychosocial evaluation, and case management. The facial burn scarring was largely a problem of disturbance of the skin contour. Although her residual facial scars were relatively flat and soft, they still were raised above the surface of her normal cheeks' skin. The deformity was impossible to cover with cosmetics. Although all of her chest and breast skin was scarred Rebecca felt that if an inframammary fold could be reestablished under both breasts, her breasts would look much more normal and she could wear her bra and overlying clothes much more normally and comfortably. Most importantly, she would no longer feel disfigured.

After a lengthy discussion of treatment options and anticipated outcomes, an operative plan was developed that consisted of resurfacing the posterior cheeks with cervicofacial rotation flaps. The forehead would be tangentially excised and resurfaced with a thick split thickness skin graft. The contractures of both of her breasts would be released and her inframammary folds reestablished using full thickness skin grafts. Although these operations would not return Rebecca to complete physical normalcy, the primary problems causing her distress would be drastically improved. She could then cover the postoperative scars with cosmetics and, thus, obtain a normal breast contour and the inframammary folds she desired.

Discussion

Rebecca is naturally outgoing and energetic but has felt compelled to inhibit these traits because of her sensitivity to stigmatizing behaviors from others (stares, personal questions, insults, avoidance). She has a strong tendency to experience intense, prolonged negative affect, especially anxious apprehension when facing novel social situations, and depression when ruminating over events in her life. She is conscientious and agreeable, which contribute to her being very concerned with the reactions of other people. The combination of unstable emotions, inhibited sociability, and overly rigid conscientiousness, often lead people to minimize their time with her, even those who are able to relate to her as a whole person and not just to her scars. Clearly, this personality style was partially developed in response to her early experience with social stigmatization, and contributes to her chronic dissatisfaction with her appearance, her discomfort with other people, and her expectation that others will be uncomfortable with her.

From Rebecca's perspective, the primary reason for her CBR consultation was to improve her self-confidence by improving her appearance. Unfortunately, although the plan outlined above will greatly improve aspects of her appearance, there are no currently available procedures that will restore her appearance to within normal limits. Therefore, in addition to scar revision, the team recommends physical and occupational therapy training in appearance enhancing techniques (58) to assist Rebecca in handling a broader range of social challenges. To help further these goals, Rebecca was put in contact with the New Life Burn Survivors Support Group and the Phoenix Society.

Because of her chronic body image disturbance and recurrent major depression, cognitive-behavioral therapy (CBT) was also recommended. The therapist helped Rebecca to increase the frequency of her exposure to new social situations, reduce her time ruminating over her appearance and unpleasant interactions, and limit the effect that depressed mood has on her physical activities. Part of this CBT work will involve learning and applying new social skills that are quite useful in handling a broad range of challenging social interactions (55). For Rebecca, the highest quality of life can be obtained through a combination of surgical interventions, social skills training focusing on issues related to her disfigurement, as well CBT to address issues specific to her psychosocial rehabilitation.

CONCLUSIONS

Clinical experience and empirical research give ample room for optimism for the recovery of satisfying levels of health and function for the majority of those who survive a major burn injury. However, there are important complications that, when present, can cause prolonged impairment and role disruption following major burn injury. The preponderance of studies cited in this chapter suggest that complementing standard medical care with assessment and interventions designed to reduce psychological distress and enhance social support may accelerate both physical and psychosocial recovery of individuals who sustain these often horrific injuries.

Key Psychosocial Issues in Assessment of Burn Reconstruction Patients

How much do you agree with the following statements?

Body Image

1. Overall, I like what I see when I look in the mirror.
   I disagree a lot   1   2   3   4   5   6   7   I agree a lot
2. My burn scars have ruined my physical appearance.
   I disagree a lot   1   2   3   4   5   6   7   I agree a lot
3. I am satisfied with the appearance of my burn scars that are being evaluated for reconstructive surgery.
   I disagree a lot   1   2   3   4   5   6   7   I agree a lot
4. My physical activities are not limited by my burn scars that are being evaluated for reconstructive surgery.
   I disagree a lot   1   2   3   4   5   6   7   I agree a lot

Social Comfort

5. I feel like I don't fit in with other people because of my burn scars.
   I disagree a lot   1   2   3   4   5   6   7   I agree a lot
6. I avoid certain social situations or events because of how my burn scars look.
   I disagree a lot   1   2   3   4   5   6   7   I agree a lot
7. It is easy for me to blend in with other people in spite of my burn scars.
   I disagree a lot   1   2   3   4   5   6   7   I agree a lot

Rumination and Hopelessness

8. I often worry about how the burn scars affect my life.
   I disagree a lot   1   2   3   4   5   6   7   I agree a lot
9. Right now, I feel that improved appearance is impossible.
   I disagree a lot   1   2   3   4   5   6   7   I agree a lot
10. Right now, I feel that improved function is impossible.
    I disagree a lot   1   2   3   4   5   6   7   I agree a lot

Intent to Adhere

11. How much do you intend to follow your doctor's recommendations for preparing for surgery?
    No intention at all   1   2   3   4   5   6   7   I intend to do exactly as recommended
12. How much do you intend to follow your doctor's recommendations for taking care of your wounds after surgery?
    No intention at all   1   2   3   4   5   6   7   I intend to do exactly as recommended

QUESTIONNAIRE 7-1 *(continued)*

Outcome Efficacy for Surgery to Achieve Goals and Satisfaction

13. How much of an improvement in your appearance do you expect to achieve with re-constructive surgery?

    No change at all   1   2   3   4   5   6   7   Look completely normal

14. How much of an improvement in your function do you expect to achieve with recon-structive surgery?

    No change at all   1   2   3   4   5   6   7   Look completely normal

15. How satisfied with the results of reconstructive surgery do you expect to be if you follow your doctor's advice exactly?

    Not satisfied at all   1   2   3   4   5   6   7   Completely satisfied

Mood

16. In the past 7 days I have felt sad most of the time.

    I disagree a lot   1   2   3   4   5   6   7   I agree a lot

17. In the past 7 days I have not been able to enjoy anything.

    I disagree a lot   1   2   3   4   5   6   7   I agree a lot

18. In the past 7 days I have been very upset by memories, images, or dreams of how I was burned.

    I disagree a lot   1   2   3   4   5   6   7   I agree a lot

19. In the past 7 days I have been avoiding thoughts, feelings, places, or people that remind me of how I was burned.

    I disagree a lot   1   2   3   4   5   6   7   I agree a lot

20. In the past 7 days I have had a lot of trouble trying to sleep or relax.

    I disagree a lot   1   2   3   4   5   6   7   I agree a lot

21. In the past 7 days I have often used alcohol or drugs.

    I disagree a lot   1   2   3   4   5   6   7   I agree a lot

REFERENCES

1. American Burn Association. Burn incidence fact sheet [American Burns Association Web site]. Available at: http://ameriburn.org/pub/BurnIncidenceFactSheet.htm. Accessed January 25, 2004.
2. Blakeney PE, Fauerbach JA, Meyer WJ, Thomas CR. Psychosocial recovery and reintegration of patients with burn injuries. In: Herndon D, ed. *Total Burn Care*. 2nd ed. Philadelphia: WB Saunders, 2002:783–798.
3. Herndon DN, ed. *Total Burn Care*. 2nd ed. Philadelphia: WB Saunders, 2002.
4. Patterson DR, Ptacek JT, Cromes F, et al. The 2000 clinical research award. Describing and predicting distress and satisfaction with life for burn survivors. *J Burn Care Rehabil* 2000;21:490–498.
5. Wenger NK, Mattson ME, Furberg CD, Ellinson J, eds. *Assessment of Quality of Life in Clinical Trials of Cardiovascular Disease*. New York: LeJaq, 1984.
6. Jacobson AM, De Groot M, Samson J. Quality of life research in patients with diabetes mellitus. In: Dimsdale J, Baum A, eds. *Quality of Life in Behavioral Medicine Research*. Hillsdale, NJ: Lawrence Erlbaum Associates, 1995:241–262.
7. Ware JE, Snow KK, Kosinski M, Gandek B. *SF-36 Health Survey: Manual and Interpretation Guide*. Boston: Nimrod Press, 1993.
8. Van Loey NE, Van Son MJ. Psychopathology and psychological problems in patients with burn scars: epidemiology and management. *Am J Clin Dermatol* 2003;4:245–272.
9. Fauerbach JA, Lawrence J, Haythornthwaite J, et al. Preinjury psychiatric illness and postinjury adjustment in adult burn survivors. *Psychosomatics* 1996;37:547–555.
10. Fauerbach JA, Lawrence JW, Bryant AG, Smith JH. The relationship of ambivalent coping to depression symptoms and adjustment. *Rehabil Psychol* 2002;47:387–401.
11. Fauerbach JA, Heinberg LJ, Lawrence JW, et al. Effect of early body image dissatisfaction on subsequent psychological and physical adjustment after disfiguring injury. *Psychosom Med* 2000;62:576–582.
12. Fauerbach JA, Lawrence JW, Munster AM, et al. Prolonged adjustment difficulties among those with acute posttrauma distress following burn injury. *J Behav Med* 1999;22:359–378.
13. Fauerbach JA, Heinberg LJ, Lawrence JW, et al. Coping with body image changes following a disfiguring burn injury. *Health Psychol* 2002;21:115–121.
14. Fauerbach JA, Richter L, Lawrence JW. Regulating acute posttrauma distress. *J Burn Care Rehabil* 2002;23:249–257.
15. Fauerbach JA, Lawrence JW, Schmidt CW Jr, et al. Personality predictors of injury-related posttraumatic stress disorder. *J Nerv Ment Dis* 2000;188:510–517.
16. Gilboa D. Long-term psychosocial adjustment after burn injury. *Burns* 2001;27:335–341.
17. Patterson DR, Finch CP, Wiechman SA, et al. Premorbid mental health status of adult burn patients: comparison with a normative sample. *J Burn Care Rehabil* 2003;24:347–350.
18. Browne G, Byrne C, Brown B, et al. Psychosocial adjustment of burn survivors. *Burns Incl Therm Inj* 1985;12:28–35.
19. Munster AM, Fauerbach JA, Lawrence J. Development and utilization of a psychometric instrument for measuring quality of life in burn patients, 1976 to 1996. *Acta Chir Plast* 1996;38:128–131.
20. Kimmo T, Jyrki V, Sirpa AS. Health status after recovery from burn injury. *Burns* 1998;24:293–298.
21. Sheridan RL, Hinson MI, Liang MH, et al. Long-term outcome of children surviving massive burns. *JAMA* 2000;283:69–73.
22. Altier N, Malenfant A, Forget R, Choiniere M. Long-term adjustment in burn victims: a matched-control study. *Psychol Med* 2002;32:677–685.
23. Pallua N, Kunsebeck HW, Noah EM. Psychosocial adjustments 5 years after burn injury. *Burns* 2003; 29:143–152.
24. Wiechman SA, Ptacek JT, Patterson DR, et al. Rates, trends, and severity of depression after burn injuries. *J Burn Care Rehabil* 2001;22:417–424.
25. Cronin-Stubbs D, de Leon CF, Beckett LA, et al. Six-year effect of depressive symptoms on the course of physical disability in community-living older adults. *Arch Intern Med* 2000; 160:3074–3080.
26. Fauerbach JA, Lezotte D, Hills RA, et al. Burden of burn: a norm-based inquiry into the influence of burn size and distress on recovery of physical and psychosocial function. *J Burn Care Rehabil* 2005;26:21–32.
27. DeRogatis LR. *The SCL-90-R Manual I: Scoring, Administration, and Procedures for the SCL-90R*. Baltimore: Clinical Psychometric Research, 1977.
28. DeRogatis LR, Spencer PM. *The Brief Symptom Inventory (BSI) Administration, Scoring and Procedures Manual-I*. Baltimore: Clinical Psychometric Research, 1982.
29. Patterson DR, Everett JJ, Bombardier CH, et al. Psychological effects of severe burn injuries. *Psychol Bull* 1993;113:362–378.
30. Pruzinsky T, Doctor M. Body images and pediatric burn injury. In: Tarnowski KJ, ed. *Behavioral Aspects of Pediatric Burns* 1994:169–191.
31. Beuf A. *Appearance-Impaired Children in America*. Philadelphia: University of Pennsylvania Press, 1990.
32. Macgregor FC. Facial disfigurement: Problems and management of social interaction and implications for mental health. *Aesthetic Plast Surg* 1990;14:249–257.
33. Thompson JK, Heinberg LJ. The media's influence on body image disturbance and eating disorders: we've reviled them, now can we rehabilitate them? *J Soc Iss* 1999;55:339–353.
34. Bull RHC, Rumsey N. *The Social Psychology of Facial Appearance*. New York: Springer-Verlag, 1988.
35. Davidson TN, Bowden ML, Tholen D, James MH, Feller I. Social support and post-burn adjustment. *Arch Phys Med Rehabil* 1981;62:274–278.
36. Orr DA, Reznikoff M, Smith GM. Body image, self-esteem, and depression in burn-injured adolescents and young adults. *J Burn Care Rehabil* 1989;10:454–461.
37. Lawrence JW, Fauerbach JA, Heinberg L, Doctor M. Visible versus hidden scars and their relation to body esteem. *J Burn Care Rehabil* 2004;25:25–32.

38. Rumsey N, Clarke A, White P. Exploring the psychosocial concerns of outpatients with disfiguring conditions. *J Wound Care* 2003;12:247–252.
39. Lawrence JW, Heinberg LJ, Roca R, et al. Development and validation of the satisfaction with appearance scale: assessing body image among burn-injured patients. *Psychol Assess* 1998;10:64–70.
40. Cash TF, Stachan MD. Cognitive-behavioral approaches to changing body image. In: Cash TF, Pruzinsky T, eds. *Body Image: A Handbook of Theory, Research, and Clinical Practice.* New York: Guilford Press, 2002:478–486.
41. Stormer SM, Thompson JK. Explanations of body image disturbance: a test of maturational status, negative verbal commentary, social comparison, and sociocultural hypotheses. *Int J Eat Disord* 1996; 19:193–202.
42. Winzelberg AJ, Abascal L, Taylor CB. Psychoeducational approaches to the prevention and change of negative body image. In: Cash TF, Pruzinsky T, eds. *Body Image: A Handbook of Theory, Research, and Clinical Practice.* New York: Guilford Press, 2002:487–496.
43. American Psychiatric Association. *The Diagnostic and Statistical Manual of Mental Disorders-TR.* Washington, DC: American Psychiatric Association, 2000.
44. Fauerbach JA, Lawrence J, Haythornthwaite J, et al. Preburn psychiatric history affects posttrauma morbidity. *Psychosomatics* 1997;38:374–385.
45. Powers PS, Cruse CW, Daniels S, Stevens B. Posttraumatic stress disorder in patients with burns. *J Burn Care Rehabil* 1994;15:147–153.
46. Bryant RA, Harvey AG. *Acute Stress Disorder: A Handbook of Theory Assessment and Treatment.* Washington, DC: American Psychological Association, 2000.
47. Perry S, Difede J, Musngi G, et al. Predictors of posttraumatic stress disorder after burn injury. *Am J Psychiatry* 1992;149:931–935.
48. Roca RP, Spence RJ, Munster AM. Posttraumatic adaptation and distress among adult burn survivors. *Am J Psychiatry* 1992;149:1234–1238.
49. Taal LA, Faber AW. Burn injuries, pain and distress: exploring the role of stress symptomatology. *Burns* 1997;23:288–290.
50. Kiecolt-Glaser JK, Williams DA. Self-blame, compliance, and distress among burn patients. *J Pers Soc Psychol* 1987;53:187–193.
51. Costa PT, McCrae RR. *The Revised NEO Personality Inventory (NEO PI-R) and NEO Five Factor Inventory (NEO-FFI) Professional Manual.* Odessa, FL: Psychological Assessment Resources, 1992.
52. Roesch SC, Weiner B. A meta-analytic review of coping with illness: do causal attributions matter? *J Psychosom Res* 2001;50:205–219.
53. Ptacek JT, Patterson DR, Montgomery BK, Heimbach DM. Pain, coping, and adjustment in patients with burns: preliminary findings from a prospective study. *J Pain Symptom Manage* 1995;10:446–455.
54. Jaffe SE, Patterson DR. Treating sleep problems in patients with burn injuries: practical considerations. *J Burn Care Rehabil* 2004;25:294–305.
55. Partridge J. *Changing Faces: The Challenge of Facial Disfigurement.* London, England: Penguin Books, 1998.
56. Blakeney PE, Thomas C, Holzer C, et al. Efficacy of a short-term, intensive social skills training program for burned adolescents. *J Burn Care Rehabil.* In press.
57. The Phoenix Society, www.phoenix-society.org. Accessed June 15, 2005.
58. Kammerer Quayle B. *The Book of Image Enhancement for Burn Survivors: A Common Sense Guide to Creating Your BEST Image.* Washington, DC: International Association of Firefighters and IAFF Burn Foundation, 2004.
59. Foa EB, Keane TM, Friedman MJ. *Effective Treatments for PTSD.* New York: Guilford Press, 2000.
60. Foa EB, Rothbaum BO. *Treating the Trauma of Rape.* New York: Guilford Press, 1997.
61. Craske MG, Barlow DH. *Mastery of Your Anxiety and Panic-Third Edition (MAP-3): Client Workbook.* San Antonio, TX: The Psychological Corporation, 2000.
62. Heatherton TF, Kleck RE, Hebl MR, Hull JG. *The Social Psychology of Stigma.* New York: Guilford Press, 2000.
63. Carver CS, Scheier MF, Weintraub JK. Assessing coping strategies: a theoretically based approach. *J Pers Soc Psychol* 1989;56:267–283.
64. Beck AT, Ward CH, Mendelson M, et al. An inventory for measuring depression. *Arch Gen Psychiatry* 1961;4:561–571.
65. Beck AT, Steer RA, Garbin MG. Psychometric properties of the Beck Depression Inventory: twenty-five years of evaluation. *Clin Psychol Rev* 1988;8:77–100.
66. Davidson JR, Book SW, Colket JT, et al. Assessment of a new self-rating scale for post-traumatic stress disorder. *Psychol Med* 1997;27:153–160.
67. Lawrence J, Fauerbach JA, Richter D, Munster AM. *Construct Validity of the Davidson PTSD Scale in an Inpatient Burn Population.* St. Louis: Mosby–Year Book, 1996.
68. Lawrence JW, Doctor M, Heinberg L, Fauerbach JA. *Assessing Perceived Social Stigmatization Among Burn Survivors.* Chicago: American Burn Association, 2002.
69. Rohe DE. Psychological aspects of rehabilitation. In: DeLisa JA, Gans BM, eds. *Rehabilitation Medicine: Principles and Practice.* 3rd ed. Philadelphia: Lippincott–Raven Publishers, 1998:189–212.

Chapter 8

Facial Trauma and Facial Cancer

Thomas Pruzinsky, PhD, Elie Levine, MD, John A. Persing, MD, Jeffrey T. Barth, PhD, and Robert Obrecht, PhD, LCDR/MSC/USN

Learning to live with a change in the appearance of one's face as a result of injury or disease is profoundly challenging. The range of variables (medical, psychological, and social) influencing the process of adaptation is far from fully understood (1). However, the plastic surgery treatment team—including the surgeon, nurses, and professionals from other disciplines—can be certain that the ultimate goal of their work, improving patient quality of life, will be determined not only by their surgical skills, which clearly have a profound positive effect on patient well-being, but also by a range of social and psychological factors. The primary goal of this chapter is to encourage development of higher standards of care for patients with acquired facial disfigurement, which includes giving routine attention to psychosocial rehabilitation (2).

Currently, the psychological and social suffering of patients with acquired facial disfigurement often goes unaddressed by the plastic surgery treatment team. There are many reasons for this, including the obvious fact that the plastic surgery team's primary goal is to provide patients with the highest standards of surgical care. Most members of the team have not been given adequate training to address patients' psychosocial concerns. Furthermore, compared to other areas of plastic surgery (e.g., in burn injury [Chapters 6 and 7]) or congenital facial disfigurement (Chapter 5) there has not been a great deal of research elucidating psychosocial responses to the forms of acquired disfigurement addressed in this chapter (1).

This chapter addresses two separate and distinct forms of facial disfigurement acquired during adulthood: disfigurement acquired from trauma (though we will not discuss disfigurement caused by burn injuries as this topic is addressed in Chapter 7) and facial disfigurement acquired through disease—primarily cancer occurring on the face (e.g., skin cancers and other forms of head and neck cancer). There is reason to believe that psychological responses to acquired disfigurement are, at least to some degree, different and perhaps even more pronounced than the psychological responses to congenital disfigurement (1). Furthermore, while patients with disfigurement acquired through trauma and those who acquire facial disfigurement from cancer share many commonalities, they also are likely to have some unique psychological characteristics. We review what is currently known about the psychological adaptation specific to facial trauma and facial cancers. This is followed by a discussion of the psychosocial aspects of adaptation shared by individuals with acquired facial disfigurement, including challenges in social functioning, body image adaptation, experience of depression, and possible substance abuse. The goal of the chapter is to provide the plastic surgery treatment team with enough information so they can more readily identify those patients having difficulties in psychosocial adjustment that can be addressed with proper referrals to mental health professionals who can help them with the process of psychosocial rehabilitation.

PSYCHOLOGICAL CHARACTERISTICS OF INDIVIDUALS SUSTAINING FACIAL TRAUMA

The psychological characteristics of facial trauma patients have received only limited empirical attention (3). The extant data clearly suggest that these individuals can experience a wide range of psychosocial concerns. For example, Shetty et al. (3) found that patients with orofacial injuries were much more likely to report symptoms of depression, anxiety, and hostility when compared to a matched control group. Many patients continued to report significant psychological problems for 12 months postinjury (4). Similarly, Shepherd et al. (5) documented patient experiences of anxiety, depression, and psychological distress within 3 months of sustaining mandible fractures.

Many of the orofacial injury patients in the study by Shetty et al. (3) had significant psychosocial problems including lack of health insurance, high levels of unemployment (approximately 75%), and relatively low levels of education (approximately 40% had not finished high school). Most of the injuries were the result of interpersonal assault (83%) and almost one-third of patients had previously sustained a traumatic injury, both of which may be indicative of significant social problems. Repeated experience of physical trauma is relatively common among these individuals (6) and they also frequently experience significant difficulties in return to pre-injury levels of occupational functioning (7).

Levine et al. (8), evaluating many of the critical variables reported in previous studies, compared the psychosocial functioning of adult patients who sustained traumatic facial injury with an age-matched, gender-matched, and race-matched control group of non-injured persons across a variety of psychosocial domains. Facial trauma patients reported higher rates of depression, substance abuse problems, posttraumatic stress disorder symptoms, body image concerns, and a lower overall satisfaction with life as compared to controls. In addition, facial trauma patients reported more problems in marital and occupational functioning and higher rates of contact with the legal system. Not surprisingly, they were rated as having a more negative facial appearance by independent raters, although the patients themselves did not rate their posttrauma appearance more negatively than their pretrauma appearance. Though the number of patients in this study was small (n = 20), it nevertheless documents significant group differences on a wide range of psychosocial variables.

Interestingly, while it has been frequently clinically observed that there is no necessary correlation between the degree of disfigurement and the extent of psychological response (1,9–10) (see Cash's chapter on body image and all three chapters on cosmetic surgery for a discussion of related issues), a recent empirical investigation of the psychological effects of minor facial lacerations documented that such injuries can have significant psychosocial effects (including self-consciousness and social anxiety) and that the degree of such disturbance was more pronounced the larger the scar (11).

PSYCHOLOGICAL RESPONSES SPECIFIC TO FACIAL TRAUMA: POSTTRAUMATIC STRESS DISORDER AND NEUROPSYCHOLOGICAL SYMPTOMS

Next, we review two areas of concern particularly relevant to facial trauma: (i) the occurrence of posttraumatic stress disorder (PTSD) symptoms; and (ii) the possible neuropsychological consequences of facial trauma.

Posttraumatic Stress Disorder (PTSD)

The primary symptoms of posttraumatic stress disorder include (i) re-experiencing of the trauma (e.g., having intrusive and distressing thoughts and/or distressing images and dreams); (ii) avoidance of thoughts, emotions, or situations related to the trauma; and (iii) autonomic nervous system hyperarousal, including difficulties with sleeping, having an exaggerated startle response, and experiencing increased irritability and tension (12). In some instances, these symptoms are not reported by the patients, but are described by individuals close to the patients. (PTSD is also described in the chapters on pediatric and adult burn injury as well as the chapter on hand trauma.)

There have been at least three studies documenting evidence of PTSD symptoms in adult facial trauma patients (8,13–14). Similar findings of high rates of PTSD in trauma induced facial disfigurement have been reported in pediatric plastic surgery populations (15). In an investigation of the prevalence of acute PTSD symptoms in 336 patients presenting to an urban hospital with orofacial trauma (midfacial or mandibular fractures) (14), 25% of patients met the diagnostic criteria for acute PTSD. Two other studies have found prevalence rates of 27% and 30% (8,13). It is also quite possible that a substantial portion of patients might experience subclinical forms of PTSD (i.e., not meeting the full diagnostic criteria) that can nevertheless substantially undermine the patient's quality of life.

Several factors may suggest to the plastic surgeon that a patient is suffering from PTSD. Individuals with orofacial trauma who reported PTSD symptoms were more likely to also report pre-injury psychological problems, increased levels of pre-injury social stress, lower levels of social support, and pre-injury "exposure to and distress" with respect to prior trauma (14). Those with PTSD also were more likely to be older, female, and have experienced more injury-related pain (14). Thus, evaluating post-surgical facial trauma patients in light of the variables predictive of PTSD may help identify patients at increased risk for experiencing other forms of postinjury psychological distress (14). Identification of PTSD symptoms can lead to a further exploration and uncovering of previously unrecognized additional psychological symptoms (e.g., depression, substance abuse).

To conduct a brief screening for PTSD in facial trauma patients seeking reconstructive surgery, we suggest that the plastic surgery team use the four-item Primary Care PTSD Screen (PC-PTSD) published by The National Center for PTSD (http://www.ncptsd.org/screen_disaster.html). We have reprinted the four items in the *Quality of Life Assessment for Facial Trauma Patients* in Questionnaire 8-1 at the end of this chapter. We recommend administering these items to all facial trauma patients in combination with the items in Questionnaire 8-2 (General Quality of Life Assessment) described later.

Potential Neuropsychological Deficits

Any patient who has sustained an injury to the face significant enough to result in facial disfigurement also may have sustained a trauma to the brain. A concussion could result in possible long-term brain-injury related neuropsychological deficits, including cognitive, emotional, and behavioral sequelae that warrant attention (16–17). Although concussion has been variously defined, its essential features include immediate and transient posttraumatic mental status (neural function) alterations, and may or may not include loss of consciousness (LOC). In general, headaches, nausea, dizziness, diplopia, confusion, slowed mental processing, attention problems, and/or amnesia/memory disturbances are the acute sequelae. In a global sense, the severity of a head injury can be categorized by using the Glasgow Coma Scale (GCS) (18). The GCS is a universal system of quantifying the level of consciousness or mental intactness following traumatic brain injury (TBI) by differentially rating an individual's best motor, verbal, and eye opening responses. On a 3 to 15 point scale, a head injury is considered mild if the GCS score is greater than or equal to 13, moderate if the GCS score is between 9 and 12, and severe if the GCS score is less than or equal to 8 (19).

Other issues to be considered in the evaluation of head injury severity are evidence of, and duration of, LOC, retrograde amnesia (loss of memory for events prior to the injury), and posttraumatic amnesia (PTA: loss of memory for events after the injury) (20–21). In a general sense, more extreme impairment suggests a more severe head injury. Moderate and severe brain injuries have obvious sequelae and are treated in the Emergency Department (ED). A mild head injury or mild traumatic brain injury (mTBI), also referred to as a concussion, is less obvious to the ED physician and may be overlooked during initial hospital treatment.

The primary mechanisms of TBI (particularly following facial trauma) include impact deceleration of the brain within the skull and impact injury to the anterior, frontal and temporal lobes, and diffuse axonal shearing (i.e., twisting, stretching, and tearing of axonal fibers from deceleration and rotational torque). These mechanisms either result in, or are associated with, a pathophysiological cascade of secondary events, including intracellular influx of calcium, reduction in potassium, and vascular and related glucose insufficiencies (20). In mTBI and concussion, these same processes may be expressed in a less identifiable form (and may not be realized on neuroimaging). Mild TBI often goes unrecognized because the more noticeable medical emergency is the facial trauma.

The Effects of Mild Head Injury

Mild head injury or concussion, particularly without LOC, was previously believed to be insufficient to cause neurologic injury. Poor outcomes and persisting symptoms were thought to be related to psychological problems and not the head trauma itself (22). Clinical research has since revealed that mild neuropsychological deficits do occur in many mild head injuries (23). While most mild head injury patients demonstrate rapid, spontaneous recovery within several days or weeks, a small percentage experience prolonged postconcussion symptoms lasting 3 months or longer. This lack of recovery following a mild head injury is referred to as postconcussive syndrome (PCS) (23).

Evaluating Patients with Head Injury

As part of the plastic surgeon's initial presurgery assessment, the patient should be evaluated for presence and severity of head injury (LOC, retrograde amnesia, and PTA) and for PCS symptoms (see Table 8-1). Being aware of their patient's functional (cognitive, psychological, and physical) changes, is critical to appropriate care. Certain memory problems may interfere with the patient's ability to take medications as directed, or the patient may not process information or recall instructional procedures. If the patient has trouble concentrating, the treatment process may be much more challenging and require more patience on the part of the plastic surgery team. Assessing for and identifying these postconcussive syndrome symptoms will help reconstructive surgeons to modify the aftercare procedures they use. Sometimes, repeating and writing down presurgical and postsurgical care plans and including significant others during these discussions so that they can help remind and explain the surgeon's plans to the patient, can be critical to treatment compliance.

To conduct a screening for possible neuropsychological deficits associated with facial trauma, we have included 13 self-report items (in addition to the four PTSD-related items) in Questionnaire 8-1 at the end of this chapter (Quality of Life Assessment for Patients Sustaining Facial Trauma). We recommend that the plastic surgeon consider administering this measure to all patients who have sustained a facial trauma to help assist in the identification of patients who may be experiencing neuropsychological problems. More clearly understanding the patient's neuropsychological functioning (as well as their overall psychological functioning) also has implications for determining the patient's ability to process information regarding

▶ **TABLE 8-1 Head Injury Taxonomy**

Presence and Severity of Head Injury	Postconcussive Syndrome (PCS) Symptoms

Glasgow Coma Scale (GCS) Score
☐ Severe Range Scores
  3 4 5 6 7 8
☐ Moderate Range Scores
  9 10 11 12
☐ Mild Range Scores
  13 14 15
	Neurocognitive Symptoms
	☐ Slowed mental processing
	☐ Inattentive
	☐ Poor concentration
	☐ Impaired memory
	☐ Poor planning
	☐ Disorganized

Loss of Consciousness (LOC)? ☐ No ☐ Yes Duration:_____	Psychological and Behavioral Symptoms ☐ Depression ☐ Anxiety ☐ Irritability/impatience ☐ Disinhibition ☐ Poor judgment ☐ Amotivation
Retrograde Amnesia? ☐ No ☐ Yes Duration:_____	
Posttraumatic Amnesia (PTA)? ☐ No ☐ Yes Duration:_____	Physical Symptoms ☐ Headache ☐ Nausea ☐ Dizziness ☐ Diplopia ☐ Tinnitus

surgical procedures and expected surgical outcomes and may help to prevent any misunderstanding that can result in disappointment postoperatively.

Neuropsychological Assessment

In cases where several PCS symptoms are present, a neuropsychological evaluation is warranted. A plastic surgeon, after referring his or her patient to a clinical neuropsychologist, should expect a comprehensive evaluation. These assessments typically include a concise description of the presenting condition (based on available medical records and input from the patient and/or family members during the clinical interview part of the assessment battery), a medical and psychosocial history, and a detailed summary of the results of the formal neuropsychological testing.

The patient's abilities and behavior that are typically assessed in any head injury neuropsychological evaluation include the following: orientation, attention/concentration, language functions, intellectual abilities, abstract reasoning, concept formation, new problem solving, mental flexibility, executive functions, learning, verbal, and spatial memory, information processing capacity and speed, visuospatial abilities, motor and sensory skills, and emotional and personality status [21]. These functional areas are evaluated using paper–pencil, mechanical, and sensory–motor tests, thereby allowing the neuropsychologist to study the impact of the patient's head injury. Computerized and Web-based neurocognitive assessment procedures can offer new precision and efficiencies in some of these evaluations and screening procedures.

The reconstructive surgeon should also expect the clinical neuropsychologist to provide feedback to the patient and/or family members. This is considered to be an integral part of the evaluation process [20]. The feedback typically includes practical, supportive, and educative information about the patient's cognitive, behavioral, and emotional strengths and weaknesses. In addition, information is given to the patient to assist in the development of realistic expectations about their time course of recovery, coping strategies, and follow-up neuropsychological evaluations (i.e., to track neurocognitive changes).

PSYCHOLOGICAL RESPONSES TO FACIAL CANCER

The psychological experience of facial cancer patients has received even less empirical or clinical attention than the experiences of facial trauma patients (24–25). Based on the extensive body image and physical appearance scholarship (Chapters 3 and 4), as well as clinical and published reports of patients' experience (26–28), the psychological effects of facial cancers are believed to be quite extensive and at least as disruptive as facial trauma.

We are aware of only one study explicitly comparing plastic surgery patients undergoing treatment for facial cancer (basal cell carcinomas, squamous cell carcinomas, and malignant melanomas) with patients undergoing reconstruction for scarring resulting from injury (29). Facial cancer patients (who were no longer undergoing cancer treatment) reported lower levels of depression, anxiety, social concern, and concern about their appearance as compared to the facial trauma patients. However, despite experience with many significant problems, including disfigurement, difficulties with swallowing and eating, pain, speech problems, and dry mouth, patients with head and neck cancer nevertheless report that their overall quality of life is not significantly compromised (30–31). Rybarczyk and Behel (32), describing the psychological adjustment to acquired disability, report that disabilities resulting from lifesaving interventions often are associated with better psychological adjustment than disabilities that occur as a result of accidents. Trauma induced disabilities are often perceived to be "random, unnecessary and unfair" resulting in blaming and anger towards one's self or others as well as being associated with idealizing one's pre-injury physical appearance (32) all of which serve to make the adjustment process more difficult.

Therefore, though no definitive empirical conclusions currently exist, there is some reason to believe that the psychological effects of facial cancers may be less psychologically disruptive than facial trauma. However, the clinical observation that patients with facial cancer are more likely to be older, married, and have greater concerns regarding whether they will live or die must be taken into consideration when making this comparison. Additionally, facial cancer patients who have particular predisposing personality traits may be at increased risk for compromised quality of life. For example, in patients with head and neck squamous cell carcinoma, higher levels of neuroticism were associated with lower quality of life (33) and higher levels of alcohol consumption (34). Such problems would unquestionably complicate the process of psychologically adapting to a cancer diagnosis, facial disfigurement, and surgical reconstruction.

A wide range of variables are thought to influence psychological adjustment to head and neck cancer (35). These include the nature and extent of the patient's social support, the existence of pre-existing psychological and/or substance abuse problems, the nature of the treatment (surgery, radiation, and/or chemotherapy), and the extent of pain, as well as postoperative fatigue. Actively seeking out social support is believed to be a highly adaptive method of coping (36). In contrast, the use of passive styles of coping with the stress of the disease (e.g., through denial or avoidance) is more likely to result in more compromised quality of life (36). Patients who are willing and able to engage in self-care (e.g., keeping their wounds clean) are more likely to experience reductions in their overall level of anxiety, at least in the initial post-operative adjustment period (37). Whatever the coping style of the patient, the challenges of living with changes in appearance and function are quite profound (38–39).

Importantly, patient perceptions of the quality of life outcomes are not necessarily correlated with clinician perceptions of quality of life (40). This finding underscores the need to explicitly ask patients about their experiences with head and neck cancer. Additionally, the experience of partners of facial cancer patients may also be quite different than that of the patient, with partners, at times, reporting greater levels of distress (31). Finally, all facial cancer patients obviously have the specter of cancer recurrence, which can clearly affect quality of life. Head and neck cancer patients may experience such understandable fears more commonly than individuals with other forms of cancer (41).

Similar to other areas of research on gender differences in body image, women with facial cancers have a more difficult time adjusting to facial disfigurement than do men (42). Women frequently report higher levels of depression and lower levels of overall happiness, especially if they have greater disfigurement and lower levels of social support (29). Some patients with facial cancers are reluctant to undergo tumor resection out of fear of disfigurement.

PSYCHOSOCIAL RESPONSES COMMON TO PATIENTS WITH FACIAL TRAUMA AND FACIAL CANCER

The review of the scholarship regarding psychosocial adaptation to acquired facial disfigurement presented thus far emphasized the unique characteristics of the facial trauma and facial cancer populations. However, concerns that many patients with all forms of acquired facial disfigurement may have in common, include (i) challenges in social functioning; (ii) body image adaptation; (iii) depression; (iv) alcohol related problems; and (v) the possibility for psychological growth related to acquiring a facial disfigurement.

Additionally, in this section, practical suggestions for identifying the psychological concerns of patients with acquired facial disfigurement (beyond the PTSD and neuropsychological issues discussed above) are provided. The primary goal of the screening process is to determine if there are significant psychosocial problems affecting quality of life. If no such (or minimal) problems are evident, then the plastic surgery treatment team can exclusively focus on the patient's surgical rehabilitation. However, if significant psychosocial problems are observed, the plastic surgery team ideally should provide appropriate feedback to the patient regarding how psychological factors can influence quality of life and be prepared to provide referrals to mental health professionals. Many patients struggling with the psychosocial aspects of rehabilitation will never seek help for such problems until and unless given assistance by the plastic surgery team.

Questionnaire 8-2 at the end of this chapter provides the plastic surgery team with a written series of questions that they can routinely administer to patients to screen for potential psychosocial problems. It addresses the primary areas of concern reviewed in this section of the chapter including questions related to problems in social functioning, body image adaptation, depression, and alcohol abuse.

Challenges in Social Functioning

The greatest psychosocial challenge for most patients with any kind of facial disfigurement is learning to cope with the social response to their facial appearance (43–47). It is quite likely that neither patients nor their families will spontaneously report these difficulties to the plastic surgery team. Nevertheless, the plastic surgery team can be certain that many patients with facial disfigurement are regularly struggling with the stress of routine violations of their social privacy as well as constant strain in their social relations.

Macgregor studied the adaptation of individuals with facial disfigurement for over 40 years and vividly described the social experience of these patients. "In their efforts to go about their daily affairs they are subjected to visual and verbal assaults and a level of familiarity from strangers . . . [including] naked stares, startle reactions, 'double takes,' whispering, remarks, furtive looks, curiosity, personal questions, advice, manifestations of pity or aversion, laughter, ridicule, and outright avoidance. Whatever form the behaviors may take, they generate feelings of shame, impotence, anger, and humiliation in their victims" (46, p. 250).

For many individuals, these constant social challenges inevitably and eventually lead to social withdrawal. Many disfigured individuals narrowly limit their range of social interactions to immediate family members and to those social contacts required for occupational functioning. In its most extreme form, social withdrawal can result in what Macgregor (45) has termed "social death."

On the basis of 40-plus years of intensive qualitative research Macgregor observed, counterintuitively, that individuals with more severe forms of facial disfigurement often have an easier time adapting to social interactions than individuals with less marked forms of disfigurement. Those with obvious disfigurements are able to reliably predict the social response to their facial appearance. They can definitely expect a negative response. However, individuals with less obvious forms of disfigurement are never sure if their disfigurement will provoke a negative social response. As a result, they experience a persistent sense of uncertainty and unpredictability in social situations, which inevitably results in heightened anxiety and social tension.

Several extensive assessment tools have been designed to assess social functioning, including those specific to living with facial disfigurement (48). In the context of the plastic surgery consultation the assessment of social functioning should be rather brief and pointed. The questionnaire presented in Questionnaire 8-2 asks patients to report their greatest difficulties in coping with their changed appearance in an open-ended manner. We also have adapted eight items from Cash's Body Image Quality of Life Inventory (described in detail in Chapter 4), four of which specifically address social functioning.

Body Image Adaptation

Whereas we have learned a great deal about the body image concerns of cosmetic surgery patients over the past decade (Chapters 14–16), we know far less about the body image issues of patients with acquired facial disfigurement (1). Individuals with an acquired facial disfigurement likely experience a long-term and ever-evolving process of body image adaptation that significantly affects their quality of life (1,49). Many variables influence this adaptation including factors related to the individuals' predisfigurement body image and overall psychological functioning, the patients' gender and culture, as well as the nature and extent of disfigurement (e.g., the cause, location, and degree of disfigurement) and surgical reconstruction (1). These issues are discussed in detail in Chapter 4 as well as the work of White (50–51) and Rumsey et al. (52).

In one of the few empirical studies examining body image, Levine et al. (8) found that facial trauma patients, as compared to control subjects, reported higher rates of negative body image thoughts, although they did not rate their overall body image more negatively nor did they report greater body image dysphoria in social situations. These patients also did not rate themselves as being less attractive posttrauma, even though they were rated as less attractive by lay and physician observers.

The body image concerns of disfigured people, like the body image concerns of most individuals, likely fall on a continuum (2). This continuum ranges from those having "no psychological concerns" to those patients who have an "extreme" level of body image concern. In the middle of this continuum are those patients who have what are best labeled as having a "normative" or "average" degree of body image concern. Those patients who fall into the middle of the continuum are likely to be the vast majority of individuals who present for reconstructive surgery. They are able to function normally and yet still experience some body image experiences that negatively affect their quality of life (e.g., periodic self-consciousness).

This "middle" group of patients is perhaps better understood by understanding the poles of the continuum. On the "positive" pole of the continuum are those individuals who have acquired a facial disfigurement but who have "no discernible body image concerns." These are patients who despite having objective disfigurement resulting from facial trauma or facial cancer report having no significant concerns regarding their appearance. This may be the result of psychological denial, a lack of investment in their facial appearance, or a deep appreciation of the "good" that has been able to come from the disfigurement (2), a phenomena discussed later. The "negative" pole of the body image concern continuum is characterized by those individuals who have an "extreme" level of body image concern that significantly affects their overall quality of life. Such individuals are likely to be experiencing a range of mental health problems that are clearly evident to the plastic surgery treatment team. Such individuals require mental health intervention.

Cash has developed many psychometrically sound measures of body image functioning. Several of these are detailed in Chapter 4 and can be of use in the assessment of persons with a facial disfigurement. In the context of routine screening of patients with acquired facial disfigurement, we recommend using the eight items from the Body Image Quality of Life Inventory (BIQLI) (53) mentioned earlier and reprinted in Questionnaire 8-2. Routinely reviewing patient responses to these eight items provides a method by which the plastic surgery team can refine their understanding of the continuum of patients' body image concerns and can provide a basis for initiating a conversation regarding referral for psychological rehabilitation for those patients who express body image concerns. This brief body image assessment, conducted preoperatively and postoperatively, can also provide a method for measuring the psychological effects of surgical reconstruction.

Depression

There is a considerable body of empirical data and clinical experience pointing to the occurrence of depression in the context of medical illness in general (54) and in cancer specifically (55). Though there has been minimal research done on people with acquired facial disfigurement, there is reason to believe that these individuals are at some increased risk for experiencing depression (56–57). However, the challenge, even for specifically trained mental health professionals, is to differentially diagnose clinical depression from a range of other reactions that individuals with an acquired facial disfigurement may experience. These reactions may include normative sadness, grief over the losses they have experienced, reactions to medications they may be taking, and fatigue that results from treatment, among other variables. Depression can obviously dramatically undermine the patient's (and family's) quality of life. Depression also places the patient at increased risk for suicide. Additionally, patients who are depressed are less likely to comply with the medical treatment recommendations of the plastic surgery team. It is fair to say that the experience of depression will compromise, in significant ways, the ability of the patient to maximize their rehabilitation.

The plastic surgery treatment team can provide at least a rudimentary screening for depressive symptoms. Though there are important differences in opinion regarding the most efficacious form of assessment, it is reasonable to use a brief screening measure (58). Therefore, in Questionnaire 8-2 we have included three items assessing three common symptoms of depression (change in mood, change in sleeping patterns, and thoughts of suicide). If the patient reports experiencing these symptoms, the plastic surgery team can inquire about them and decide if a referral for mental health consultation is needed.

Alcohol-related Problems

It is important to assess the alcohol use of patients who have sustained facial trauma (3,8) as well as those who have head and neck cancer (33). More than half of the patients with orofacial injuries in one study had symptoms of alcohol-related problems while approximately 31% reported problems indicative of alcohol dependence (3). Compared to a matched control group, these patients were "five times more likely" to have clinically significant problems with alcohol. Levine et al. (8) documented similar findings in their study of facial trauma patients. Additionally, alcohol abuse is a well-known and significant cause of some forms of head and neck cancer (33). Therefore, for some patients in the acquired facial disfigurement population there is reason to assess if pre-existing alcohol-related problems existed. Other patients may use alcohol in an attempt to cope with the range of emotions and problems that can emerge subsequent to their disfigurement. Continued alcohol use and abuse may adversely affect the surgical treatment and rehabilitation of the patient as they go through the process of surgical reconstruction.

A common clinical method for screening patients for alcohol-related problems is via use of the CAGE questions (59), which we have incorporated into Questionnaire 8-2. These four questions request that patients report their experience of **C**utting down on their use of alcohol (Have you ever felt that you should cut down on your drinking of alcohol?); their feelings of **A**nnoyance when criticized for their alcohol use (Have people annoyed you by criticizing your drinking of alcohol?); their feelings of **G**uilt about drinking alcohol (Have you felt bad or guilty about your drinking of alcohol?) as well as their use of alcohol upon awakening from sleep (i.e., consuming an **E**ye opener; Do you ever have a drink of alcohol when you first get up from sleeping in order to steady your nerves?). A positive (yes) answer to any one of these questions is cause for a discussion of the role that alcohol may play in the patient's overall rehabilitation.

Post-disfigurement Psychological Growth

When discussing psychological responses to acquired facial disfigurement it is easy to exclusively focus on the range of negative psychological responses that patients may experience. However, it is important to reiterate that these negative psychological responses are not evident in all patients. Additionally, there is now a compelling and ever-growing body of scientific literature documenting psychological growth in response to highly traumatic experiences (60–61).

In the context of congenital facial disfigurement, Eiserman (62) has described with great eloquence and insight the fact that facial disfigurement, in addition to the suffering we assume to be inherent in the experience, can result in often unexpected and profoundly deep "blessings in disguise." It is important to note that, at least to our knowledge, there is not any empirical documentation of these types of responses in patients with acquired facial disfigurement. However, it has been clearly evident in our personal contact with some individuals who have sustained a facial disfigurement. While more attention needs to be given to evaluating and treating the suffering of patients with acquired facial disfigurement, it should also be kept in mind that some patients will demonstrate not only remarkable resilience, but also growth in the face of their experience.

CASE EXAMPLES

The following case examples are illustrative of many of the psychological issues outlined above.

Case 1: Mr. Smith: Facial Trauma

Mr. Smith is a 42-year-old European–American male who experienced a facial trauma involving the upper third of his face while working as a self-employed mason. He sustained a comminuted fracture of the outer table of the frontal sinus with gross contour deformity and sustained soft tissue injuries that included a complex 10-cm laceration with some soft tissue loss. He had no loss of consciousness, had a Glasgow Coma Scale of 15 at all times, and experienced no brain trauma. His soft tissue lacerations were repaired in the emergency room. The following day after fine cut axial and coronal CT scanning was performed, Mr. Smith was taken to the operating room for repair of the fractured frontal bone. His postoperative course was uneventful and he was discharged from the hospital and returned home. At no time was there any evidence of postconcussive symptoms.

Mr. Smith was interviewed 18 months after he sustained his facial trauma and had undergone his initial reconstruction. Mr. Smith believed that prior to the trauma he was "average" in appearance. After the trauma he felt that he was moderately disfigured and found himself assessing his appearance in the mirror much more often. A lay panel and a panel of physicians who assessed his pretrauma and posttrauma photos concurred that his appearance had changed from not disfigured to being moderately disfigured. Furthermore, he has consulted a plastic and reconstructive surgeon for possible scar revision. He was concerned about the cost and had not yet made a decision about revising his scar.

Mr. Smith has reported that although he had fully physically healed by about 6 weeks after his injury, he was depressed about his appearance, was concerned that it might change the relationship with his spouse, and had begun fighting with his wife and children. Prior to the trauma he stated that his relationship with his family was close and strong. He also reported that it was only after marital and family counseling that he was able to reconcile with his family.

There are many possible explanations for Mr. Smith's psychological changes postinjury. One of these was his concern for his appearance, which was quite marked. He also reported an extended period of being out of work. He indicated that the longer that he was out of work, the more depressed he became, which in turn made it still harder to return to work. He also reported that his level of alcohol consumption increased significantly after his injury and that this caused problems for him.

Mr. Smith believes that his work-related injury significantly impacted his life. He feels that the trauma itself was mildly disruptive, but that the subsequent events severely damaged his relationship with his wife, hurt him financially, and endangered his well-being and social standing. While his relationship with his family has been rebuilt, he believes that it will never be like before. Nevertheless, it is clear that this patient, while experiencing significant psychological disruption posttrauma, has benefited from his reconstructive surgery and has been able to return to a reasonable level of functioning.

Case 2: Mrs. Smith: Facial Cancer

Mrs. Smith is a 49-year-old European–American woman with a recurrent morpheiform basal cell carcinoma in her right nasolabial fold. She had previously undergone two resections of this tumor over the course of the previous 5 years. At the time of this surgical consultation the lesion was approximately 2 cm in diameter.

Mrs. Smith was previously a fashion model and is currently married to a high ranking official in a foreign government. While she was understandably motivated to remove the cancer from her face she also was very fearful of the disfigurement that might result from aggressive surgical excision. She reported that she recognized that her concerns about her appearance were "superficial," but she had used her beauty to get along in the world for so long, that she felt that compromise of this might negatively affect her quality of life as well as her marriage.

Mrs. Smith readily recognized that she needed to have the tumor removed because the consequences of not having it excised could ultimately result in much worse facial disfigurement, and, in the worst case scenario, threaten her life. She indicated, with some trepidation and apparent guilt, that her concerns about her appearance may have negatively influenced her former surgeon into doing less than what was necessary to eradicate the tumor at the time of the previous excisions.

She achieved an excellent cosmetic result and has resumed her preoperative lifestyle with no apparent major disruption or distress. However, as would be expected of most females with similar types of scars, she used makeup to lessen their visibility. Overall, here again, the patient benefited greatly from the surgical skills of the plastic surgery team as well as the sensitive management of the patient's anxiety and preoperative concerns. However, it is easy to imagine that she would have had a much more difficult postoperative had her surgical outcome not been less than ideal.

GENERAL PRINCIPLES OF PSYCHOLOGICAL MANAGEMENT

Pruzinsky and Edgerton (63) presented some general principles for the psychological management of patients undergoing reconstructive surgery that are helpful to reiterate here, including (i) setting realistic surgical expectations; (ii) assessing and addressing each patient's unique concerns; and (iii) developing and refining a range of responses to patients' psychological concerns.

Set Realistic Surgical Expectations

The plastic surgery team needs to do whatever is necessary to allow the patients and families to create realistic expectations for the anticipated surgical outcome. The team should be as clear as possible regarding the length of time it will take to "complete" the reconstruction, the total number of surgeries anticipated, as well as how much pain and life disruption will likely occur.

Assess and Address Each Patient's Unique Concerns

One of the most important contributions that the plastic surgery team can make to the care of patients is to take time to closely listen to their unique concerns, and those of their family members, about the surgery, the outcome of surgery, or their experience living with disfigurement. In the time-pressured practice of medicine today, one of the greatest gifts that health care providers can give to patients and families is their full and undivided attention. What is needed is an understanding of each patient's unique concerns so that these can be addressed.

Develop a Range of Responses to Patient's Psychological Distress

Many patients require little by way of extra psychological care from the plastic surgery team other than the routine attention given to providing adequate informed consent and clear communication regarding surgical planning. However, there are others who are considerably more anxious and who benefit from extra time, attention, and reassurance from the plastic surgery team. The plastic surgery team is clearly able, in most instances, to adequately respond to the needs of these patients.

However, problems can arise when it becomes evident that a particular patient is in need of mental health consultation. The team members do not want to offend the patient by making such a referral and are often uncomfortable broaching the topic. Three specific points will help make it easier for the team to make this kind of referral: (i) provide an explanation to the patient that having acquired a facial disfigurement places an unusual burden of stress on the patient and the family, even if the disfigurement is quite modest in nature; (ii) make it clear to the patient that the symptoms they are experiencing can be addressed, just like any other problem, by seeking out the help of an expert in that area; and (iii) identifying a trusted mental health professional as a consultant. (Chapter 16 also provides suggestions for making referrals to mental health professionals.)

PSYCHOSOCIAL REHABILITATION AND TREATMENT

A major premise of this chapter is that there is help we can offer individuals with acquired facial disfigurement if they encounter psychosocial challenges during the course of their rehabilitation. It is heartening that there has been some progress made in addressing the specific psychosocial concerns of individuals with facial disfigurement, including (i) addressing the critical need for social skills development to learn how to adaptively cope with persistently negative social response to disfigured individuals (64); (ii) applying the particularly efficacious cognitive-behavioral forms of intervention to the specific concerns of those living with disfigurement (65); (iii) developing and disseminating effective psycho-educational materials (66–68); (iv) providing important connections to our current knowledge of body image adaptation (69–70); (v) developing forms of assessment that can identify those patients who have concerns regarding their appearance (48); and (vi) enlisting the involvement of nursing professionals (71) in addressing the concerns of these individuals. In sum, there is growing empirical documentation for relatively brief psychosocial interventions to have a significantly positive effect on increasing the overall quality of life of patients with facial disfigurement.

Additionally, there is still a great deal of work to be done to make these kinds of resources routinely available to patients with acquired disfigurement. Providing these services are not currently a part of the standard of care for patients in most countries, although, they appear to be somewhat more common in the U.K. Furthermore, it is critically important to develop a better understanding of the willingness of patients with acquired facial disfigurement to engage in an active program of psychosocial rehabilitation. The social stigma attached to psychological services that still exists for many people may prevent those who may benefit from partaking of these services. To maximize patient participation in such programs we believe it is essential that the provision of psychosocial services be "framed" in terms of rehabilitation interventions specifically designed to cope with the consequences of the facial disfigurement in contrast to being presented to patients as "psychological services" for individuals who have psychiatric problems.

CONCLUSIONS

In conclusion, it is imperative to emphasize that the most important ways in which the plastic surgery treatment team can enhance patients' psychosocial rehabilitation is to become familiar with the published empirical and clinical literature on the psychosocial adaptation process of patients with acquired facial disfigurement. This will help to make it clear that a significant number of these patients are suffering, for the most, in silence. It is also important to routinely ask patients how they are coping with the changes that have occurred since the change in their facial appearance, and, if possible, to also have a sense of the family's view of this adaptation process. Contact with the plastic surgery team is likely the only way that the vast majority of patients will ever have to address their quality of life concerns. Finally, the single most important step that plastic surgery treatment teams can make to ensure that their patients attain the highest level of psychosocial rehabilitation is to develop a consistent and trusting relationship with a mental health professional to whom you can confidently and enthusiastically refer your patients. Becoming comfortable with the process of referral, treating it is a regular part of your practice, and obtaining feedback on the efficacy of these referrals, over time, will build confidence in the unique role that these consultations can play in maximizing the patient's overall level of rehabilitation and quality of life.

Quality of Life Assessment for Patients Sustaining Facial Trauma

In relation to your facial injury, have you ever had any of the following experiences during the past month?[a]

1. Have had nightmares about it or thought about it when you did not want to?
   Yes   No

2. Tried hard not to think about it or went out of your way to avoid situations that reminded you of it?
   Yes   No

3. Were constantly on guard, watchful, or easily startled?
   Yes   No

4. Felt numb or detached from others, activities, or your surroundings?
   Yes   No

Since the time my face was injured I have noticed that:

■ I have more frequent headaches	Yes	No	Not Sure
■ I have ringing in my ears	Yes	No	Not Sure
■ I feel sick to my stomach more often	Yes	No	Not Sure
■ I feel dizzy more often	Yes	No	Not Sure
■ I have double vision	Yes	No	Not Sure
■ My thinking seems slower than it used to be	Yes	No	Not Sure
■ My concentration is not as good as it was	Yes	No	Not Sure
■ My memory is not a good as it used to be	Yes	No	Not Sure
■ I seem to be more disorganized	Yes	No	Not Sure
■ I feel sadder than I used to	Yes	No	Not Sure
■ I am more anxious than I used to be	Yes	No	Not Sure
■ I am more irritable	Yes	No	Not Sure
■ I am more impatient	Yes	No	Not Sure

[a](PTSD Screen [Primary Care-PTSD] developed and published by The National Center for PTSD. Items reprinted by permission from: http://www.ncptsd.org/facts/disasters/fs_screen_disaster.html)

General Quality of Life Assessment

Name: _____

We are interested to know how your quality of life has been affected by the changes in your appearance that have brought you to see the plastic surgeon. Please complete the following questions so that we can better serve you.

■ For me, the hardest part of experiencing the change in my facial appearance has been . . .

_____
_____
_____

■ Since the change in the appearance of my face, the people who know me best would say that the hardest part of this experience for me has been . . . .

_____
_____
_____

Different people have different feelings about their physical appearance. Some people are generally satisfied with their looks, while others are dissatisfied. Listed below are various ways that your facial appearance may influence your life. For each item, circle how much your feelings about your appearance affect that aspect of your life.

−3	−2	−1	0	+1	+2	+3
Very Negative Effect	Moderate Negative Effect	Slight Negative Effect	No Effect	Slight Positive Effect	Moderate Positive Effect	Very Positive Effect

■ How confident I feel in my everyday life. −3 −2 −1 0 +1 +2 +3
■ How happy I feel in my everyday life. −3 −2 −1 0 +1 +2 +3
■ My basic feelings about myself—feelings of self-worth. −3 −2 −1 0 +1 +2 +3
■ My experiences when I meet new people. −3 −2 −1 0 +1 +2 +3
■ My experiences at work or at school. −3 −2 −1 0 +1 +2 +3
■ My relationships with friends. −3 −2 −1 0 +1 +2 +3
■ My relationships with family members. −3 −2 −1 0 +1 +2 +3
■ My day-to-day emotions. −3 −2 −1 0 +1 +2 +3

During the past two weeks:
■ I have felt sad/blue. Often Sometimes Never
■ I have had difficulty sleeping. Often Sometimes Never
■ I have had thoughts of suicide. Often Sometimes Never

(continued)

QUESTIONNAIRE 8-2 *(continued)*

During my life I have had treatment for the following emotional problems.

■ Depression	Yes	No
■ Anxiety	Yes	No
■ Substance abuse	Yes	No
■ Have you ever felt that you should cut down on your drinking of alcohol?	Yes	No
■ Have people annoyed you by criticizing your drinking of alcohol?	Yes	No
■ Have you felt bad or guilty about your drinking of alcohol?	Yes	No
■ Do you ever have a drink of alcohol when you first get up from sleeping in order to steady your nerves?	Yes	No

The last four items above are reprinted from Ewing JA. Detecting Alcoholism: The CAGE Questionnaire. *JAMA* 1984;252:1905–1907.

REFERENCES

1. Pruzinsky T. Body image adaptation to reconstructive surgery for acquired disfigurement. In: Cash TF, Pruzinsky T, eds. *Body Image: Handbook of Theory, Research, and Clinical Practice.* New York: Guilford Press, 2002:440–449.
2. Pruzinsky T. Enhancing quality of life in medical populations: a vision for body image assessment and rehabilitation as standards of care. *Body Image: An International Journal of Research.* 2004;1:71–81.
3. Shetty V, Glynn S, Brown KE. Psychosocial sequelae and correlates of orofacial injury. *Dent Clin North Am* 2003;47:141–157.
4. Lento J, Glynn S, Shetty V, et al. Psychologic functioning and needs of indigent patients with facial injury: a prospective controlled study. *J Oral Maxillofac Surg* 2004;62:925–932.
5. Shepherd JP, Qureshi R, Preston MS. Psychological distress after assaults and accidents. *BMJ* 1990;301:849–850.
6. Laski R, Ziccardi VB, Broder HL, et al. Facial trauma: a recurrent disease? The potential role of disease prevention. *J Oral Maxillofac Surg* 2004;62:685–688.
7. Girotto JA, MacKenzie E, Fowler C, et al. Long-term physical impairment and functional outcomes after complex facial fractures. *Plast Reconst Surg* 2001;108:312–327.
8. Levine E, Degutis L, Pruzinsky T, et al. Quality of life and facial trauma: psychological and body image effects. *Ann Plast Surg* 2005;54:502–510.
9. Rumsey N, Clarke A, White P, et al. Altered body image: appearance related concerns of people with visible disfigurement. *J Adv Nurs* 2004;43:23–27.
10. Thompson A, Kent G. Adjusting to disfigurement: processes involved in dealing with being visibly different. *Clin Psychol Rev* 2001;21:663–682.
11. Tebble NJ, Thomas DW, Price P. Anxiety and self-consciousness in patients with minor facial lacerations. *J Adv Nurs* 2004;47:417–426.
12. American Psychiatric Association. *The Diagnostic and Statistical Manual of Mental Disorders-TR.* Washington, DC: American Psychiatric Association, 2000.
13. Bisson JI, Shepherd JP, Dhutia M. Psychological sequelae of facial trauma. *J Trauma* 1997;43:496–500.
14. Glynn SM, Asarnow JR, Asarnow R, et al. The development of acute post-traumatic stress disorder after orofacial injury: a prospective study in a large urban hospital. *J Oral Maxillofac Surg* 2003;61:785–792.
15. Rusch MD, Grunert BK, Sanger JR, et al. Psychological adjustment in children after traumatic disfiguring injuries: a 12-month follow-up. *Plast Reconstr Surg* 2000;106:1451–1458.
16. Hohlrieder M, Hinterhoelzl J, Ulmer H. Maxillofacial fractures masking traumatic intracranial hemorrhages. *Int J Oral Maxillofac Surg* 2004;33:389–395.
17. Ozolins M, Parsons O, Ozolins D. Postconcussive symptoms in craniofacial trauma. *J Craniomaxillofac Trauma* 1996;2:8–13.
18. Teasdale G, Jennett B. Assessment of coma and impaired consciousness: a practical scale. *Lancet* 1974;2:81–84.
19. Gronwall D. Behavioral assessment during the acute stages of traumatic brain injury. In: Lezak MD, ed. *Assessment of the Behavioral Consequences of Head Trauma.* New York: Alan R. Liss, 1989:19–36.
20. Smith RJ, Barth JT, Diamond R. Evaluation of head trauma. In: Goldstein G, Nussbaum PD, Beers SR, eds. *Neuropsychology.* New York: Kluwer Academic Publishers, 1998:135–170.
21. Broshek DK, Seegmiller RA, Diamond R, et al. The neuropsychological sequelae and assessment of head trauma. In: Anchor KA, Felicetti TC, eds. *Disability Analysis in Practice: Framework for an Interdisciplinary Science.* Dubuque, IA: Kendall/Hunt, 1998:131–158.
22. Barth JT, Freeman JR, Winters JE. Management of sports-related concussions. *Adv Sports Dentistry* 2000;44:67–83.
23. Alves WM, Macciocchi SN, Barth JT. Post concussion symptoms after uncomplicated mild head injury. *J Head Trauma Rehabil* 1993;8:48–59.
24. Hughes MJ. *The Social Consequences of Facial Disfigurement.* Brookfield, VT: Ashgate Publishing, 1998.
25. Pruzinsky T. Psychosocial aspects of facial deformity for advanced skin cancer of the head and neck. In: Weber RS, Miller M, Goepfert H, eds. *Basal and Squamous Cell Skin Cancers of the Head and Neck.* Philadelphia: Lea & Febiger, 1994.
26. Grealy L. *Autobiography of a Face.* Boston: Houghton Mifflin, 1994.
27. Piff C. *Let's Face It.* London, England: Victor Gollancz, 1985.
28. Piff C. A patient's perspective: living with facial cancer. *J Tissue Viability* 2001;11:64–66.
29. Newell R. Psychological difficulties amongst plastic surgery ex-patients following surgery to the face: *Br J Plastic Surg* 2000;53: 386–392.
30. List MA, Lee Rutherford J, Stracks J, et al. An exploration of the pretreatment coping strategies of patients with carcinoma of the head and neck. *Cancer* 2002;9:98–104.
31. Vickery LE, Latchford G, Hewison J, et al. The impact of head and neck cancer and facial disfigurement on the quality of life of patients and their partners. *Head Neck* 2003;25: 289–296.
32. Rybarczyk BD, Behel M. Rehabilitation medicine and body image. In: Cash TF, Pruzinsky T, eds. *Body Image: A Handbook of Theory, Research and Clinical Practice.* New York: Guilford Press, 2002:387–394.
33. Aarstad HJ, Aarstad AK, Birkhaug EJ, et al. The personality and quality of life in HNSCC patients following treatment. *Eur J Cancer* 2003;39:1852–1860.
34. Aarstad HJ, Heimdal JH, Aarsta AKH, et al. Personality traits in head and neck squamous cell carcinoma patients in relation to the disease state, disease extent and prognosis. *Acta Otolaryngol* 2002;122:892–899.
35. Moadel AB, Ostroff JS, Shantz SP. Head and neck cancer. In: J Holland, ed. *Psychooncology* London, England: Oxford University Press, 1999:314–323.
36. Baker CA. Factors associated with rehabilitation in head and neck cancer. *Cancer Nurs* 1992;15:395–400.
37. Dropkin MJ. Anxiety, coping strategies, and coping behaviors in patients undergoing head and neck cancer surgery. *Cancer Nurs* 2001;24:143–148.

38. Dropkin MJ. Body image and quality of life after head and neck cancer surgery. *Cancer Pract* 1999;7:309–313.
39. Dropkin MJ. Coping with disfigurement/dysfunction and length of hospital stay after head and neck cancer surgery. *ORL Head Neck Nurs* 1997;15:22–26.
40. Kwok HC, Morton RP, Chaplin JM, et al. Quality of life after parotid and temporal bone surgery for cancer. *Laryngoscope* 2002;112:820–833.
41. Humphris GM, Rogers S, McNally D, et al. Fear of recurrence and possible cases of anxiety and depression in orofacial cancer patients. *Int J Oral Maxillofac Surg* 2003;32:486–491.
42. Katz MR, Irish JC, Devins GM, et al. Psychosocial adjustment in head and neck cancer: the impact of disfigurement, gender and social support. *Head Neck* 2003;25:103–112.
43. Lansdown R, Rumsey N, Bradbury E, et al. *Visibly Different: Coping with Disfigurement.* Oxford, England: Butterworth-Heinemann, 1997.
44. Macgregor FC. *Transformation and Identity the Face and Plastic Surgery.* New York: New York Times Book Company, 1974.
45. Macgregor FC. *After Plastic Surgery: Adaptation and Adjustment.* New York: Praeger Publishers, 1979.
46. Macgregor FC. Facial disfigurement: problems and management of social interaction and implications for mental health. *Aesthetic Plast Surg* 1990;14:249–257.
47. Rankin M, Borah GL. Perceived functional impact of abnormal facial appearance. *Plast Reconstr Surg* 2003;14:2140–2146.
48. Carr A, Harris D, James C. The Derriford Appearance Scale: a new scale to measure individual responses to living with problems of appearance. *Br J Health Psychol* 2000; 5;201–215.
49. Sarwer DB, Whitaker LA, Pertshuk MJ, et al. Body image concerns of reconstructive surgery patients: an under recognized problem. *Ann Plast Surg* 1998;40:403–407.
50. White CA. Body image dimensions and cancer: a heuristic cognitive-behavioural model. *Psychooncology* 2000; 9:183–192.
51. White CA. Body images in oncology. In: Cash TF, Pruzinsky T, eds. *Body Image: A Handbook of Theory, Research and Clinical Practice.* New York: Guilford Press, 2002:379–386.
52. Rumsey N, Harcourt D. Body image and disfigurement: issues and interventions. *Body Image: An International Journal of Research.* 2004:1,83–97.
53. Cash TF, Fleming EC. The impact of body image experiences: development of the Body Image Quality of Life Inventory. *Intl J Eating Disord* 2002;31:455–460.
54. Palmer SC, Coyne JC. Screening for depression in medical care: pitfalls, alternatives and revised priorities. *J Psychosom Res* 2003;54:279–287.
55. Trask PC. Assessment of depression in cancer patients. *J Natl Cancer Inst Monogr* 2004;32:80–92.
56. Rumsey N, Clarke A, White P. Exploring the psychosocial concerns of outpatients with disfiguring conditions. *J Wound Care* 2003;12:247–252.
57. Katz MR, Kopek N, Waldron J, et al. Screening for depression in head and neck cancer. *Psychooncology* 2003;13: 269–280.
58. Berwick DM, Murphy JM, Goldman PA, et al. Performance of a five-item mental health screening test. *Med Care* 1991;29:169–176.
59. Ewing JA. Detecting alcoholism: The CAGE Questionnaire. *JAMA* 1984;252:1905–1907.
60. Cordova MJ, Cunningham LLC, Carlson CR, et al. Posttraumatic growth following breast cancer: a controlled comparison study. *Health Psychol* 2001;20:176–185.
61. Brickman P, Coates D, Janoff-Bulman R. Lottery winners and accident victims: is happiness relative? *J Pers and Soc Psych* 1978;36:917–927.
62. Eiserman W. Unique outcomes and positive contributions associated with facial difference: expanding research and practice. *Cleft Palate Craniofac J* 2000;38:236–244.
63. Pruzinsky T, Edgerton MT. Psychological understanding and management of the plastic surgery patient. In: Georgiade NG, Georgiade GS, Riefkohl R, Barwick WJ, eds. *Essentials of Plastic, Maxillofacial, and Reconstructive Surgery.* Baltimore: Williams & Wilkins, 1997.
64. Robinson E, Rumsey N, Partridge J. An evaluation of the impact of social interaction skills training for facially disfigured people. *Br J Plast Surg* 1996;49:281–289.
65. Kleve L, Rumsey N, Wyn-Williams M, et al. The effectiveness of cognitive-behavioural intervention provided at outlook: a disfigurement support unit. *J Eval Clin Practice* 2002;8:387–395.
66. Changing Faces. *Facing Disfigurement with Confidence.* London, England: Changing Faces, 2001.
67. Clarke A. Managing the psychological aspects of altered appearance: the development of an information resource for people with disfiguring conditions. *Patient Educ Couns* 2001;43:305–309.
68. Newell R, Clarke M. Evaluation of a self-help leaflet in treatment of social difficulties following facial disfigurement. *Int J Nurs Stud* 2000;37:381–388.
69. Rumsey N. Body image and congenital conditions with visible differences. In: Cash TF, Pruzinsky T, eds. *Body Image: Handbook of Theory, Research, and Clinical Practice.* New York: Guilford Press, 2002:226–233.
70. Rumsey N. Optimizing body image in disfiguring congenital conditions: surgical and psychosocial interventions, In: Cash TF, Pruzinsky T, eds. *Body Image: Handbook of Theory, Research, and Clinical Practice.* New York: Guilford Press, 2002:431–439.
71. Clarke A, Cooper C. Psychological rehabilitation after disfiguring injury or disease: investigating the training needs of specialist nurses. *J Adv Nurs* 2001;3;18–26.

Chapter 9

Hand Trauma

Brad K. Grunert, PhD

In the United States, there are approximately 16 million hand injuries every year (1–2). Of these injuries, 16,000 result in amputations of digits, hands, or arms (2). In addition, many other hand traumas result in loss of function due to crushes, nerve lacerations and transections, and significant scarring. Hand injuries are often both functionally and psychologically devastating.

Several factors contribute to the psychological sequelae of hand injuries. Hands are the individual's primary means of interacting with the world. They are critical to both accomplishing tasks and interacting socially. Our hands, unlike our faces, are almost constantly in our line of vision and, thus, have a high degree of salience in one's day-to-day life. For an individual with a hand injury, it is nearly impossible to avoid viewing the disfigured hand, which is a different experience than, for example, someone with a disfigurement of the body or even the face. Mutilating hand injuries often produce functional and cosmetic deficits that can be overwhelming for the individual experiencing them.

Family members and associates may become guarded, self-conscious, or overly protective of the individual with the injury. The disfigured hand is obvious to most people who come in contact with the affected individual, as the hand is a "public" part of the body rarely concealed. In addition to the clumsiness or altered function created by the injury to the hand, public exposure of the mutilated extremity creates a situation in which the individual is repeatedly called upon to explain how the injury occurred by many individuals who are, at best, only casually known by the injured person. Friends and family often move into a protective role by buffering these interactions that can further contribute to the loss of personal efficacy. The loss of efficacy is magnified by the fact that the individual's capacity to engage in skilled and habitual tasks is compromised by the functional deficits secondary to the injury. The performance of these activities in public often draws even further attention to the injured extremity, resulting in even greater feelings of stigmatization and social conspicuousness. In the most extreme cases, onlookers may respond with socially inappropriate comments regarding the appearance of the hand, with looks of horror or revulsion, or with staring at the injured extremity. Each of these reactions serves to further alienate and ostracize the injured individual.

This chapter will review the psychological aspects of traumatic hand injuries. The first part will discuss the most frequently occurring psychological reactions to these injuries. As compared to other areas of plastic surgery discussed in this book, the empirical literature in this area is currently less well developed. The second half of the chapter draws heavily from clinical experience and discusses the psychological management and treatment of patients who suffer these often devastating and disruptive injuries.

Psychological and Behavioral Symptom Patterns

The psychological sequelae of hand injuries have been described in the hand surgery literature for over 25 years (3–9). Many of these factors can be understood in the context of Post Traumatic Stress Disorder (PTSD), which has emerged as the most frequent type of psychopathology associated with hand trauma (10–11).

PTSD is a well-defined disorder with a distinct pattern of symptoms. First, the individual must have been exposed to an event in which they experienced an injury or circumstance that threatened their bodily integrity or life. The second is that they experience repetitive reliving of the event in a distressing manner (i.e., flashbacks, nightmares). The third is that they avoid reminders of the event in order to prevent triggering of their flashbacks or nightmares. They also experience physiologic arousal including such symptoms as hyperarousal, hypervigilance, and concentration deficits. These symptoms must persist for at least 30 days and must be disruptive to the individuals' normal daily activities. (PTSD also has been discussed in Chapters 7 and 8). In addition, avoidance of work, appearance-related concerns, sleep disruption, pain, and impairments in social functioning postinjury are other significant psychological responses to hand trauma.

Flashbacks

Flashbacks associated with hand injuries can begin as early as 15 minutes after the injury and are one of the most common psychological responses to hand trauma (12). The occurrence of flashbacks appears to be related to attributions the patient makes regarding the cause of the injury. Individuals attributing their injuries to external causes over which they had little or no control were more likely to experience ongoing flashbacks, as well as avoidance of stimuli associated with the injury, than those believing that the cause of their injury was internal.

Both work-related and nonwork-related hand injury victims have been found to have similar rates of flashback occurrence in the emergency department immediately after their injuries (12). However, at a 6-month follow-up, the work-related patients had a significantly higher percentage of flashbacks than nonwork-related patients. Individuals injured in nonwork settings were much more likely to accept responsibility for being a causal agent of the accident than were the work-injured victims. Hand-injured workers who blamed their coworkers or their equipment for their injury were more likely to resist returning to their previous work than workers who judged themselves to be responsible for their accidents (13). Thus, attribution of cause of injury emerges as a key prognostic indicator for resumption of normal activities following hand injury.

There appear to be three distinct components of flashbacks following hand trauma: (i) replay; (ii) projected; and (iii) appraisal. They appear to be associated with postinjury prognosis.

Replay Flashbacks

The replay flashback consists of the replaying of the entire accident. The person experiencing this often visually re-experiences all of the images from the time of the accident. They may also experience auditory memories (e.g., the sound of their bones shattering), kinesthetic memories (e.g., the feeling of their hand trapped in the machine), and olfactory memories (e.g., the smell of their skin burning). Regardless of the nature of the memory stimuli, they re-experience the accident in a manner very similar to that in which it occurred. Individuals with this type of flashback are the most successful at processing it psychologically. They also returned to work at a much higher rate than did individuals having other types of flashback components (14).

Projected Flashbacks

In this type of flashback, the individual not only replays the flashback but also views a more catastrophic injury as occurring. For instance, the victim may replay an accident in which the finger of the hand was amputated. Rather than the injury flashback ending there, however, the images go on to ones in which the entire arm is pulled into the machine. This type of flashback is more complicated to treat as it involves not only desensitization to the injury that actually occurred, but also cognitive reprocessing of an accident component that never happened. The return to work success rate for these individuals was found to be lower than for those with replay flashbacks alone (14).

Appraisal Flashbacks

In this type of flashback, the individual experiences a snapshot-like recollection of the trauma, without all of the detail of the replay or projected flashback. This almost always consists of an image of the hand as it was first seen after the injury. This type of flashback is generally accompanied by feelings of horror and surreality. This flashback also may involve a projected element, in which the snapshot image of the injury transforms into an even more extensive and traumatic image.

Both the projected and appraisal flashback require much more complex psychological interventions. Imagery techniques used for intervention with these flashbacks are most successful when the patient is able to redevelop the context of the injury (i.e., create a replay-type flashback). Processing the feelings of surreality or dissociation is also necessary. These two types of flashbacks are the most resistant to treatment and have the poorest outcomes associated with them in terms of return to previous employment (14–15). Specific psychological interventions for dealing with these issues are discussed later in this chapter.

Avoidance

Avoidance symptoms are predictive of return to the activity at which one was injured. At the time of an initial evaluation conducted by a nurse in the emergency room, most injured workers felt that they would be able to return to work (12,15). This was also true for the nonwork-injured patients. At a 6-month follow-up, however, many of the work-injured patients no longer felt able to return to their previous jobs. This was not true for the nonwork-related individuals, the majority of whom reported no significant symptoms of avoidance.

One of the factors that may influence this outcome is the fact that the injured workers received compensation for their injuries. Because the patient is provided with a weekly monetary payment for their injury throughout the recovery time may suggest to the injured individual that someone else is culpable for the injury. Most patients fail to understand that the Workers Compensation system is a "no-fault" insurance (i.e., there is no blame assigned for the cause of the injury), which requires payment even if the injury was intentionally incurred by the worker. Therefore, such payments may create a degree of cognitive dissonance for the worker, which leads them to believe that they had little or no blame for the accident. That is, many feel absolved of blame by the mere fact that they are receiving compensation and, therefore, must have been injured through some form of negligence. This was seen in the pattern of attributions in workers, the majority of whom at 6 months postinjury, were attributing their injuries to external causes such as a lack of safety guards or improper maintenance on the machines on which they were injured. Individuals who suffered nonwork-related injuries displayed a much more stable pattern of attributions as to injury cause and were much more likely to accept personal responsibility for their injury.

Appearance-related Concerns

Regardless of the cause of the injury, concerns about appearance are a major factor in the long-term functioning of the hand-injured patient. Appearance deficits can be divided into two categories: (i) personal or self-appearance and (ii) social appearance. Self-appearance pertains to the individual's own perceptions of the hand. People are often uncomfortable with the altered appearance of the hand, which can then trigger intrusive thoughts and recollections of the trauma. This negative appraisal of the injured hand can have a variety of effects including shame over the mutilation, camouflaging behaviors, and even significant alterations in sexual desire and performance (11,16). Keeping one's hand in a pocket, avoiding viewing the hand during physical therapy, or using dressings on the hand long after adequate healing has taken place are frequent indicators of self-appearance concerns. A gradual process of desensitizing the individual to the appearance of the hand often helps to address these concerns and to diminish their impact.

Social-appearance concerns also exist. Often the mutilation accompanying severe hand injuries causes the person to feel socially unacceptable. This can result in a loss of self-confidence and feelings of social inadequacy. It is important to normalize these responses and to encourage the patient to use the hand as normally as possible when in public. This serves two purposes. The first is that the hand injury itself is less conspicuous when the hand is used normally. The second is that even when the mutilation is noticed, the fact that the hand is being used normally (i.e., to gesture during a conversation) conveys to other individuals that the patient has accommodated the injury.

Many hand injury patients are unsure how to respond when someone asks them what happened to their hand. This often causes the injured person to feel uncomfortable, vulnerable, and angry. Assertiveness training can be helpful in re-establishing the personal boundaries of the injured party. Often by simply giving them permission to decline to answer or to tell others that they would prefer not to talk about it can enhance their feelings of control and of their personal boundaries. It is also helpful to normalize the fact that some people will stare at their injured hand and that this is merely a reflection of that person's curiosity (or rudeness). Often, it is beneficial to have the injured individuals begin their exposure of their hand to public viewing in a controlled manner. For example, they can first show the injury to family members and then progress to having it uncovered while in the clinic and waiting room setting. In this gradual manner, they can become more comfortable with both the personal and social aspects of their hand injury.

Sleep Problems

Sleep problems are frequently present following severe hand injuries. These often begin shortly after the initial injury. Many patients experience a high level of pain and discomfort after the accident. The pain, or diminished effectiveness of pain medication over time, often interrupts their sleep. As patients move into lighter stages of sleep, nightmares of the trauma appear more readily. Individuals are often startled awake from re-experiencing of the accident. Heart palpitations, hyperventilation, and profound hyperhidrosis often accompany the startle reaction to these intrusive thoughts. It is not uncommon for the nightmare to resume once the individual returns to sleep, leading to further sleep disruption.

As this pattern develops, individuals often begin to attempt to avoid sleep as a means of coping. Sleep onset becomes disrupted and the individual's mood begins to deteriorate as sleep deprivation persists. Individuals frequently describe the time just before they fall asleep as one in which they are more likely to experience flashbacks or recurrent thoughts about the accident. This often occurs because they are not as active and able to distract themselves from thoughts of the trauma as when they are busy during the day. Patients often opt to begin watching television in bed as they wait to fall asleep in order to keep their mind away from the accident memories, further contributing to poor sleep habits. Many patients benefit from a sleeping aid or anti-depressant to facilitate the resumption of a more normalized sleep pattern. As they progress through the treatment of their intrusive thoughts, the need for these medications generally disappears. We also recommend that these individuals practice a regimen of good sleep hygiene. This includes going to bed at a regular time each night, no napping during the day, using the bed only to sleep in rather than for watching television or reading, and getting out of bed if they fail to fall asleep within 20 minutes and then returning to bed in another half hour.

Pain Problems

Pain is another major concern for most hand-injured patients. As noted above, pain initially following the injury can be very disruptive to sleep. It also produces a generalized sense of irritability and discomfort when poorly controlled. One of the more challenging clinical distinctions to make is determining when the patients' pain is of a type that will respond to pain medication and when is it more "psychological" in origin suggesting that anti-depressant medication or nonpharmacologic methods may serve as more effective treatments. A combination of both medication and active coping strategies are most effective at providing pain control. This is particularly true with phantom pain occurring after an amputation. The instruction in cognitive coping strategies, discussed in detail below, helps to restore a sense of self-efficacy that further benefits the patient.

Unfortunately, some patients resort to self-medicating with alcohol or illicit drugs in order to control both their physical pain and psychological symptoms. This causes major problems with the rehabilitation process. Due to the emotional numbing from these agents, patients are often unable to benefit from exposure and cognitive re-processing techniques to assist in the psychological desensitization to their accident. While the numbing of the symptoms may provide some relief in the short term, over time, patients often become even more avoidant and prone to alcohol or drug abuse. A pattern of dependence and noncompliance with treatment can rapidly develop, which only further complicate rehabilitation. In these cases, treatment of the dependence and abuse issues are paramount before any other psychological intervention related to the trauma can be successful.

As also discussed in the chapter on acquired disfigurement, pre-injury substance abuse is a significant risk factor for the development of PTSD. Individuals abusing substances often have a predisposition for avoidant behavior that markedly decreases their response to psychological intervention. It is important for the health care providers working with these patients to destigmatize their need for intervention for their substance abuse and to focus on this as a necessary prerequisite to the rehabilitation of the hand injury.

Social Functioning

Another area of concern is social functioning. Following hand injuries, patients often become isolated and withdrawn. While some of this is due to their appearance discomfort and reduced ability to function as before the injury, some is also due to feelings of depression, vulnerability, and worthlessness. Often, the individuals experience a major life disruption as they become dependent on others to accomplish seemingly simple tasks such as cutting their meat or tying their shoes. They become fearful of what the future will hold for them and how others will view them. The easiest solution often seems to be one in which they simply withdraw and become socially isolated. This tends to heighten their feelings of worthlessness, as they are no longer performing in pre-injury social roles as family member, friend, or neighbor. This can detrimentally affect other relationships, as injured individuals become dependent on family members to assist them in activities of daily living.

For these reasons and others, hand injuries can have a detrimental affect on marital and sexual functioning. A spouse can become resentful of the extra workload that he or she must carry at home and at work. The injury, and resulting changes in the dynamic of the marital relationship, can lead to the deterioration of the sexual relationship. Approximately, 12% of men continue to have problems with erectile dysfunction secondary to their hand injuries 6 months later (16). Many men and women report clumsiness during foreplay as a major factor in inhibiting their sexual response and libido following an upper extremity injury. An open discussion of these topics by the treating surgeon or consulting psychologist can help to normalize these feelings and lead to improved resolution of intimacy problems.

Additional Concerns

The loss of a sense of personal control and efficacy is often a primary source of psychological disruption following a major hand injury. For those individuals experiencing a sense of helplessness over the circumstances of their injury, fear and anxiety are generally the predominant postinjury emotions. Guilt more frequently occurs when the injured person feels a sense of having contributed to the accident either through engaging in risky behavior or through an error that resulted in the injury. In addition, many individuals experience feelings of shame and vulnerability as secondary emotional states. From a psychotherapeutic standpoint, it is important to process each of these issues in order for the patient to function in a maximally effective manner following the injury. The nature of the intervention, however, must be tailored to the experiences and emotional states of the individual (17–18). While PTSD is believed to be the most prevalent reaction documented in hand-injured patients, a variety of other reactions occur including panic disorder, depressive disorders, and social anxiety disorder.

Summary

This section has reviewed the most common psychological sequelae of traumatic upper extremity injuries. Questionnaire 9-1 at the end of this chapter can be of great help in identifying patients experiencing these symptoms. The rating scale allows for the identification of the most debilitating symptoms and allows for intervention to be directed to the most pertinent areas of dysfunction. These questions should be asked in the context of providing patients with the most comprehensive care of their injuries possible. In addition, it is often useful for the treating surgeon to remind patients that many of the long-term effects of the injury may be psychological as well as physical. With this as a prelude, patients will often share their concerns with the surgeon. Simply by discussing the issue in a general manner, the surgeon communicates to the patient that this is not a taboo subject and that they genuinely care about the total welfare of their patients.

TREATMENT OF PSYCHOLOGICAL AND BEHAVIORAL SYMPTOMS

Several studies have examined various interventions for the psychological sequelae of hand injuries (19–23). One of the clearest findings from these studies is that early psychological intervention has a major, positive influence upon subsequent recovery. This section will review several topics thought to be related to successful psychological outcome, including (i) teaching patients about normal psychological responses to hand injury; (ii) shaping patients' expectations regarding surgical reconstruction; (iii) using imaginal exposure to assist in coping with the memory of the injury; and (iv) counseling to assist patients in recovering pre-injury physical functioning. As discussed throughout this book, an established collaborative relationship between the treating surgeon and mental health professional is an important part of the management of these issues.

Teaching Patients about "Normal" Psychological Responses to Hand Injury

The first component of early psychological intervention generally consists of normalization of the trauma response. It is important for the patient to know that intrusive thoughts, sleep disruption, fears for the future, and concentration or attentional difficulties are frequent accompaniments of traumatic hand injuries. This information often has a soothing and anxiety-reducing effect on the patient, who may have been feeling that, in addition to a devastating hand injury, they may be "losing their minds." Very few patients have experienced flashbacks prior to their injuries and, as a result, the new flashbacks can be quite anxiety provoking for them. By normalizing these experiences, the patient recognizes that they are part of the injury process, which instills confidence that the flashbacks can be successfully treated.

Shaping Treatment Expectations

A second important component is to help the patients understand the nature of their injury and of the process of reconstructive surgery. Patients are often unduly optimistic about regaining total function in their hands following surgery. This appears to be particularly true when the patient has undergone a replant or revascularization procedure. Patients often believe that because the hand has been restored surgically, they also will regain complete function and sensation. It is important for the mental health professional working with the patient to be knowledgeable regarding the procedures that have been performed and to be able to discuss these with the individual. This allows the patient to explore the implications of the surgery in a manner not often allowed for with the surgeon due to the time constraints under which the surgeon works. Additionally, being knowledgeable about the surgical and hand therapy that the patient has or will undergo enhances the formation of rapport with the mental health professional. This is invaluable as the next phases of treatment are initiated.

Imaginal Exposure

A number of psychotherapeutic techniques can be implemented early in treatment that will assist the patient in reducing intrusive thoughts and future avoidance. The foremost among these is imaginal exposure. This procedure consists of having the patients close their eyes and basically "relive" the accident by providing a detailed description to the mental health professional. The process of imaginal exposure often begins by having the patient recall a point earlier in the day on which the injury occurred. The patient tells the story of the accident complete with the accompanying emotional reactions. Subjective units of distress (SUDS) ratings are obtained to judge the degree of affective distress experienced by the patient. These are typically rated on a scale of 0 to 10, with 0 being no distress and 10 being severe distress. As the imagery progresses, the patient proceeds through the events of the accident itself, as well as the "rescue" or arrival of medical personnel. The rescue phase is critical to the imagery as patients frequently curtail their intrusive thoughts at the moment of greatest distress. As a result, they may fail to process the fact that others did intervene and come to their assistance.

As discussed above, imaginal exposure appears to be particularly helpful at converting appraisal or projected flashbacks into a more complete recollection resembling the replay flashbacks. These flashbacks are associated with a much better outcome in terms of longer-term occurrence of intrusive thoughts or avoidance (14–15,17).

Imaginal Exposure with Reprocessing

Imaginal exposure appears to be particularly effective with those patients experiencing fear and anxiety as their predominant posttraumatic emotions (17–18). For individuals experiencing anger, shame, or guilt, imaginal exposure coupled with cognitive reprocessing seems to be more efficacious (17–18). Imaginal exposure with reprocessing also relies on reliving the accident, as described above. The difference from simple imaginal exposure, however, is that the patient engages in a Socratic dialogue with the mental health professional, which assists in restructuring the manner in which the patient experiences the traumatic event. For instance, a patient injured in a machine malfunction may feel completely helpless when re-experiencing the injury. In this case focusing on the fact that the patient was able to extricate the hand from the machine and to go and seek medical help may help to restore a sense of control and self-efficacy that had been previously overlooked. This may help the patient to move from the perception of being a victim to being a survivor who has successfully coped with adversity.

Employing cognitive restructuring in the presence of imaginal exposure serves to activate the affect that accompanied the trauma and to allow for more complete processing of the event. As such, the patient actually becomes capable of developing empowering beliefs that promote an element of mastery over the accident itself. These empowering beliefs can take a variety of forms. They can range from understanding the role that the patient had in the rescue by giving instructions to confronting a coworker who was responsible for causing the accident. These cognitive restructurings serve to both empower the victim and to promote resolution of the underlying affective content (17).

Recovery of Behavioral Functioning

While affective processing through imaginal exposure is critical in overcoming the psychological factors which occur following hand trauma, one of the major behavioral goals is to return the patient to as functional a lifestyle as possible. Many hand injuries occur within the work setting. As previously mentioned, avoidance is a frequent symptom for many individuals. A variety of techniques have been developed to facilitate return to work with the same employer. All of these entail in vivo exposure and desensitization.

The typical approach to treating a hand-injured patient via in vivo exposure and desensitization begins by constructing a hierarchy of anxiety-provoking stimuli with the patient in order to formulate a graded program of exposure. This often begins with the patient simply going to the workplace and parking in the employee parking lot. The patient may do this for a week, after which he or she is asked to exit the car and walk up to the door or, if possible, enter the building in a safe area, such as the human resources office. Following this, the patient progresses to observing work in the area in which the injury was sustained and where they may be working again in the future. Once the patient has become comfortable in the work setting, a graded return to work (within the physical restrictions determined by the physician) is initiated.

Since it is uncommon for the injured worker to tolerate a return to the same machine or job at which they were injured, we usually restrict our patients from doing so. In those cases where the patient is too fearful to return to the employer, we attempt an on-site therapy session in which the mental health professional accompanies the worker back to the employer. During this procedure, the psychologist models and instructs the patient in coping techniques. This often facilitates initiating the graded exposure work previously described. Despite the implementation of all of these techniques, some patients are unable or unwilling to return to their previous employers. We estimate the rate of failure to return to work to be between 4 and 6%.

A variety of factors can influence a patient's response to treatment. As discussed previously in this chapter, substance abuse can greatly reduce the patient's ability to respond to exposure techniques due to the level of avoidance present. Thus, the patient with an alcohol/drug dependency problem should receive treatment for that condition prior to more specific psychotherapy designed to facilitate the return to work. Comorbidity of other psychological disorders can negatively impact psychological treatment of the hand trauma. Symptoms of depression often have to be treated conjointly with the PTSD symptoms. These patients, thought to represent approximately 15% of those engaged in psychological treatment, often benefit from an anti-depressant medication following a psychiatric evaluation.

The typical course of psychological treatment is 8 to 16 sessions for the PTSD symptoms, with an additional 6 to 10 sessions if issues involving sexual dysfunction, physical appearance, or familial issues need to be addressed. In most cases, this coincides well with the course of physical rehabilitation. Interestingly, intellectual ability and age appear to have little effect on the response to psychological treatment.

This treatment approach has been used for a variety of hand conditions including disfiguring injuries such as thermal and chemical burns, tendon lacerations, nerve injuries with resultant loss of function and cosmetic disfigurement from muscle atrophy, and minor injuries resulting in reflex sympathetic dystrophy (complex regional pain syndrome, type I). Interestingly, little work has been done at our clinic with children or adults with birth defects resulting in hand disfigurement. This is certainly an area which would benefit from more intensive study.

CASE EXAMPLES

The first case portrays a rather typical hand trauma case. It demonstrates the role of the surgeon in the detection of PTSD symptoms and the utility of an early referral of a mental health professional. The case also highlights a course of desensitization with cognitive restructuring in helping the patient cope with both the injury and then the return to work. The second case study is more complex and less typical of most hand-injured patients.

Case 1: Jack

Jack is a middle-aged male who has been employed at his present job for nearly 30 years. He has worked a punch press for the past 6 years and was very familiar with its operation and setup. Prior to his injury, Jack had reported to his boss that the machine was not functioning properly. His boss had inspected the machine declaring that there was nothing that he could detect that was wrong with it, so Jack should go ahead and continue to operate it.

At the time of the accident, Jack had reached into the press in order to take out a part that had just been made. The press came down unexpectedly, closing on his fingers. He was caught in the press for about 15 seconds as it completed its cycle. During this time Jack was in excruciating pain and knew that he was badly injured. When the press opened and he was able to extricate his hand, he looked at it and saw the bones of his fingers extruded from his hand, the crushed fragments of his three fingers in the press, and his little finger dangling from his hand. He also vividly recalled the sound and sensation of his finger bones bursting. He described almost fainting and wondering what his life would be like as a one-handed individual. He was able to call for help from his fellow workers, several of whom came to his assistance. The remnants of his fingers were retrieved and sent with him to the hospital. His index, middle, and ring fingers were amputated and crushed so severely that they could not be re-attached. In addition, his little finger was crushed but was able to be revascularized. His thumb was lacerated but able to be repaired.

Jack was initially referred for treatment at his initial outpatient follow-up visit after questioning by his surgeon revealed that he was having daily flashbacks of his injury. When seen for psychological evaluation, Jack was having replay flashbacks five or six times per day. These would last for approximately 10 minutes and he would re-experience the entire accident with the accompanying sound and sensations of his bones breaking. The flashbacks would cause him to dissociate and he would lose track of whatever he had been doing. He attributed his accident to his employer, believing that if they had been safety conscious, they would have stopped the press from running and had maintenance check it out. His feelings of distrust for his employer grew as he continued to have flashbacks. He was fearful of returning to his job, as he felt that there were no guarantees that this would not happen again. He found himself feeling fearful and bitter about what had happened.

Physical therapy for his hand proved difficult as Jack refused to look at his hand after surgery. He kept his hand wrapped at all times and insisted that the therapists and his physician keep his hand covered so that he could not see it when he was in the clinic. His avoidance also resulted in his minimizing of his symptoms during his first few sessions of psychotherapy. He admitted to feeling "weak" because he was not able to cope with things on his own. Additionally, he experienced profound sleep disruption with nightmares, a startle response that woke him in the middle of the night, and avoidance of even attempting to fall asleep until he was exhausted. He was often tearful and admitted to grieving for his missing fingers. He denied any history of substance abuse.

Intervention was initiated with Jack with the immediate goals of reducing his thought intrusions and desensitizing him to the appearance of his hand. Photographs of his hand were taken in order for him to look at these before he actually saw his hand. These were taken with various parts of his hand uncovered and were presented to him over several sessions in a graded manner, beginning with photos in which his thumb was the only part exposed and progressing eventually to his entire hand being uncovered. Jack took one photo home with him between each treatment session and was instructed to view it at least three times daily for 10 minutes. He was told to keep a log of his thoughts and feelings each week. He did this and these were reviewed with him at each session. This phase of treatment lasted for six sessions.

Cognitive restructuring techniques were used to assist him in reconceptualizing what the appearance of his hand was actually like. Questions such as "How much is your hand actually bleeding right now?" were asked to help him comprehend that his hand had healed and was no longer freshly injured. This cognitive restructuring allowed him to reduce his feelings of horror and helplessness. He admitted that despite the improbability of it, he really thought of his hand as it had been the last time he saw it prior to surgery. By gradually exposing him to a series of photos he was able to reconceptualize the appearance of his hand to more closely conform to its actual appearance. Once this was completed, he proceeded with in vivo desensitization in which he was gradually exposed to more and more of his hand. He was tearful when he finally viewed his hand with nothing covering it and admitted that it had been much worse in his mind than it was in actuality.

Once the desensitization to the appearance of his hand was complete, treatment progressed to addressing his flashbacks. This was initiated by having him close his eyes and imagine himself back at work on the day of the accident. He was then instructed to describe the accident in as much detail as he could with respect to both the events as they unfolded as well as his thoughts and feelings regarding what he was describing. Special emphasis was given to developing a perception of control and mastery over many of his reactions. For example, he recalled the profound sense of helplessness and despair while trapped in the machine. By focusing on his thoughts at the time (i.e., that he would need to control his bleeding and call for help when the machine opened) he was able to recapture a sense of self-efficacy even in the face of his accident. He found as this progressed that his sleep problems and nightmares diminished. He no longer experienced profound startle reactions and noticed a marked improvement in his memory and concentration. He was able to focus his efforts on his rehabilitation rather than on his psychological symptoms. This phase of psychotherapy consisted of ten sessions.

The next major step was to assist Jack in returning to work. A graded desensitization program was established. Jack was instructed to begin this by simply driving down to his employer's parking lot and parking in it for 20 minutes. While he initially thought that this was foolish, he found that he was highly anxious when he actually carried this out. He proceeded with this for 2 weeks before he was ready for the next step. He then was instructed to proceed to the door of the plant and to arrange for several of his coworkers to talk with him outside of the building while they were on their breaks. He did this for 2 weeks and then proceeded to enter the building, going to the personnel office. After completing this step, he began to enter the plant in an area where he had worked in the past. Over several weeks he progressed to actually entering his department at the time of his injury and, ultimately, went up to the machine on which he had been injured. Due to his physical limitations he was not able to do his previous job. However, he did reach the point where he was comfortable being in the part of the plant where he had been injured. His company was able to place him in an alternate position and he was able to successfully return to full-time work without any significant psychological symptoms. He was seen weekly during this 10-week period of treatment. During the entire course of treatment, his progress was reviewed at least monthly with his surgeon, hand therapist, psychologist, and Workers Compensation rehabilitation nurse.

Case 2: Kim

Kim had been employed for 10 years as a punch press operator. She worked at a company where her husband was responsible for the safety of all of the equipment. She was recently recruited by another employer and decided to take a position with them as it would allow her to work hours that would be better for caring for her children and increase her pay. On her third day at work at the new job, her punch press malfunctioned and she sustained amputations to her ring and little fingers of her left hand.

She underwent successful replantation of her little finger but her ring finger remained amputated at the PIP joint level. She experienced frequent projected flashbacks and nightmares of the accident. She had a great deal of difficulty concentrating that worsened as she became progressively more sleep deprived. She refused to look at her finger, having her mother care for her wounds, and would not allow her husband to see it. She lost all interest in any sexual activity and was convinced that her husband found her unattractive and "disgusting." She was highly avoidant and would not even drive down the street that led to her employer. She blamed herself for the accident as she felt that if she had not changed jobs she would never have been injured.

Psychological treatment was initiated with a course of imaginal exposure in which Kim re-experienced the accident. Due to her avoidance, she had great difficulty with this and would not discuss it in the present tense. It took several sessions before this was able to be accomplished. The session in which she was able to accomplish this was tape-recorded and she was given the tape with the instructions that she listen to it daily. It became quickly apparent, however, that she was not compliant with this request. She was also provided with a course of graded exposure for viewing her finger that went somewhat more successfully. After several weeks she was able to look at her hand during therapy and to keep her dressings off at home. Whenever she was in public, however, she still kept her fingers wrapped. At this point a referral was made for her to be evaluated for a finger prosthetic for her ring finger. After a few months she obtained this and was able to wear it in public. This greatly reduced her discomfort around other individuals.

When Kim was physically able to return to work, a course of in vivo desensitization was initiated. This began with an attempt to have her return to her employer for an initial conference in the human relations office. She attempted to do so but had a panic attack in the office after about 5 minutes and had to leave. Following this, she was not able to go back to the building. A second attempt was made to return her to work at another plant with the same employer. This time she was accompanied by her psychotherapist. She was able to accomplish this visit although her affect seemed to be blunted. A schedule for her to visit this worksite over the next week was set up at the conclusion of the on-site visit. She was able to complete this for the next 2 days but on the third day again had a severe panic attack. She then revealed that she had begun consuming alcohol as a means of controlling her emotional upset. She had been regularly drinking for several weeks since the accident. She was strongly encouraged to refrain from alcohol abuse and to resume her imaginal exposure in order to more effectively control her intrusive thoughts. She was not willing to do this and discontinued treatment at that time. Her husband encouraged her to follow through with her treatment, but she refused. Eventually she went through a detoxification program and was able to maintain her sobriety. She was unable to work, however, for 4 years after her accident. At that point she returned for a follow-up session.

At the time of follow-up Kim continued to be symptomatic for PTSD. She has been started on 30 mg of Paxil by the psychiatrist treating her alcohol abuse, which had improved her mood and controlled her panic attacks. She was willing to again attempt imaginal exposure to assist her in controlling her thought intrusions. This was initiated and she made some progress in reducing her fear and anxiety but continued to have flashbacks at the same rate and severity.

Cognitive restructuring was added to the imaginal exposure Kim was again directed to close her eyes and to re-experience the accident. She was then instructed, however, to picture herself as a survivor 4 years after the accident. She went on to discuss her feelings of guilt over deciding to take a different job that resulted in her injury. By doing this in a state in which all of her trauma memories were activated by the imagery, she was able to process through the roadblocks to her recovery. After six sessions of cognitive restructuring, she was able to eliminate the thought intrusions that she had experienced for over the past 4 years. Her sleep also stabilized and her concentration improved. She began to talk about resuming work and looked at several job opportunities. Within 4 months, she was able to obtain a job as a punch press operator with a new employer. Presently, she has been back at work for over 10 years. She no longer needs her finger prosthesis to go out in public and feels that her relationships with her children and husband are better than they ever were.

This case was atypical for several reasons. Clearly, Kim's initial imaginal exposure course was nonbeneficial and may have been detrimental to her recovery. Similarly, first course of in vivo exposure also failed. Certainly, Kim's decision to resort to alcohol in order to self-medicate likely contributed to these initial failures. Unlike other patients, Kim had no previous history of alcohol abuse. It was not until these obstacles were addressed through a combination of antidepressant medication and abstinence that the second course of exposure with cognitive restructuring helped her to return to a normal lifestyle.

CONCLUSIONS

This chapter has reviewed the typical symptoms and interventions for individuals sustaining traumatic hand injuries. These symptoms included flashbacks, nightmares, concerns with personal appearance, avoidance of reminders of the trauma and physiologic arousal such as hypervigilance and an easy startle response. Social effects of these injuries were also examined including marital and familial issues and return to work issues. Treatment interventions reviewed were imaginal and in vivo exposure with and without cognitive restructuring. The two case studies illustrated these diagnostic and treatment techniques.

While there is much that we have learned about individuals' reactions to hand trauma, there is still much work to be done. Further research into the interaction of flashback types, attributions of injury cause, and treatment techniques is crucial in order to avoid the prolonged suffering of patients. Research on the social conspicuousness of an injury and its effects on subsequent social adjustment and interpersonal functioning of the individual are lacking. Each of these areas provides fertile ground for upcoming and established researchers to explore.

Hand Injury Assessment Instrument

For each of the following items, please report how often you have had the experiences described during the past month.

	Not at All	Seldom	Moderately Often	Frequently	Almost Always
1. I have flashbacks of my accident.	0	1	2	3	4
2. My sleep is good.	0	1	2	3	4
3. My injured extremity is painful.	0	1	2	3	4
4. Others are bothered by the appearance of my arm/hand.	0	1	2	3	4
5. My concentration is good.	0	1	2	3	4
6. I feel panicky when I think about my accident.	0	1	2	3	4
7. I avoid anything that reminds me of my accident.	0	1	2	3	4
8. I socialize as much as I ever have.	0	1	2	3	4
9. I am troubled whenever I look at my injured arm/hand.	0	1	2	3	4
10. My sexual functioning has not been affected by my injury.	0	1	2	3	4
11. I startle easily.	0	1	2	3	4
12. I am always watchful that something else does not harm me.	0	1	2	3	4
13. I blame myself for my accident.	0	1	2	3	4
14. My accident makes me feel angry.	0	1	2	3	4
15. I am depressed about what happened to me.	0	1	2	3	4

REFERENCES

1. Krieger N, Kelsey JL, Harris C, Pastides H. Injuries to the upper extremity: patterns of occurrence. *Clin Plast Surg* 1981;8:13–19.
2. U.S. Department of Health and Human Services. *Injury Control: Setting the National Agenda for Injury Control in the 1990s*. Washington, DC: U.S. Department of Health and Human Services, 1991.
3. Cohney BC. Some psychological aspects of hand injuries. *Prog Surg* 1978;16, 4–6.
4. Bear-Lehman J. Factors affecting return to work after hand injury. *Am J Occup Ther* 1983;37:189–194.
5. Chau N, d'Houtaud A, Gruber N, et al. Personality self-representations of patients with hand injury, and its relationship with work injury. *Eur J Epidemiol* 1995;11:373–382.
6. Cheng YH. Explaining disablement in modern times: hand-injured workers accounts of their injuries in Hong Kong. *Soc Sci Med* 1997;45:739–750.
7. Johnson RK. Psychological evaluation of patients with industrial hand injuries. *Hand Clin* 1986;2:567–575.
8. Knorr NJ, Edgerton MT. Hand injuries: psychiatric considerations. *South Med J* 1971;64:1328–1332.
9. Hennigar C, Saunders D, Efendov A. The injured workers survey: development and clinical use of a psychological screening tool for patients with hand injuries. *J Hand Ther* 2001;14:122–127.
10. Grunert BK, Smith CJ, Devin CA, et al. Early psychological aspects of severe hand injuries. *J Hand Surg* 1988;13B:177–180.
11. Grunert BK, Devin CA, Matloud HS, et al. Psychological adjustment following work-related hand injury: 18 month follow-up. *Ann Plast Surg* 1992;29:537–542.
12. Grunert BK, Hargarten SW, Matloud HS, et al. Predictive value of psychological screening in acute hand injuries. *J Hand Surg* 1992;17A:196–199.
13. Rusch MD, Dzwierzynski WW, Sanger JR, et al. Return to work outcomes after work-related hand trauma: the role of causal attributions. *J Hand Surg* 2003;28A:673–677.
14. Grunert BK, Devine CA, Matloub HS, et al. Flashbacks after traumatic hand injuries: prognostic indicators. *J Hand Surg* 1988;13A:125–127.
15. Grunert BK, Dzwierzynski WW. Prognostic factors for return to work following severe hand injuries. *Techniques in Hand and Upper Extremity Surgery*. 1997;1:213–218.
16. Grunert BK, Devine CA, Matloub HS, et al. Sexual dysfunction following traumatic hand injury. *Ann Plast Surg* 1988; 21:46–48.
17. Grunert BK, Smucker MR, Weis JM, Rusch MR. When prolonged exposure fails: adding an imagery-based cognitive restructuring component in the treatment of industrial accident victims suffering from PTSD. *Cognitive and Behavioral Practice* 2003;10:334–347.
18. Smucker MR, Grunert BK, Weis JM. Posttraumatic stress disorder: a new algorithm for treatment model. In: Leahy RL. ed. *Roadblocks in Cognitive-Behavioral Therapy*. New York: Guilford Press, 2003,175–194.
19. Meyer TM. Psychological aspects of mutilating hand injuries. *Hand Clin* 2003;19:41–49.
20. Grunert BK, Devine CA, Smith CJ, et al. Graded work exposure to promote return to work after severe hand trauma: a replicated study. *Ann Plast Surg* 1992;29:532–536.
21. Grunert BK, Matloub HS, Sanger JR, Yousif NJ. Treatment of posttraumatic stress disorder after work-related hand trauma. *J Hand Surg* 1990;15A:511–515.
22. Grunert BK, Devine CA, McCallum-Burke S, et al. On-site work evaluations: desensitisation for avoidance reactions following severe hand injuries. *J Hand Surg* 1989;14B:239–241.
23. Weis JM. Early versus delayed imaginal exposure for the treatment of posttraumatic stress disorder following accidental injury. *Dissertation Abstracts International: The Sciences & Engineering*.1999; 60, 5-B (UMI No. 2375).

Chapter 10

Orthognathic Surgery

H. Asuman Kiyak, MA, PhD

Orthognathic surgery, also known as surgical orthodontic treatment, is designed to correct skeletal discrepancies in the orofacial region that orthodontics alone cannot modify. Although this procedure is intended primarily to improve severe dentofacial malrelations and their impact on mastication, speech, and mouth opening, most patients who seek orthognathic surgery do so in order to improve their dental and facial appearance. Indeed, the dramatic changes in appearance have significant preoperative and postoperative implications worthy of discussion.

The majority of patients in Western countries undergo orthognathic surgery for mandibular retrognathia (sometimes including a genioplasty), followed by bimaxillary procedures to correct maxillary prognathia. However, other skeletal problems are also treated through a combination of facial surgery and orthodontics. Occlusal function is less of an incentive than aesthetics for patients who are referred for this type of surgery than for the orthodontists and surgeons who treat them. Unlike most plastic surgical procedures, the surgical component is just one part in the sequence of treatment; the orthodontic phase of treatment can take up to 2 years presurgery and postsurgery. Therefore, patients' psychological responses to their posttreatment changes in appearance and function evolve over significant periods of time.

This chapter begins by reviewing the influence of dental malocclusion on judgments of physical attractiveness and the role of body image and subjective well-being in understanding patient motivations for orthognathic procedures. Subsequently, the psychological benefits of orthognathic surgery, as well as the potential adverse effects of surgical procedures on physical and psychological functioning, are discussed. Specific clinical management recommendations are provided, including the use of a brief questionnaire to assess treatment expectations of patients and their significant other.

MALOCCLUSION AND JUDGMENTS OF ATTRACTIVENESS

The face is one of the areas of the body that produces the greatest concern among most people regarding their physical attractiveness. During social interaction, it is the individual's focal point and the source of vocal and emotional communication. In one of the first large-scale surveys of body image and its association with specific body parts, Berscheid et al. (1) found that people who were satisfied with their facial features expressed greater self-confidence overall. Perhaps the most extreme examples of this are children with cleft lip and palate, who have been found to demonstrate lower self-concept and introversion than children without this condition (2–3). (This research is reviewed in detail in Chapter 5.) Even in less severe conditions, such as malocclusion, persons are rated as less attractive than those with normal occlusion. Such ratings are often associated with negative judgments regarding the intelligence level of these individuals, as well as their social desirability (4–5). Helm et al. (4) found that self-ratings were particularly negative among young adults with extreme overjet (i.e., upper front teeth protruding outward), deep bite (upper teeth covering most of the lower teeth), or crowding.

Gender differences also have been found; in most cases body image is lower among women with malocclusion than among men (4,6–8). Women score lower on self-evaluations of body image, particularly on items describing the face. However, men who undergo orthognathic surgery often report lower facial body image satisfaction than women within the first few months after surgery; it appears that it takes longer for men to adapt to changes in their physical appearance.

Body Image, Self-esteem, and Psychological Well-being

The two psychological variables explored most often among those with malocclusion are body image and self-esteem. When compared to the general population that has not been referred for orthodontic or surgical correction of a dentofacial disharmony, preoperative patients report significantly lower overall body image, as well as heightened dissatisfaction with their facial appearance (9–10). Differences are particularly striking between females in the pretreatment and no treatment groups. Members of minority groups who seek surgical orthodontic treatment generally report a more positive body image than their Caucasian counterparts; the most favorable scores were reported by Black respondents in a study of patients and age-matched nonpatients in London (10).

It is instructive to compare people with similar levels of malocclusion who do and do not seek treatment (orthodontics only or combined orthodontic and surgical procedures). An individual who is objectively judged to have a dentofacial skeletal discrepancy severe enough to recommend surgical intervention may not seek treatment because of higher levels of body image satisfaction and self-esteem. Such psychological strengths may serve as a protective barrier against external pressure to undergo treatment. In some cases, they may undergo orthodontics alone, recognizing that it will not correct the skeletal problem (11–12). In contrast, those who undergo orthognathic surgery have been found to score lower on measures of body image, but this is focused primarily on their facial appearance and profile (7–8). This finding is consistent with studies of body image concerns among cosmetic surgery patients. As reviewed in Chapter 15, women undergoing breast augmentation surgery report greater dissatisfaction with their breasts than physically similar women who are not interested in surgery.

At least one study has found differences in body image as a function of the specific type of dentofacial or skeletal discrepancy. Among patients in the Netherlands, Hakman (13) found greater dissatisfaction with facial features in individuals with mandibular retrognathia than in those with a prognathic mandible. Patients who presented with an increased lower anterior face height ("long face"), with lip incompetence and exposed maxillary incisors, reported more teasing by their peers and lower body image. Surgical treatment of patients with anterior open bite may reduce their lower facial height, and indirectly improve their satisfaction with their facial appearance (13–14).

The combined orthodontic–surgical procedure results in improvements in facial appearance, more than the changes observed for patients who elect orthodontics only, despite the benefits of surgical orthodontics for their condition. Since the early work of Kiyak et al. (7,15–16), who expanded the Secord and Jourard Body Cathexis Scale (17) to include more items describing the face, orthodontic researchers have utilized this measure to assess body image. When the items are classified as facial, profile, and general body image, facial and profile image scores show significant improvement after *both* surgery and orthodontics have been completed. In one study, pretreatment patients were compared with patients who had completed treatment 9 to 12 years earlier, and with a control group who did not need any orthodontic treatment. Facial profile and facial body image were lowest among the pretreatment group, higher in the posttreatment, and highest in the nonpatient control group (8). Overall body image satisfaction has been shown to remain relatively high in these studies and does not show significant changes following surgery (7–8,18–19). It is noteworthy that improvements in body image typically do not emerge fully until postsurgical orthodontics is completed. That is, surgery alone is insufficient to change patients' facial and profile images.

Despite earlier studies that demonstrated significantly lower levels of self-esteem among people with severe malocclusion, subsequent research has generally found scores in the normal range on measures of self-esteem (20–21). Using various measures, researchers have found few or no differences between patients and control groups not seeking orthognathic surgery, or between preoperative and postoperative patients (9,22). Even when changes are observed in the same patient population over time, improvements in self-esteem are modest and not clinically significant (23–25). Although surgical orthodontics does not dramatically improve the individual's self-esteem, this variable may be a significant predictor of postoperative outcomes. Van Steenbergen et al. (26) tested whether postoperative satisfaction with facial appearance could be predicted by self-esteem, psychological distress, demographic variables, or orthodontists' ratings of the patient's lateral and frontal facial disharmony. Although all these variables showed significant correlations with satisfaction in the bivariate analyses, the only significant predictor of patients' postoperative satisfaction with their appearance was self-esteem scores, accounting for 15% of the variance in this outcome. Those who had high self-esteem before undergoing treatment demonstrated the highest satisfaction with their facial appearance following their combined surgical and orthodontic procedures.

A sizable minority of orthognathic surgery patients may experience psychological distress. In particular, young adults anticipating treatment were found to experience slightly higher levels of distress than a group of age-matched nonpatient controls, as observed on three of the ten dimensions of the Symptom Checklist (SCL-90-R), a widely used measure of psychological symptomotology (27). The scales on which pretreatment patients scored worse than nonpatients were interpersonal sensitivity, obsessive–compulsiveness, and psychoticism. A mild elevation of distress was found for 15% to 25% of patients on these dimensions in a study of 194 adults seeking surgical orthodontic treatment in a university medical center (21). These researchers found that almost 19% of patients had an elevated Global Severity Index (GSI) score, and almost 25% met the criteria for a psychiatric diagnosis. In addition, men seeking orthognathic surgery scored higher than population norms on the phobic anxiety dimension of the SCL-90-R; women scored higher on the paranoid ideation dimension.

The authors caution clinicians that these symptoms should not disqualify a potential patient from undergoing surgical orthodontic treatment. Underscoring the recommendations of Pogrel and Scott (28), they suggest that patients with excessive symptoms and inadequate support systems should be referred for counseling between the time they initiate orthodontics and before undergoing surgery. This was subsequently echoed by Phillips et al. (29), in which a computerized treatment planning simulation was found to create more discomfort in patients with elevated scores on the SCL-90-R measure of generalized psychological distress. To date, no studies have investigated the rate of formal psychopathology, such as mood or anxiety disorders, among these patients.

MOTIVES FOR SURGICAL ORTHODONTICS

Despite gender differences in attention to and dissatisfaction with body image as a result of severe malocclusion, both men and women report that improved aesthetics is a major reason for seeking treatment. Some researchers have used an open-ended technique, asking patients to describe their primary motives for surgery. Not surprisingly, 76% to 89% of patients reported that improved appearance was a central motivation (30–31). Improved aesthetics and self-concept were more commonly expressed as motives, as compared to functional changes, in a sample of patients undergoing treatment at a university medical center (32). At least one study, however, has suggested that, for some patients, appearance concerns may not be the primary motivation for surgery. In a retrospective examination of patients who had undergone orthognathic surgery to correct an open bite, Hoppenreijs et al. (14) asked patients to list their reasons for seeking treatment. They found that the most commonly recalled motive was a desire to improve biting and chewing (61%), followed by concerns with facial appearance (47%), and temporomandibular dysfunction (TMD, 36%). The retrospective nature of this study, where patients were able to truly appreciate the postoperative improvements in biting and chewing, may account for this finding. It may also be that patients who are asked to list their motives in an open-ended manner feel compelled to give more practical motives for treatment.

Using a checklist of potential motives before surgery, Kiyak et al. (6) found a similar range of responses regarding aesthetics. More than half, 53%, of women and 41% of men listed a desire to change their appearance as a motive. Improving mastication was reported by the same percentage of men, but only 29% of women. These gender differences are consistent with the body image investigations described above, as well as other studies where women, as compared to men, typically report greater body image concerns.

Other studies that have asked respondents to select from a checklist have also found a combination of aesthetic and functional motives for surgery. In one investigation, a desire to improve the appearance of one's teeth was rated more highly than changing one's general appearance (25). A subsequent study of 100 patients in Finland used the same checklist to assess patients one month before and one year after surgery. After surgery, improved occlusion and mastication, as well as reduction in temporomandibular joint (TMJ) disorders were rated higher than a desire to improve appearance (33). Cultural differences may account for the greater emphasis on functional motives among Finnish patients, although these were relatively high in the American sample reported above. Alternatively, consistent with other retrospective studies, it may be that patients are pleasantly surprised by the functional benefits of surgery after they have undergone the procedure. Nevertheless, both studies found that dissatisfaction with the appearance of one's teeth was greater than dissatisfaction with facial or general appearance, suggesting that improvements in appearance, rather than function, likely were the strongest motivations for surgery.

Psychological Benefits of Orthognathic Surgery

As early as 1970, researchers demonstrated that patients undergoing surgery for dentofacial malrelations were more satisfied with the effects of surgery on their appearance and personality than on their oral function. Patients are more likely to report that the surgery has improved their dental and facial appearance than their general appearance (8,22). This is not surprising, given that the focus of these patients and their clinicians is on improving dentofacial harmony and function. Anecdotal reports have suggested an increase in positive life events, such as finding a desirable job, following surgery (34). Subsequent research has more or less supported these findings. Other studies have documented improvements in interpersonal confidence and social relationships (22,35–36).

Orthognathic surgery has been associated with other life changes. When patients were asked to rate their satisfaction with specific aspects of their lives before and 12 months after surgery, the most significant improvements occurred in self-reported physical and mental health, "concept of life," and personal relationships (33). The majority of patients in this study, conducted in Finland, also reported that they had achieved their motives with respect to occlusion, chewing, TMD, and teeth appearance. However, they were less likely to perceive their overall facial appearance as having improved 12 months following surgery.

Patients are more likely to report positive life changes in the early (2 to 5 years) than later postoperative years. This may reflect long-term adjustment to their dentofacial changes or declining attribution to their improved appearance as the cause of other positive life events. Nevertheless, long after undergoing surgical orthodontics, the vast majority of patients (84% to 92%) report satisfaction with the treatment, and indicate that they would undergo treatment again. However, this favorable attitude toward orthognathic surgery does not generalize to other cosmetic procedures; only 31% report that they would consider other types of cosmetic surgery (8,22,37).

Although most researchers report high levels of overall satisfaction with surgical outcomes (as high as 100% in some studies), this is not a complete picture of the full range of possible outcomes. For example, in one study 23% of patients reported dysesthesia of the alveolar nerve and 20% experienced relapse of their surgically corrected open bite (14). Nevertheless, retrospective interviews 6 years later revealed high rates of satisfaction; 75% were satisfied with their dental appearance and 85% with their facial appearance (38). The long duration of combined orthodontics and surgery may result in cognitive dissonance, that is, having made the decision to undergo this long-term procedure, patients may feel the need to justify their commitment by expressing high satisfaction with functional and aesthetic outcomes, even in cases where the physically apparent changes are minimal and/or postoperative complications such as paresthesia persist (39–40). On the other hand, patients who perceive their aesthetic changes to be less dramatic than expected tend to report less satisfaction with treatment outcomes.

Adverse Effects of Surgery and Impact on Psychological Outcomes

Some researchers who have examined the psychological outcomes of surgical–orthodontic treatment also have inquired about potential adverse effects. The most common finding is dysesthesia of the lip and tongue, which may be transitory, although some patients report experiencing it up to 10 years later (13–14,22,33). TMD has been reported by some patients following orthognathic surgery, but for other patients the surgery indirectly corrects the problem (7,14). It is also not uncommon for patients to experience a relapse of their previously corrected dental disharmony; objective assessments have found relapse rates to be as high as 20% several years after surgery (14,40). Additionally, limited mouth opening has been reported among approximately 25% of patients as many as 16 years later, but this does not appear to influence their ability to function (39). Quite surprisingly, researchers who found postsurgical complications among treated patients, such as dysesthesia, TMD, relapse, and limited mouth opening also have reported high levels of overall satisfaction with treatment outcomes (38–39). Only one published study found lower overall satisfaction scores among those with postoperative numbness (33). The majority of patients in these studies indicated that their motives for treatment had been fulfilled, in particular their desire for improved aesthetics and oral function. On the other hand, patients who report that the aesthetic outcomes of their combined orthodontics and surgery are less attractive than they had expected tend to be less satisfied overall (38).

Transient psychological problems have been identified both pre- and postoperatively. Using the Profile of Mood States (41), Kiyak et al. (42) found the highest levels of tension-anxiety scores within the few days before surgery, indicating heightened anticipation and anxiety. Not surprisingly, fatigue, confusion, and tension-anxiety were high at the immediate postsurgical stage but declined (in most cases) to presurgical levels by the 24-month assessment. Depression scores were highest just after surgery and steadily decreased for most patients within 6 weeks. The high scores observed immediately after surgery may reflect the residual effects of general anesthesia and adverse effects of pain and the medications that are prescribed for pain management during the first few days postoperatively (43). In addition, they also may have reflected the "postoperative blues," a period when patients are psychologically ready to return to preoperative levels of activity but do not yet have the stamina to do so. Among those with continued high levels of depression, most had reported higher than average expectations for improvements in their oral function and interpersonal relationships. In addition, several patients were experiencing other major life events during the postoperative period (e.g., divorce, starting college) that may have accounted for the elevated symptoms of depression, rather than their recovery from surgery and orthodontics.

The importance of assessing patients' emotional states during the period before and after surgery is underscored by the fact that complaints regarding treatment outcomes are correlated with psychological well-being (42). Patients with higher scores on depression, tension–anxiety, anger–hostility, and confusion were less satisfied overall. They also reported more pain, surgical discomfort, TMD, problems with oral function, and interpersonal relationships during the postoperative phase.

Several researchers have concluded that the best approach to preventing postoperative dissatisfaction with pain, temporary dysesthesia, and unexpected changes in facial appearance is to improve presurgical communication between the patient and surgeon (14,22,38–39). Although their long-term treatment is managed by their orthodontist, patients and their support network are faced with the immediate impact of surgery in terms of physical discomfort, pain, facial swelling, and dysesthesia. In addition, the surgeon must address the potentially dramatic changes in patients' appearance before initiating treatment. Thus, while most researchers have found that surgeons provide sufficient technical information about the reasons why surgery should accompany orthodontics for these patients, and the nature of this surgery for a particular case, surgeons have been criticized for not providing more information about the postoperative period of physical and psychological adjustment. Recommendations include developing informational brochures for patients and their significant others (22), offering opportunities to speak with patients who have undergone similar procedures, or viewing a video with such patients describing their experiences (38).

PREPARING PATIENTS FOR ORTHOGNATHIC SURGERY

The importance of good communication between the surgeon and patient is discussed in several chapters of this book and is highlighted in Chapter 19. One of the striking findings in recent research by the author is that patients seeking surgical orthodontics are not well informed about the reasons, risks, and benefits of their treatment (44). Although both surgeons and orthodontists provide patients with general information about each stage of their treatment and have them sign an informed consent statement before undergoing surgery, short-term recall of this information is poor. In one study, the preoperative meeting between the surgeon and the patient (and in some cases including a spouse, parent, or partner) was audiotaped and the specific elements of informed consent mentioned by the surgeon were documented. Patients were interviewed in person immediately after their interaction with the surgeon. On average, surgeons told their patients five reasons why they needed surgery; patients recalled fewer than three of these. Of greater concern was that, of the 6.2 risks mentioned by surgeons in the average discussion, only 1.5 of these risks was recalled by patients shortly after this interaction. Fully 52% of patients said they knew of no risks or that they could not remember them (44). Reasons for this poor recall include the heightened anxiety levels of patients during these preoperative sessions, and that patients are often focused on different concerns or expectations than what the surgeon is addressing in the meeting. These findings provide further evidence for improving preoperative communication with the patient.

One approach is to use the "Expectations Scale" in Questionnaire 10-1 at the end of this chapter during the consultation. It is a tool that has been developed in the author's previous studies and validated by self-reports of oral dysfunction and body image. Both individual items and scores on the four dimensions that the scale represents (oral function, appearance, social acceptance, and general health) provide valuable insights into the patient's expectations from the procedure. Indeed, this scale can be used to examine expectations in both patients and their significant others, as illustrated in the following case.

CASE EXAMPLE

A 32-year-old woman sought out treatment from an orthodontist because she had been dissatisfied since adolescence with her "crooked teeth and lack of a chin." When the orthodontist told her that her condition could be treated but that she would need a combined surgical and orthodontic procedure, the young woman was relieved. She rated her expectations at the highest level on all 14 items of the Expectations Scale. After 2 years of orthodontics, she saw significant improvements in her teeth but not in her jaw, which required a mandibular surgery to move the jaw forward almost one centimeter. The surgery and postoperative orthodontics were very successful, and the patient was delighted with the outcome. In fact, all her expectations had been met. Additionally, the patient changed her hairstyle, learned how to highlight her most attractive features with make-up, and even proceeded to have her first book of poetry published. Unfortunately, this dramatic improvement in body image and self-confidence was not met with enthusiasm by the woman's spouse. After the lengthy procedures were completed and the woman began this new phase of her life, her husband told her he liked her better in her former state, and that she no longer looked like the woman he had loved and married! This experience taught the clinical team that it is very important to involve significant others in the planning of each stage of treatment, and even more important, to ask these individuals to complete the Expectations Scale as well. By comparing the responses from patients and their significant others, we can determine if the patient will have support from loved ones during the extensive period of orthodontic and surgical treatment. If there are discrepancies, it is important to resolve them or at least educate both the patient and significant others about the numerous changes associated with these procedures.

CONCLUSIONS

The research reviewed in this chapter illustrates the complex interactions of cosmetic and functional objectives in orthognathic surgery, as well as the complications produced by the long-term nature of this combined orthodontic and surgical procedure. Patients who seek this procedure are most concerned about the appearance of their teeth, face, and facial profile. Most studies have found significant improvements in these specific aspects of appearance, particularly among those who sought treatment for open bite and an extreme retrognathic or prognathic mandible. For the majority of patients seeking surgical orthodontics, self-esteem is within the normal range, but those with low self-esteem at baseline are less likely to be satisfied with treatment outcomes.

These findings can be used to guide clinical care. Patients who are referred for this type of surgery frequently have a reasonably accurate self-image and feel good about themselves, with the exception of the specific orofacial features that need correction. However, it behooves the clinician to be alert for signs of low self-esteem or other symptoms that may hamper postoperative adjustment. The surgeon and the orthodontist who treat these patients must also be aware that as many as 25% of patients who seek treatment experience significant levels of psychological distress, particularly interpersonal sensitivity and obsessive–compulsive tendencies. These patients will require more attention from the clinical team and may benefit from a referral to a mental health professional during the course of their orthodontic treatment. It is unclear whether surgery should be postponed until such patients can re-establish their psychological well-being. In the absence of information on the relationship between preoperative psychological symptoms and postoperative outcomes, these decisions should be made on a case-by-case basis. Nevertheless, it is important to provide emotional support and reassurance to these patients, as well as ensuring that they have a strong social support network to assist them as they proceed through the many stages of surgical orthodontics. Indeed, the finding that patients who experience depression, anger, and confusion for several weeks following surgery are less satisfied with outcomes and report more postoperative pain and TMJ problems suggests that these patients, in particular, could likely benefit from additional emotional support (42).

The finding of most studies in the United States and Europe that the primary motive for surgical orthodontics is aesthetic makes it imperative that both the orthodontist and surgeon spend time with patients prior to treatment to explain how much change they should expect. Computerized simulations of the anticipated postoperative appearance may be helpful in this regard. For those who expect dramatic improvements in their dental occlusion and oral functions, it is especially important to inform them on how much change they should realistically expect through this combined procedure.

Of course, it is also critical that surgeons review in detail, in language patients can understand, and in an interactive rather than lecture mode, the risks and benefits of this surgical procedure. (See Chapters 17, 18, and 19 for additional discussion of issues related to informed consent.) Many studies have described patients' surprise at the level of dysesthesia and pain they experienced, as well as relapse after a number of years. The clinician may have explained these risks prior to the surgery, but it would help to repeat the most common potential problems several times preoperatively. The more realistic a patient's expectations, the more satisfied they appear to be with the treatment outcomes. For all these reasons, it is important for the surgeon and/or a member of the surgical team to provide opportunities for unhurried communication, including time to answer specific questions about the procedure, and perioperative and postoperative experiences they can expect.

Treatment Expectations Questionnaire

Whenever we decide whether or not to have some dental or medical treatment, we usually expect the treatment to result in some changes in our lives. These changes may be good or bad. Think about the idea of having orthodontics and surgery. Think about the changes that having this combined treatment might make in your life. For each of the areas below, **circle the number** that best describes how much change you would expect the combined orthodontics and surgery to make in your life. You can use any number from −3 (that area will become much worse after orthodontics) to 0 (no change expected) to +3 (that area will become much better):

	Worse after orthodontics			No change after orthodontics			Better after orthodontics	
a. Chewing	−3	−2	−1	0	+1	+2	+3
b. Biting into foods	−3	−2	−1	0	+1	+2	+3
c. Fitting back teeth together	−3	−2	−1	0	+1	+2	+3
d. Fitting front teeth together	−3	−2	−1	0	+1	+2	+3
e. Speech	−3	−2	−1	0	+1	+2	+3
f. Popping/clicking of jaw joint	−3	−2	−1	0	+1	+2	+3
g. Sinus problems	−3	−2	−1	0	+1	+2	+3
h. Appearance of teeth	−3	−2	−1	0	+1	+2	+3
i. Facial profile	−3	−2	−1	0	+1	+2	+3
j. General appearance	−3	−2	−1	0	+1	+2	+3
k. Feelings about self	−3	−2	−1	0	+1	+2	+3
l. Socializing	−3	−2	−1	0	+1	+2	+3
m. Performance in school	−3	−2	−1	0	+1	+2	+3
n. Being out in public	−3	−2	−1	0	+1	+2	+3
o. Other	−3	−2	−1	0	+1	+2	+3

Please describe:

REFERENCES

1. Berscheid E, Walster E, Bohrnstedt G. Body image. *Psychol Today* 1973;7:119–123.
2. Jones JE. Self-concept and parental evaluation of peer relationships in cleft lip and palate children. *Pediatr Dent* 1984;6:132–138.
3. Tobiasen JM. Psychosocial correlates of congenital facial clefts: a conceptualization and model. *Cleft Palate J* 1984;21:3–10.
4. Helm S, Kreiborg S, Solow B. Psychological implications of malocclusion: a 15-year follow-up study in 30-year-old Danes. *Am J Orthod* 1985;87:110–118.
5. Shaw WC. The influence of children's dentofacial appearance on their social attractiveness as judged by peers and lay adults. *Am J Orthod* 1981;79:399–415.
6. Kiyak HA, Hohl T, Sherrick P, et al. Sex differences in motives for and outcomes of orthognathic surgery. *J Oral Surg* 1981;39:757–764.
7. Kiyak HA, Hohl T, West RA, McNeill RW. Psychological changes in orthognathic surgery patients: a 24-month follow-up. *J Oral Maxillofac Surg* 1984;42:506–512.
8. Lazaridou-Terzoudi T, Kiyak HA, Moore R, et al. Long-term assessment of psychologic outcomes of orthognathic surgery. *J Oral Maxillofac Surg* 2003; 61:545–552.
9. Phillips C, Kiyak HA. Psychosocial vs. clinical responses to orthognathic surgery (NIH Grant RO1 DE10028). Final Report.
10. Cunningham SJ, Gilthorpe MS, Hunt NP. Are orthognathic patients different? *Eur J Orthod* 1990;22:195–202.
11. Bell R, Kiyak HA, Joondeph DR, et al. Perceptions of facial profile and their influence on the decision to undergo orthognathic surgery. *Am J Orthod* 1985;88:323–332.
12. Kiyak HA, McNeill RW, West RA, et al. Personality characteristics as predictors and sequelae of surgical and conventional orthodontics. *Am J Orthod* 1986;89:383–392.
13. Hakman ECJ. Psychological studies on orthognathic surgery. In: DeBeaufort I, Hilhorst M, Holm S, eds. *In the Eye of the Beholder: Ethnics and Medical Change of Appearance.* Copenhagen, Denmark: Scandinavian University Press, 1996:48–75.
14. Hoppenreijs TJM, Hakman ECJ, Van Hof MA, et al. Psychologic implications of surgical-orthodontic treatment in patients with anterior open bite. *Int J Adult Orthodon Orthognath Surg* 1999;14:101–112.
15. Kiyak HA, West RA, Hohl T, McNeill RW. The psychological impact of orthognathic surgery: a 9-month follow-up. *Am J Orthod* 1982a;81:404–412.
16. Kiyak HA, McNeill RW, West RA, Hohl T, Bucher F, Sherrick P. Predicting psychological responses to orthognathic surgery. *J Oral Maxillofac Surg* 1982b;40:150–155.
17. Secord PF, Jourard SM. The appraisal of body cathexis: Body cathexis and the self. *J Consult Psychol* 1953;17:343–347.
18. Kiyak HA. Psychological aspects of orthognathic surgery. *Psychology and Health*, 1993;8:197–212.
19. Rivera S, Hatch J, Rugh R. Psychosocial factors associated with orthodontic and orthognathic surgical treatment. *Semin Orthod* 2000;4:259–263.
20. Dann C, Phillips C, Broder HL, Tulloch JF. Self-concept, Class II malocclusion and early treatment. *Angle Orthod* 1995;65:411–416.
21. Phillips C, Bennett ME, Broder H. Dentofacial disharmony: psychological status of patients seeking a treatment consultation. *Angle Orthod* 1998;68:547–556.
22. Cunningham SJ, Hunt NP, Feinmann C. Perceptions of outcome following orthognathic surgery. *Br J Oral Maxillofac Surg* 1996;34:210–213.
23. Finlay PM, Atkinson JM, Moos KF. Orthognathic surgery: patient expectations, psychological profile and satisfaction with outcomes. *Br J Oral Maxillofac Surg* 1993;33:9–14.
24. Flanary CM, Barnwell GM, VanSickels JE, et al. Impact of orthognathic surgery on normal and abnormal personality dimensions: a 2-year follow-up study of 61 patients. *Am J Orthod Dentofacial Orthop* 1990; 98:313–322.
25. Ostler S, Kiyak HA. Treatment expectations versus outcomes among orthognathic surgery patients. *Int J Adult Orthodon Orthognath Surg* 1991;6:247–255.
26. VanSteenbergen E, Litt MD, Nanda R. Presurgical satisfaction with facial appearance in orthognathic surgery patients. *Am J Orthod Dentofacial Orthop* 1996;110:653–659.
27. Derogatis LR. *The SCL-90-R Administration, Scoring and Procedures Manual* 3rd ed. Minneapolis: National Computer Systems, 1994.
28. Pogrel MA, Scott P. Is it possible to identify the psychologically "bad risk" orthognathic surgery patient preoperatively? *Int J Adult Orthodon Orthognath Surg* 1994;9:105–110.
29. Phillips C, Bailey L, Kiyak HA, Bloomquist D. Effects of a computerized treatment simulation on patient expectations for orthognathic surgery. *Int J Adult Orthodon Orthognath Surg* 2001;16:87–98.
30. Jacobsen A. The influence of children's dentofacial appearance on their social attractiveness as judged by peers and lay adults. *Am J Orthod* 1981;79:399–415.
31. Laufer D, Glick D, Gutman D, Avigdor S. Patient motivation and response to surgical correction of prognathism. *J Oral Surg* 1976;41:309–313.
32. Phillips C, Broder HL, Bennett ME. Dentofacial disharmony: motivations for seeking treatment. *Int J Adult Orthodon Orthognath Surg* 1997;12:7–15.
33. Forssell H, Finne K, Forssel K, et al. Expectations and perceptions regarding treatment: a prospective study of patient undergoing orthognathic surgery. *Int J Adult Orthodon Orthognath Surg* 1998;13:107–113.
34. Crowell NT, Sazima HJ, Elder ST. Survey of patients' attitudes after surgical correction of prognathism: a study of 33 patients. *J Oral Surg* 1970; 28:818–822.
35. Barbosa ALB, Marcantonio E, Barbosa CE, et al. Psychological evaluation of patients scheduled for orthognathic surgery. *J Nihon Univ Sch Dent* 1993;35:1–9.
36. Garvill J, Garvill H, Kahnberg KE, Lundgren S. Psychological factors in orthognathic surgery. *J Craniomaxillofac Surg* 1992;20:28–33.

37. Flanary CM, Barnwell GM, Alexander JM. Patient perceptions of orthognathic surgery. *Am J Orthod* 1985;88:137–145.
38. Kiyak HA, Bell R. Psychosocial considerations in surgery and orthodontics. In: Proffit WR, White RP, eds. *Surgical-Orthodontic Treatment*. St. Louis: Mosby–Year Book, 1991:71–91.
39. Cunningham SJ, Crean SJ, Hunt NP, Harris M. Preparation, perceptions, and problems: a long-term follow-up study of orthognathic surgery. *Int J Adult Orthodon Orthognath Surg* 1996;11:41–47.
40. Hoppenreijs TJM, Van der Linden FPGM, Freihofer HPM, et al. Occlusal and functional conditions after surgical correction of anterior open bite deformities. *Int J Adult Orthodon Orthognath Surg* 1996;11:29–39.
41. Lorr M, McNair DM. *Manual for the profile of mood states*. San Diego, CA: EDITS; 1971.
42. Kiyak HA, McNeill RW, West RA. The emotional impact of orthognathic surgery and conventional orthodontics. *Am J Orthod* 1985;88:224–234.
43. Neal CE, Kiyak HA. Patient perceptions of pain, paresthesia and swelling after orthognathic surgery. *Int J Adult Orthodon Orthognath Surg* 1991;6:169–181.
44. Kiyak HA, Iseri H, Kayaalp F, Altug A. Informed consent in orthodontics and orthognathic surgery. *J Dent Res* 2002;81:Abstract 159.

Chapter 11

Breast Reconstruction

Georita M. Frierson, PhD, and Barbara L. Andersen, PhD

The successful use of cancer screening has resulted in earlier diagnoses, less radical surgeries, and more treatment options for women with breast cancer (1). When diagnosis comes, however, it is an emotionally traumatic experience (2). While women with breast cancer share the same concerns of most other cancer patients, they particularly fear the significant body image changes that will result from their treatments. Such concerns are common and are not specific to particular treatments. For example, women treated with, or without, breast-conserving surgery may share the same worries about the disease and its effects on their quality of life.

This chapter discusses psychological and behavioral aspects of adjustment to breast cancer, with an emphasis on the issues and stressors relevant to breast change. Body change stress is the subjective stress that accompanies women's negative and distressing thoughts, emotions, and behaviors specifically relevant to their body change as a result of having breast cancer and subsequent treatment (3). Women's responses to breast change must be also considered in the context of other responses, such as psychological adjustment, social adjustment, relationships with sexual partners, physical symptoms, and related concerns (4).

We begin with an overview of women's psychological responses to the diagnosis of cancer. We next consider women's responses to changes to the breast wrought by surgeries and other cancer treatments. A clinical vignette illustrates the concerns of one such patient. It is in this difficult context that the consultation with the plastic surgeon usually occurs. We discuss the consultation from the patient's perspective, and also note the circumstances under which women may not be offered or not choose to receive reconstruction. We then review the psychological and behavioral outcomes for women receiving reconstruction. In general, the literature suggests that women who are able to receive breast-conserving techniques have more positive attitudes about their bodies and better sexual adjustment than those women who undergo mastectomy. For the latter, breast reconstruction can bring improvements, but it is, unfortunately, not a panacea (4–5). Still, many factors may influence women's satisfaction with the final surgical result and have implications for easing the difficult, but essential, consultation process.

THE BREAST: PHENOMENOLOGY AND THE DISTRESS OF CHANGE

For centuries, descriptions have been offered of the influence that women's breasts have on their self-identity, interpersonal relationships (including sexual ones), and other important aspects of their lives. Not surprisingly, the impact of breast cancer has been extensively discussed. For example, Moyer and Salovey (4) state that the disfigurement associated with breast cancer treatment forces a woman to address the cultural connection of the breast to her femininity, sexuality, and physical intactness (3,6).

Some women may grieve or mourn the loss of her preoperative breast(s) (7). The grieving process may be pronounced and lengthy, particularly when treatment involves radical surgery such as mastectomy (8–9). It can include a wide range of thoughts, feelings, and behaviors. For example, a breast cancer survivor may purchase loose fitting clothes to hide the appearance of her breasts, thereby reflecting her physical self-consciousness (10). She may be less comfortable engaging in sexual behavior because of her body changes, which in turn can result in less frequent or less satisfying sexual experiences. Whereas such behaviors may diminish with time, they may also be the circumstances that eventually motivate women toward breast reconstruction.

A woman's adaptation to breast reconstruction may be hindered if the surgery is immediate rather than delayed. In these circumstances, the mourning of the loss of the breast may be short-circuited. Interestingly, some urge women to "complete" the grieving process prior to reconstruction surgery (7). Winder and Winder (11) comment that when ample time is given, a woman will be more able to integrate the reconstructed breast into her new body image. However, it is important to note that these are clinical perspectives only, and they remain to be examined empirically.

We view women's responses to changes to the breast following cancer surgery as being similar to those of persons who experience traumatic life stressors (3). The Breast Impact of Treatment Scale (BITS) (see Questionnaire 11-1) is a 15-item questionnaire designed specifically for use with breast cancer patients to assess their level of body image distress attributed to the breast cancer surgery. Within the measure, body image distress is conceptualized as a breast cancer survivor's thoughts and behaviors (that tend to reflect anxiety like symptoms) toward her new altered body image following the stressor (i.e., surgery for breast cancer).

The BITS format is similar to that of the Impact of Events Scale (IES) (12–13). The IES is a self-report measure that subjectively assesses anxiety symptoms such as avoidance and intrusion responses to a significant life event (e.g., cancer). Similarly the BITS items are scored on a scale of 0 = not at all, 1 = rarely, 3 = sometimes, and 5 = often. The BITS consists of 15 items where four items are characterized as Avoidance (scores ranging from 0 to 20) and the remaining 11 items are Intrusion (scores ranging from 0 to 55). The Avoidance and Intrusion items reflect the two factors of this measure. Intrusive responses are worded to evaluate pervasive thoughts (e.g., "Things I see or hear remind me that my body is different"), troubling images (e.g., "How my body changed pops into my mind"), and troubled dreams and strong feelings ("I think about how my treatments may affect my sex life"). Avoidant responses include thoughts (e.g., "I think about how my body looked before I was treated"), denial surrounding the event (e.g., "I avoid looking at and or touching my scar"), and behaviors (e.g., "I turn away when I have to undress in front of my partner").

The BITS has satisfactory reliability and validity (14) as demonstrated in studies of breast cancer samples. For example, women receiving mastectomy report higher body change stress on the BITS than do women receiving breast-conserving treatment following surgery (4) as well as 12 months later (14). The BITS appears to be a clinically useful and relevant measure for a breast cancer team.

As discussed in Chapter 4, body image is a multidimensional concept that refers to how persons perceive their physical appearance, with all associated thoughts, feelings, and behaviors (15). In the breast cancer literature, Hopwood (16) has commented on the similarities between body image and related topics, such as self-concept, attractiveness, self-confidence, sexuality, and self-esteem. Unfortunately in this literature, some researchers have used the term body image, when in fact they were measuring sexual functioning, self-esteem, or body integrity (17). With this confusion, integrating findings and arriving at definitive conclusions regarding the role of body image in breast reconstruction is difficult (6,16–19). Further complicating the issue is the fact that many different "body image" measures have been used in past research. These include the *Body Image Scale* from the Derogatis Sexual Functioning Inventory (20); *Body Satisfaction Scale* short version (21); *Body Image Visual Analogue Scale* (6); *Tennessee Self Concept Scale* (22); *Body Cathexis Scale* (23); Homonyms Test (24); and the *Body Esteem Scale* (25), among others. Some of these measures, unfortunately, have relatively undocumented reliability and validity, thus limiting their utility (8,26). Both clinicians and researchers need to be mindful of these issues when selecting measures. Chapter 4 provides a more detailed discussion of body image assessment tools.

Case 1: Jane

Jane is a 47-year-old woman who underwent a complete mastectomy of her left breast. As she recovers, she repeatedly thinks: "This is horrible; my body is destroyed." A year ago she was satisfied with her body. Somehow, though, it has turned on her, "gotten" cancer, and now she is left disfigured. She can barely stand to look at herself in the mirror or look down when she takes a shower. The complete body hair loss makes it worse; "I am an alien from the planet Chemo." Her thoughts reveal her encompassing, negative self-view (i.e., a negative schema) (27). Her thoughts also suggest the possibility of other negative sequelae. She feels anxious and depressed, has become increasingly self-conscious, and now avoids sexual contact with her husband. She camouflages her appearance in baggy, loose fitting shirts. These and related changes can, in turn, limit opportunities for improvements in emotions, thoughts, and actions, and a downward spiral ensues.

PSYCHOSOCIAL RESPONSES TO CANCER DIAGNOSIS

An early clinical study suggested that the diagnosis of cancer produces an "existential plight," meaning that the news brings shock, disbelief, and emotional turmoil (28). For the individual, the manner in which the information regarding the diagnosis is disclosed is important. Physicians who communicate hope have patients who are, in turn, more hopeful and have a more favorable emotional adjustment. Alternatively, communicating "false hope" is unwelcome (29). In a study of gynecologic cancer patients, for example, Roberts et al. (30) found that, although patients expect compassion from their physicians, the majority (89%) also prefers "straight-talk" about their prognosis. This points to the need for physicians and other health professionals to be effective communicators with their patients (31–32).

Illustrating this point, a study by Rutter et al. (33) evaluated physician communication training as a strategy to reduce patient distress. Physicians received 1 hour and 15 minutes of training and a handbook regarding ways to improve the structure and style of their patient interactions. Based on Ley's work (34), training included aids to enhance cognitive understanding (e.g., simplification, repetition) and emotional understanding (e.g., conveying warmth, listening, giving feedback). Trained physicians also provided patient information booklets describing adjuvant treatments to encourage patient participation and enhanced feelings of control. All patients were assessed before and after their physician consultation for adjuvant chemotherapy. Three physicians, prior to their communication skills training, saw a consecutive series of 18 patients who served as controls. Then, physician training was completed, and data were gathered from the next 18 patients of the same physicians. All patients reported reductions in anxiety (35) following their physician visit. More importantly, patients seen following physician training reported fewer depressive symptoms (36) and higher levels of satisfaction and personal control. After training, physicians were also evaluated by their patients as more skilled.

The importance of physician communication training is underscored by the clinical context of sadness (depression), fear (anxiety), and anger, which characterized patients' responses at the time of diagnosis. A patient's level of distress exists along a continuum from normal feelings to those including profound vulnerability, sadness, fear, anxiety, panic, and social isolation (37). Depressive symptoms are the most common emotional problem. In a recent review of studies (38), as many as 23% of cancer patients met the criteria for major depressive disorder; much higher than the rate of 5% to 6% in the general population (38). When major depression and depressed mood are considered, prevalence rates are comparable—21% in Bodurka-Bevers et al. (39), 16% in Derogatis et al. (40), 17% in Kornblith et al. (41), and 25% in a review by Massie and Holland (42). Lower rates of depression have been found when patients are ambulatory with good physical functioning rather than in the midst of or recovering from treatments (41–43). For example, in a study of Latina cervix cancer patients undergoing radiotherapy (44), depressive symptoms were predicted by lower levels of support from the family, stress, physical symptoms from the treatment, and practical barriers to receiving treatment (e.g., transportation difficulties). In general, depression is more common for newly diagnosed patients with pain or other disturbing symptoms rather than not, those in active treatment (e.g., chemotherapy), and/or those with a history of affective disorder or substance abuse (41,45–46).

Anxiety-related problems also can be significant. For some patients, anxiety is severe. Studies report, for example, that diagnostic rates of cancer-related Post Traumatic Stress Disorder (PTSD) are low (3% to 10%) (47–49), but sub-syndromal PTSD symptoms occur in up to 50% of patients (50,51). PTSD symptoms include cognitive (e.g., images of re-experiencing the traumatic events), behavioral (e.g., avoidance of reminders of the event), emotional (e.g., a "numbing" or blunting of affect), and physiological (e.g., hyperarousal, alertness) responses. Importantly, the BITS assesses the magnitude of women's posttraumatic stress responses specific to their breast changes.

Psychological variables appear to play a role in the magnitude of emotional distress. Individuals who perceive their illness as severe (52), or who have a sense of pessimism about one's life (53), tend to have greater mood disturbance. In fact, Carver et al. (53) found that general pessimism (versus optimism) at diagnosis predicted poorer well being (mood and life satisfaction), not only one day before surgery but at 3-month, 6-month, and 12-month follow-ups as well. Miller et al. (54) reported similar results at 2-month and 4-month follow-ups. Alternatively, when patients use positive ways to cope, such as seeking social support and assistance from friends and family, they have less anxiety and depression; when they use avoidance, their moods worsen (55).

The clinical problem of diagnostic and treatment-related distress can be alleviated through psychological interventions (56–57). Even modest, early efforts can significantly reduce patients' distress as they approach cancer treatments. For example, McQuellon et al. developed a brief oncology clinic orientation program in the hopes of reducing anxiety, distress, and uncertainty in newly diagnosed cancer patients (58). The same principles shown in this study could be applied when devising a patient orientation for reconstructive surgery. The standardized program was designed to minimize the appraisal of threat in the new and unfamiliar setting. The 20-minute intervention included a tour of the oncology clinic, a verbal description of clinic administrative procedures, a handout of information (telephone numbers, map to the clinic, etc.), and a brief question and answer session. Patients were encouraged to address all medical questions to the medical staff. One hundred fifty patients were randomized into the treatment and control (no orientation) groups. One week after their initial visit, anxiety and mood disturbance decreased significantly for patients who received the intervention, whereas mood disturbance increased for control patients.

Improvements such as these are all the more impressive because they can be achieved with brief, cost-effective interventions delivered by nonphysicians (56).

PSYCHOSOCIAL RESPONSES TO CANCER SURGERY

Of course, a certain component of the emotional distress that occurs at the time of the breast cancer diagnosis is due to the patient's anticipation of treatments. Consider the multiple "stops" the breast cancer patient makes on the way to surgery. There are radiology studies, biopsy, physical examinations, tumor surveys, laboratory studies, and other requirements. Thus, the process of learning about and selecting the appropriate therapy, and waiting for it to occur, represents multiple medical stressors for patients. And then, there is the reconstruction consultation.

As discussed below, the data are consistent in their portrayal of increased distress (particularly fear and anxiety) among cancer patients. There are slower rates of emotional recovery, and, perhaps, higher rates of other behavioral difficulties (e.g., food aversions, continued fatigue, and malaise) among surgery patients relative to healthy individuals undergoing medical treatment. There have been few psychosocial investigations of cancer surgery, per se, but there are numerous descriptive and intervention studies of the reactions of healthy individuals undergoing surgery for benign conditions. The latter studies are consistent in their portrayal of (i) high levels of self-reported preoperative anxiety predictive of lowered postoperative anxiety and (ii) postoperative anxiety predictive of recovery (e.g., time out of bed, pain reports). What may distinguish cancer surgery patients are higher overall levels of distress and slower rates of emotional recovery. For example, Andersen, Anderson, and De-Prosse reported significantly worse negative moods for cancer patients than those with benign disease, as both awaited surgical treatment (59). Also, negative moods for both groups were higher than those for a matched group of healthy women. Following surgery, distress can continue. Gottesman and Lewis found greater and more lasting feelings of crisis and helplessness among cancer patients in comparison to benign surgery patients for as long as 2 months following discharge (60).

As noted above, there has been considerable research on the psychological and behavioral aspects of surgery. Many effective interventions designed to address these issues have been tested (61). Components of these interventions include procedural information (i.e., how the surgery is to be performed as well as preoperative and postoperative events from the perspective of the patient); sensory information on the actual physical sensations of preparatory procedures and the surgery per se (e.g., the specific nature of postsurgical pain); behavioral coping instructions; cognitive coping interventions; relaxation; hypnosis; and emotion focused interventions. In a meta-analysis of this literature, Johnston and Vogele reported that providing procedural information and behavioral instructions showed consistent and strong positive effects on postoperative recovery (61). Effects are significant for a broad band of measures, including ratings of negative affect and pain, amount of pain medication, length of stay, behavioral recovery, and physiological indices (61).

Psychological interventions have focused on a variety of methods to improve patient adjustment. The physician communication training intervention of Rutter, Iconomou, and Quine (33) discussed above and related efforts to provide additional information (e.g., orientation to the reconstruction consultation) can be cost effective. These interventions, as well as relaxation therapy (62), could be implemented with breast cancer patients. Further, with adequate training and supervision, peers or volunteers could be successfully used as "therapists." With a triage model, intensive (and expensive) efforts, such as psychiatric referral, could be provided selectively to moderate to high risk/high distress patients. Whether delivered to individual patients or to patient groups, these interventions are multimodal and include components consisting of stress reduction (progressive muscle relaxation training), disease/treatment information, cognitive-behavioral coping strategies, and social support (56).

RECONSTRUCTION: WHEN IS IT NOT PERFORMED?

According to statistics reported by the American Society for Plastic Surgery, in 2000 approximately 80,908 breast reconstruction procedures were performed, whereas 62,930 breast reconstruction surgeries were performed in 2004 (63). This decline may reflect the impact of limits on insurance reimbursement, more surgeries performed by nonspecialists, or declining rates of referral. Among some physicians and patients alike, there remain concerns that reconstruction may adversely affect treatment of the primary tumor or detection of cancer recurrence (65–72). Additionally, there are concerns that reconstruction prior to radiotherapy might result in later morbidities (e.g., delayed tissue healing) (66–67). However, other literature suggests that there are no additional complications when reconstruction precedes radiation treatment nor are there problems with detecting a recurrent cancer in the reconstructed breast (71–73).

Of course, the most influential factor determining whether breast reconstruction is recommended for any particular patient is the patient's medical history. For example, a patient's current cigarette smoking or obesity may be clear contraindications (74). If surgery proceeds, these factors may have continuing, adverse effects on the rate and severity of postsurgical complications. Indeed, a patient's risk for postsurgical complications increases threefold with one risk factor and 10-fold with two (74).

The majority of women receiving reconstruction are between the ages of 35 years and 64 years (63). Rates of reconstruction for older patients are low. For example, Morrow et al. (75) report that 8% of their patients were between 50 years and 69 years but only 1% was 70 or older. Panieri et al. (76–79) report similar findings of an inverse relationship between age and breast reconstruction. There are several factors that likely contribute to lower rates of reconstruction among older women, including higher rates of medical comorbidities (e.g., diabetes) that raise the risk for complications beyond what is considered prudent. Older patients may not be presented with the option for breast reconstruction and may not receive sufficient information about the available procedures. Some suggest that older women may not be as concerned about having an altered breast (80), although this is certainly not the case for all (81).

Other sociodemographic factors appear to be related to reconstruction rates. Interesting data comes from analyses of over 68,000 women in the National Cancer Database (75). Data were expressed in terms of odds ratios (OR); an odds ratio of 1.0 would indicate no effect of the variable, yet one >1.0 indicates a greater likelihood of the factor having a positive impact on the performance of reconstruction. Rates of reconstruction were 4.3-fold greater if a woman was age 50 or younger. Also, rates were higher among women with an income greater than $40,000 (OR = 2.0), an ethnicity other than African–American (OR = 1.6), who obtained treatment at a National Cancer Institute designated center (OR = 1.4), or who lived in geographic regions other than the midwest or southern United States (OR = 1.3).

THE RECONSTRUCTION CONSULTATION

Discussions between patients and surgeons regarding the indications for and the type and timing of breast reconstruction often occur within days of receiving a diagnosis of breast cancer. As detailed above, extreme levels of emotional distress characterize this period. In fact, stress levels during this period have been found to have an adverse effect on women's immunity (82). Women later describe these days as the worst of their lives. They are experiencing the highest levels of distress and confusion that are likely to occur throughout their cancer treatment (80–82). Indeed, the magnitude of stress at the time of diagnosis relates to the severity of concurrent depressive symptoms and also predicts quality of life, long after all cancer treatments have ended (85–86). Thus, it is not surprising that for some women, their attention is focused only on comprehending their diagnosis and treatment options, making it very difficult to adequately consider the complex issues involved in making decisions about breast reconstruction.

In view of the factors that need consideration, consultation is best viewed as a process rather than something to be accomplished in one visit. One consultation with the treatment team is a minimum. To the extent that time permits, patients should be allowed the opportunity to process the information and to consider the implications and outcomes of choosing or declining reconstruction. Should the patient wish, a spouse, partner, or close friend or relative might be included in the consultation process (77). Including another individual in the consultation can usually contribute to supportive atmosphere and thereby decrease a patient's stress. Another individual can help to recall the detailed information discussed. Suggesting that the patient audiotape the session can be similarly helpful (87).

The consultation team often consists of the oncology and plastic surgeons and perhaps a nurse. From a clinical perspective, preoperative consultation should provide, at the least, realistic expectations regarding reconstruction outcomes (88) including expectations about breast appearance, the feel of the reconstructed breast, symmetry of the breasts, and any need for additional surgeries (e.g., breast reduction/augmentation on the unaffected side) (89). This also includes review of the types of reconstruction procedures available to the patient as well as the types of implants which might be used, including their associated risks (77,88). Similarly, women may be unaware of the possibility of nipple reconstruction, as well as the possible options for it, including use of skin from the opposite nipple, local (star) flap, or tattooing (12).

Pictures of breast(s) before and after surgery to illustrate the chosen reconstruction method are an important aid for patients. Pictures depicting the range of clinical outcomes (e.g., ideal outcomes versus average outcomes versus less than average outcomes) informs and, hopefully, prompts patients to consider realistically how their body might change (87). Patient expectations for the surgical outcome require an assessment. Misperceptions regarding postoperative breast size or the appearance of the breast can easily occur. For example, patients need to understand that the type of reconstruction may predetermine breast size rather than personal preference (77).

Because financial concerns affect patients' choices regarding surgical reconstruction, it is also important to review costs in detail, including the cost of follow-up visits and any additional surgeries that might be needed or offered beyond the initial reconstruction (13,90–93). Of course, discussion of wound healing/care, recovery, and related issues is essential to providing the patient with fully informed consent.

Women need encouragement to engage actively in the consultation rather than being quiet recipients of information. The team may need to facilitate the patient's expression of her personal reasons for reconstruction. Conducting a consultation that allows the patient to make the best personal decision may require considerable time, skill, and patience on the part of the treatment team.

A number of researchers have examined the decision-making process for reconstruction (94–97). For example, Harcourt and Rumsey (98) studied 93 patients, 37 of whom elected breast reconstruction. The researchers identified three styles of decision making. The first style was one in which patients' decisions were immediate (82%), and one in which they expressed confidence and their mood was positive.

One-third of the women with this decision-making style elected breast reconstruction, whereas the others did not. The second most common decision-making style was focused on information seeking (15%). This style was similar to the first, but these women actively sought and used information in their decision making. A larger percentage of these women (71%) opted for reconstruction. Only 3% of women were indecisive. For them, providing additional information only seemed to add to their confusion and anxiety. Additionally, these patients took a longer period of time to arrive at a decision and when they finally did, they expressed low confidence in it. While this is a clinically useful report, these "styles" have not been empirically validated.

PSYCHOSOCIAL OUTCOMES FOLLOWING CANCER TREATMENTS

Quality of life issues are important to recovery from treatment and return to one's "normal" life. It is this larger context within which women undergoing reconstruction are functioning. At times their responses to reconstruction may take precedence, but it may be more typical that reconstruction is just one of many life circumstances with which patients are trying to cope.

As individuals recover and resume their lives, there may be residual emotional distress and difficulties that require continued coping. Lingering emotional distress from the trauma of diagnosis, treatment, and, more generally, life threat may occur for perhaps 5% to 7% of cancer patients (99). However, it is unlikely that such extreme distress will occur for the "average" breast cancer patient. This may be more likely for those who have undergone the most difficult and radical treatments, such as bilateral mastectomy. Longitudinal studies provide a glimpse of the mood, social adjustment, employment, and marital adjustment outcomes following treatment. For example Andersen, Anderson, and deProsse followed women for one year following their diagnosis (83). Although there were significant elevations of depression, anxiety, and confusion at the time of diagnosis, these traits stabilized within normal ranges during the posttreatment year. Similarly there was no significant disruption of social relationships or activities during recovery, and women gradually returned to their pretreatment levels.

Not surprisingly, there is a high incidence of sexual disruption among breast and gynecologic cancer patients alike (100). This has, in part, prompted concern about the risk of marital disruption. For example, one of the first clinical studies of women receiving radical mastectomy noted the realistic feelings of body disfigurement that both the women and spouses would feel, with the view that it would prompt sexual retreat, emotional estrangement, and, not surprisingly, marital disruption (101). Yet, despite the emotional distress and, for some, accompanying sexual disruption, data indicate that marriages remain intact, satisfactory, and occasionally stronger (102). Other data suggests that breast cancer patients who are more optimistic also feel more attractive and this, in turn, promotes perceptions that their partners are available for support (103). More recent data indicate that when marital breakdown occurs, it is most likely among those couples with precancer difficulties (104).

Stress may become significant for those closest to the patient, such as one's spouse or children (105). Problems facing the family members of a cancer patient can include loneliness, isolation, and role overload. As reviewed by Sales et al. (106), family strain appears to be affected by patient characteristics (e.g., prognosis, duration of illness, care giving demands, patient's distress), family variables (e.g., age and gender of family members, socioeconomic status, other family stressors), and relational factors (e.g., quality of marriage, marital communication, family stage, and social support). Young families, in which the wife/mother has cancer and young children are in the home, may be at heightened risk for relational difficulties (107). In addition, Ell, Nishimoto, Mantell, and Hamovitch (108) found that those relatives who were functioning poorly (e.g., lower perceived personal control, less adequate emotional support from close others, and greater stress unrelated to cancer) when the patient was diagnosed, or who lost personal and social resources during the patient's treatment and recovery, tended to function poorly at follow-up. In sum, a subset of partners and family members appear to be at psychosocial risk.

The impact of a breast cancer diagnosis and its treatment on quality of life is well documented (109–110). Late onset sequelae from cancer treatments have the potential to impact intimate relationships, social support, and heighten emotional distress (109,111–114). Cancer survivors report these problems and others, such as fatigue, somatic complaints, and loss of stamina (115–116). A cancer history can also result in financial difficulties, jeopardize insurance coverage, and narrow employment options. Indeed, one fifth of cancer survivors report chronic, stressful, and economic difficulties (117). These common sequelae can befall any cancer patient, including women undergoing breast reconstruction.

PSYCHOSOCIAL OUTCOMES UNIQUE TO BREAST RECONSTRUCTION

Research on psychological outcomes in breast reconstruction have primarily focused on three types of comparison studies: (i) outcomes for lumpectomy and mastectomy patients, with or without reconstruction; (ii) outcomes for women receiving immediate versus delayed reconstruction; and (iii) outcomes for women receiving different reconstruction procedures.

Prior to reviewing the literature it is important to provide the context for considering these psychosocial outcomes. That is, women who undergo mastectomy, in contrast to wide local excision, have more difficult sexual and body image adjustment. They complain of more physical symptoms related to their surgery and are more likely to report that their surgery had a negative impact on their sex lives (118–120). It is also the case that the vast majority (if not all) of mastectomy patients also receive adjuvant chemotherapy. The administration of chemotherapy is predictive of greater psychosocial distress, body image disturbance, and sexual dissatisfaction (120). In fact, Taylor et al. (121) analyzed their data controlling for the effects of chemotherapy. When groups were equated for receipt of chemotherapy, sexual attractiveness was equivalent for lumpectomy and mastectomy groups. Thus, the crucial question regarding reconstruction is the following: In view of the negative scenario anticipated for mastectomy patients, does reconstruction offer any possibility of lessening this burden?

Thus far, the literature suggests that breast reconstruction is not a panacea for the challenges faced by these patients. For example, Rowland et al. (119) studied 1,957 breast cancer survivors who had been treated with lumpectomy or mastectomy, with or without reconstruction. Women in both mastectomy groups compared to the lumpectomy group reported significantly higher levels of physical complaints and higher body image distress. Interestingly, women who received reconstruction noted that breast cancer had a more negative impact on their sexual functioning compared to women receiving lumpectomy or mastectomy alone. The reason for this latter effect is unclear. Certainly one possibility is that reconstruction patients may more easily attribute their dissatisfactions to their reconstruction per se, because of its salience.

Similarly, Yurek, Farrar, and Andersen (3) examined both body change stress and sexual functioning outcomes of 78 previously sexually active women who received lumpectomy/breast-conserving treatment and women who received modified radical mastectomy, 29 with and 79 without reconstruction. In this study, all women were assessed immediately following surgery but prior to beginning adjuvant therapy. Significantly poorer body image outcomes were revealed for all women receiving a mastectomy compared to women receiving a lumpectomy. Poorer body image outcomes were conceptualized as body change stress (e.g., avoidant behaviors such as looking at their body) and situational distress (e.g., feeling uncomfortable in a bathing suit). Women receiving mastectomy also engaged in significantly less frequent sexual activity than women treated with lumpectomy. Interestingly, women who underwent mastectomy and breast reconstruction reported less sexual activity and sexual responsiveness than women in the mastectomy and lumpectomy groups. Regarding the latter differences, the longer period of operative recovery that usually occurs for reconstruction patients may have been an important factor. Finally, 40% of the reconstruction group and 30% of the mastectomy group had not yet resumed sexual activity one month following surgery. These rates were significantly different from the 13% estimate for the lumpectomy patients.

Many authors have described the range of concerns patients can have after treatment. Harcourt and Rumsey (98) provide a discussion of patients' experiences and complex responses. The majority of women undergoing reconstruction may report disappointment with the reconstruction outcome per se, yet still report satisfaction with their decision to undergo reconstruction. Disappointment can come from continuing problems such as pain, the need for additional operations, lack of breast symmetry, and the absence of sensation in reconstructed breast, among others. The disease-free breast may also require surgery—breast reduction, augmentation, or mammoplasty—to match the reconstructed one (12,89).

Other studies have reported similar effects (122). Despite there being no obvious advantages to reconstruction with regards to sexuality or body image, there are important clinical benefits of reconstruction that women commonly report. Perhaps one of the most important is the positive impact of reconstruction on simple, day-to-day circumstances, such as clothing choice and fit. Also, the timing of reconstruction may be important for enhancing patient outcomes. For example, Al-Ghazal et al. (123) compared women who received immediate (IR; n = 38) versus delayed (DR; n = 83) breast reconstruction. Ninety-five percent of the IR patients preferred their timing where as only 24% of the DR group did. IR women also reported significantly lower levels of anxiety and depression and more positive body image, self-esteem, and feelings of sexual attractiveness. This same pattern of differences has been reported in other studies (76–77,124–125).

Finally, there are some data to suggest that there may be different psychosocial outcomes with regards to type of reconstruction performed. Wilkins et al. (125) examined the psychosocial outcomes of 250 reconstruction surgery patients who underwent one of three surgical procedures—tissue/implant expander (n = 56), pedicle TRAM flap (n = 128), or free TRAM flap (n = 66). The patients were assessed prior to, and one year following, reconstruction. Considering the patients who had received immediate reconstruction (regardless of type), there were no differences between surgical groups in psychosocial outcomes. However, for women receiving delayed reconstruction, the findings were mixed. Women electing expanders/implants reported significantly greater social well-being than the TRAM flap groups. Conversely, women receiving either type of TRAM flap reported more positive body image than did the women receiving an expander/implant. Another study comparing unipedicled and bipedicled TRAM flap groups reported no differences in daily activities or satisfaction with surgery, whereas Alderman et al. (126) reported greater satisfaction among women receiving pedicle flaps in contrast to those receiving free TRAM flaps.

In summary, our literature review emphasizes that women receiving mastectomy have a more difficult psychosocial course than women able to receive breast-conserving surgeries. Reconstruction does not appear to lessen this difficult outcome with regards to body image or sexuality. Even so, the practical advantages to reconstruction are considerable. When reconstruction is performed, women who receive it early do appear to have psychosocial advantages in comparison to cases that are delayed. There are too few studies to determine if one surgery type has advantages over others. Patient variables are potentially important factors in psychosocial outcomes. Women who are young, come to reconstruction with a poor preoperative body image, or have histories of a mood disorder have higher risk for distress and dissatisfaction following reconstruction (5,124).

CONCLUSIONS

Breast reconstruction is an option for many breast cancer patients. However, clinical practice patterns suggest reconstruction is not equally available to all patients. Furthermore, there is some reason to believe that reconstructive surgery may not achieve a goal of fully restoring a woman's preoperative body image, and it cannot, of course, resolve other psychosocial problems, such as mood disorders.

With the complexities surrounding breast reconstruction (e.g., timing, type of method, healing process, additional surgeries, medical complications), it is critical that the consultation be conducted with great care. Information regarding the details of breast reconstruction should be presented to the patient after she has had some time to assimilate and respond to her cancer diagnosis and consider options for her primary treatment. The level of distress with breast cancer diagnosis and treatment is considerable, and thus, it may be useful to conduct an assessment of the patient's current psychosocial functioning. Clinicians might administer global measures of mood (127), depressive and anxiety symptoms (128–129), and quality of life (130), as well as more specific measures like the BITS included with this chapter. This information can facilitate the care of the patient undergoing and adapting to breast reconstruction.

The Breast Impact of Treatment Scale (BITS)

Directions: Below are comments women have made following breast cancer treatments. Using the scale provided, please indicate how frequently these comments have been true in describing your experience.

Code: 0 = Not at all
                1 = Rarely
                3 = Sometimes
                5 = Often

___ 1. I feel uncomfortable about being seen naked.

___ 2. I avoid looking at and/or touching my scar.

___ 3. I am bothered by feeling or thoughts of bodily disfigurement.

___ 4. I think about how my treatments may affect my sex life.

___ 5. I feel self-conscious about letting my partner (person I am sexually intimate) see my scar. Even if you do not have a partner now, rate how you believe you would feel.

___ 6. When I see other women, I think my body appears different than theirs.

___ 7. I have waves of strong feeling about the way my body looks.

___ 8. I think about how my body looked before I was treated.

___ 9. I am reminded of my scar when I pick out clothes to wear.

___ 10. Things I see or hear remind me that my body is different now.

___ 11. I avoid letting myself get emotional when I think of how my body has changed.

___ 12. I turn away when I have to undress in front of my partner (person with whom I am sexually intimate). Even if you do not have a partner now, rate how you believe you would feel.

___ 13. How my body has changed pops into my mind.

___ 14. I don't want to deal with how my body looks.

___ 15. I try not to think about my breasts being different.

Note: Items 1, 2, 5, and 12 comprise the Avoidance Scale and items 3, 4, 6–11; items 13–14 comprise the Intrusion Scale.

REFERENCES

1. Jemal A, Murray T, Ward E, et al. Cancer statistics, 2005. *CA Cancer J* 2005;55: 10–30.
2. Andrykowski MA, Cordova MJ, McGrath PC, et al. Stability and change in posttraumatic stress disorder symptoms following breast cancer treatment: a 1 year follow-up. *Psychooncology* 2000;9:69–78.
3. Yurek D, Farrar W, Andersen BL. Breast cancer surgery: comparing surgical groups and determining individual differences in postoperative sexuality and body change stress. *J Consult Clin Psychol* 2000;68:697–709.
4. Moyer A, Salovey P. Psychological sequelae of breast cancer and its treatment. *Ann Behav Med* 1996;18:110–125.
5. Pruzinsky T. Body image adaptation to reconstructive surgery for acquired disfigurement. In: Cash TF, Pruzinsky T, eds. *Body Image: A Handbook of Theory, Research, and Clinical Practice.* New York: Guilford Press, 2002:440–449.
6. Mock V. Body image in women treated for breast cancer. *Nurs Res* 1993;42:153–157.
7. Osteen RT. Reconstruction after mastectomy. *Cancer* 1995;76:2070–2074.
8. Kemeny M, Wellisch D, Schain W. Psychological outcome in a randomized surgical trial for treatment of primary breast cancer. *Cancer* 1988;62:1231–1237.
9. Steinberg MD, Juliano MA, Wise L. Psychological outcome of lumpectomy versus mastectomy in the treatment of breast cancer. *Am J Psychiatry* 1985;142: 34–39.
10. Fallowfield LJ, Hall A. Psychosocial and sexual impact of diagnosis and treatment of breast cancer. *Br Med Bull* 1991;47:388–399.
11. Winder AE, Winder BD. Patient counseling: clarifying a woman's choice for breast reconstruction. *Patient Educ Couns* 1985;7: 65–75.
12. Antoniuk PM. Breast reconstruction. *Obstet Gynecol Clin North Am* 2002;29:209–223.
13. Desch CE, Penberthy LT, Hillner BE, et al. A sociodemographic and economic comparison of breast reconstruction, mastectomy, and conservative surgery. *Surgery* 1999;125:441–447.
14. Frierson G. The Breast Impact of Treatment Scale: the Assessment of Body Image Distress for Breast Cancer Patients [dissertation]. Columbus, OH: The Ohio State University; 2003.
15. Cash TF, Pruzinsky T, eds. *Body Image: A Handbook of Theory, Research, and Clinical Practice.* New York: Guilford Press, 2002.
16. Hopwood P. The assessment of body image in cancer patients. *Eur J Cancer* 1993;29A:276–281.
17. White CA. Body image dimensions and cancer: a heuristic cognitive behavioural model. *Psychooncology* 2000;9:183–192.
18. White CA. Body images in oncology. In: Cash TF, Pruzinsky T, eds. *Body Image: A Handbook of Theory, Research, and Clinical Practice.* New York: Guilford Press, 2002:379–386.
19. Souto CM, Garcia TR. Construction and validation of a body image rating scale: a preliminary study. *Int J Nurs Terminol Classif* 2002;13:117–126.
20. Derogatis LR, Melisaratos N. The DSFI: a multidimensional measure of sexual functioning. *J Sex Marital Ther* 1979;5:244–281.
21. Berscheild G, Walster E, Bohrnstedt G. Body image: a psychology today questionnaire. *Psychol Today* 1972;6:57–66.
22. Roid GF, Fitts WH. *Tennessee Self-Concept Scale: Revised Manual.* Los Angeles: Western Psychological Services, 1988.
23. Secord P, Jourard S. The appraisal of body cathexis: body cathexis and the self. *J Consult Psychol* 1958;21:343–347.
24. Secord P. Objectification of word association procedures by use of homonyms: a measure of body cathexis. *J Pers* 1953;21:471–495.
25. Franzoli SL, Shields SA. The body esteem scale: multideminisional structure and sex differences. *J Pers* 1984;48:173–178.
26. Hopwood P, Lee A, Shenton A, et al. Clinical follow-up after bilateral risk reducing ("prophylactic") mastectomy: mental health and body image outcomes. *Psychooncology* 2000;9:462–472.
27. Andersen BL, Cyranowski M. Women's sexual self-schema. *J Pers Soc Psychol* 1994;67:1079–1100.
28. Weisman AD, Worden JW. The existential plight in cancer: significance of the first 100 days. *Int J Psychiatry Med* 1976;7:1–15.
29. Sardell AN, Trierweiler SJ. Disclosing the cancer diagnosis. *Cancer* 1993;72:3355–3365.
30. Roberts JA, Brown D, Elkins T, et al. Factors influencing views of patients with gynecologic cancer about end-of-life decisions. *Am J Obstet Gynecol* 1997;176:166–172.
31. Sell L, Devlin B, Bourke SJ, et al. Communicating the diagnosis of lung cancer. *Respir Med* 1993;87:61–63.
32. Woodard LJ, Pamies RJ. The disclosure of the diagnosis of cancer. *Prim Care* 1992;19:657–663.
33. Rutter DR, Iconomou G, Quine L. Doctor–patient communication and outcome in cancer patients: an intervention. *Psychol Health* 1996;12:57–71.
34. Ley P. *Communicating with Patients.* London, England: Chapman & Hall, 1988.
35. Spielberger CD, Gorsuch RL, Lushene RD. *Manual for the State-Trait Anxiety Inventory (STAI).* Palo Alto, CA: Consulting Psychologists Press, 1970.
36. Beck AT, Beck RW. Screening depressed patients in family practice: a rapid technique. *Postgrad Med* 1972;52:81–85.
37. National Comprehensive Cancer Network. *Clinical Practice Guidelines for Management of Distress.* Atlanta: American Cancer Society, 2002.
38. Locke BZ, Regier DA. Prevalence of selected mental disorders. In: Taube CA, Barrett SA, eds. *Mental Health United States.* Rockville, MD: National Institute of Mental Health, 1985:1–6.
39. Bodurka-Bevers D, Basen-Engquist K, Carmack CL, et al. Depression, anxiety, and quality of life in patients with epithelial ovarian cancer. *Gynecol Oncol* 2000;78:302–308.

40. Derogatis LR, Morrow GR, Fetting J. The prevalence of psychiatric disorders among cancer patients. *JAMA* 1983;249:751–757.
41. Kornblith AB, Thaler HT, Wong G, et al. Quality of life of women with ovarian cancer. *Gynecol Oncol* 1995;59:231–242.
42. Massie MJ, Holland JC. Depression and the cancer patient. *J Clin Psychiatry* 1990;51:12–17.
43. Levin SH, Jones LD, Sack DA. Evaluation and treatment of depression, anxiety, and insomnia in patients with cancer. *Oncology* 1993;7:119–125.
44. Meyerowitz BE, Formenti SC, Ell KO, et al. Depression among Latina cervical cancer patients. *J Soc Clin Psychol* 2000;19:352–371.
45. Bukberg J, Penman D, Holland JC. Depression in hospitalized cancer patients. *Psychosom Med* 1984;46:199–212.
46. Cella DF, Orofiamma B, Holland JC, et al. The relationship of psychological distress, extent of disease, and performance status in patients with lung cancer. *Cancer* 1987;60:1661–1667.
47. Alter CL, Axelrod A, Harris H, et al. Identification of PTSD in cancer survivors. *Psychosomatics* 1996;37:137–143.
48. Cordova M, Andrykowski M, Kenady D, et al. Frequency and correlates of posttraumatic-stress-disorder-like symptoms after treatment for breast cancer. *J Consult Clin Psychol* 1995;63:981–986.
49. Green B, Rowland J, Krupnick J, et al. Prevalence of posttraumatic stress disorder in women with breast cancer. *Psychosomatics* 1998;39:102–111.
50. Butler L, Koopman C, Classen C, et al. Traumatic stress, life events, and emotional support in women with metastatic breast cancer: cancer-related traumatic stress symptoms associated with past and current stressors. *Health Psychol* 1999;18:555–560.
51. Cella D, Mahon S, Donovan MI. Cancer recurrence as a traumatic event. *Behav Med* 1990;16:15–22.
52. Marks G, Richardson JL, Graham JW, et al. Role of health locus of control beliefs and expectations of treatment efficacy in adjustment to cancer. *J Pers Soc Psychol* 1986;51:443–450.
53. Carver CS, Pozo-Kaderman C, Harris SD, et al. Optimism versus pessimism predicts the quality of women's adjustment to early stage breast cancer. *Cancer* 1994;73:1213–1220.
54. Miller DL, Manne SL, Talyor K, et al. Psychological distress and well-being in advanced cancer: the effects of optimism and coping. *J Clin Psychol Med Settings* 1996;3:115–130.
55. Lutgendorf SK, Anderson B, Rothrock N, et al. Quality of life and mood in women receiving extensive chemotherapy for gynecologic cancer. *Cancer* 2000;89:1402–1411.
56. Andersen BL. Psychological interventions for cancer patients to enhance the quality of life. *J Consult Clin Psychol* Year 60:552–568.
57. Andersen BL. Biobehavioral outcomes following psychological interventions for cancer patients. *J Consult Clin Psychol* 2002;70:590–610.
58. McQuellon RP, Wells M, Hoffman S. Reducing distress in cancer patients with an orientation program. *Psychooncology* 1998;7:207–217.
59. Andersen B, Lachenbruch P, Anderson B, et al. Sexual dysfunction and signs of gynecologic cancer. *Cancer* 1986;57:1880–1886.
60. Gottesman D, Lewis M. Differences in crisis reactions among cancer and surgery patients. *J Consult Clin Psychol* 1982;50:381–388.
61. Johnston M, Vogele C. Benefits of psychological preparation for surgery: a meta-analysis. *Ann Behav Med* 1993;15:245–256.
62. Larsson G, Starrin B. Relaxation training as an integral part of caring activities for cancer patients: effects on well-being. *Scand J Caring Sci* 1992;6:179–186.
63. American Society of Plastic Surgeons. *2004 Breast Surgery Statistics.* Arlington Heights, IL: American Society of Plastic Surgeons, 2004.
64. Sarwer DB. Cosmetic surgery and changes in body image. In: Cash TF, Pruzinsky T, eds. *Body Image: A Handbook of Theory, Research, and Clinical Practice.* New York: Guilford Press, 2002:422–430.
65. Williams JK, Carlson GW, Bostwick J, et al. The effects of radiation treatment after TRAM flap breast reconstruction. *Plast Reconstr Surg* 1997;100:1153–1160.
66. Kraemer O, Andersen M, Siim E. Breast reconstruction and tissue expansion in irradiated versus not irradiated women after mastectomy. *Scand J Plast Reconstr Surg Hand Surg* 1996;30:201–206.
67. Forman DL, Chiu J, Restifo RJ, et al. Breast reconstruction in previously irradiated patients using tissue expanders and implants: a potentially unfavorable result. *Ann Plast Surg* 1998;40:360–363.
68. Allweis TM, Boisvert ME, Otero SE, et al. Immediate reconstruction after mastectomy for breast cancer does not prolong the time to starting adjuvant chemotherapy. *Am J Surg* 2002;183:218–221.
69. Deutsch MF, Smith M, Wang B, et al., Immediate breast reconstruction with the TRAM flap after neoadjuvant therapy. *Ann Plast Surg* 1999;42:240–244.
70. Yule GJ, Concannon MJ, Croll G, et al. Is there liability with chemotherapy following immediate breast construction? *Plast Reconstr Surg* 1996;97:969–973.
71. Shaikh N, LaTrenta G, Swistel A, et al. Detection of recurrent breast cancer after TRAM flap reconstruction. *Ann Plast Surg* 2001;47:602–607.
72. Slavin SA, Love SM, Goldwyn RM. Recurrent breast cancer following immediate reconstruction with myocutaneous flaps. *Plast Reconstr Surg* 1994;93:1191–1207.
73. Schain WS, Wellisch DK, Pasnau RO, et al. The sooner the better: a study of psychological factors in women undergoing immediate versus delayed breast reconstruction. *Am J Psychiatry* 1985;142:40–46.
74. Lin KY, Johns FR, Gibson J, et al. An outcome study of breast reconstruction: presurgical identification of risk factors for complications. *Ann Surg Oncol* 2001;8:586–591.
75. Morrow M, Scott SK, Menck HR, et al. Factors influencing the use of breast reconstruction postmastectomy: a National Cancer Database study. *J Am Coll Surg* 2001;192:1–8.
76. Panieri E, Lazarus D, Dent DM, et al. A study of the patient factors affecting reconstruction after mastectomy for breast carcinoma. *Am Surg* 2003;69:95–97.

77. Tebbetts J, Tebbetts T. An approach that integrates patient education and informed consent in breast augmentation. *Plast Reconstr Surg* 2002;1:971–978.
78. Greenfield S, Blanco DM, Elashoff RM, et al. Patterns of care related to age of breast cancer patients. *JAMA* 1987;257:2766–2770.
79. Polednak AP. Geographic variation in postmastectomy breast reconstruction rates. *Plast Reconstr Surg* 2000;106:298–301.
80. Schain WS. Breast reconstruction. Update of psychosocial and pragmatic concerns. *Cancer* 1991;68:1170–1175.
81. Rowland JH. Psychological impact of treatments for cancer. In: Spear SL, ed. *Surgery of the Breast: Principles and Art.* Philadelphia: Lippincott–Raven Publishers, 1998.
82. Andersen BL, Farrar WB, Golden-Kreutz D, et al. Stress and immune responses after surgical treatment for regional breast cancer. *J Natl Cancer Inst* 1998;90:30–36.
83. Andersen BL, Anderson B, deProsse C. Controlled prospective longitudinal study of women with cancer: II. Psychological outcomes. *J Consult Clin Psychol* 1989;57:692–697.
84. Andersen BL, Anderson B, deProsse C. Controlled prospective longitudinal study of women with cancer: I. Sexual functioning outcomes. *J Consult Clin Psychol* 1989;57:683–691.
85. Golden-Kreutz DM, Andersen BL. Depressive symptoms after breast cancer surgery: relationships with global, cancer-related, and life event stress. *Psychooncology* 2004;13:211–220.
86. Golden-Kreutz D, Thorton LM, Wells-Di-Gregorio S, et al. Stress at initial breast cancer diagnosis/surgery: a predictor of psychological and physical quality of life. *Health Psychol* 2005. (In press.)
87. Wolf L. The information needs of women who have undergone breast reconstruction. Part I: decision-making and sources of information. *Eur J Oncol Nurs* 2004;8:211–223.
88. Baker C, Johnson N, Nelson J, et al. Perspective on reconstruction after mastectomy. *Am J Surg* 2002;183:562–565.
89. Wickman M. Breast reconstruction—past achievements, current status and future goals. *Scand J Plast Reconstr Surg Hand Surg* 1995;29:81–100.
90. Elkowitz A, Cohen S, Slavin S, et al. Various methods of breast reconstruction after mastectomy: an economic comparison. *Plast Reconstr Surg* 1998;101:964–970.
91. Scanlon EF. The role of reconstruction in breast cancer. *Cancer* 1991;68:1144–1147.
92. Khoo A, Kroll S, Reece G, et al. A comparison of resources costs of immediate and delayed breast reconstruction. *Plast Reconstr Surg* 1993;92:77–83.
93. Franchelli S, Leone MS, Berrino P, et al. Can the cost affect the choice of various methods of postmastectomy breast reconstruction? *Tumori* 1998;84:383–386.
94. Reaby LL. The quality and coping patterns of women's decision-making regarding breast cancer surgery. *Psychooncology* 1998b;7:252–262.
95. Pierce PF. Deciding on breast cancer treatment: a description of decision behavior. *Nurs Res* 1993; 42:22–28.
96. Reaby LL. Breast restoration decision making: enhancing the process. *Cancer Nurs* 1998a;21:196–204.
97. Broadstock M, Michie S. Processes of patient decision making: theoretical and methodological issues. *Psych Health* 2000;15:191–204.
98. Harcourt D, Rumsey N. Mastectomy patients' decision-making for or against immediate breast reconstruction. *Psychooncology* 2004;13:106–115.
99. Smith MY, Redd WH, Peyser C, et al. Post-traumatic stress disorder in cancer: a review. *Psychooncology* 1999;8:521–537.
100. Andersen BL, Jochimsen PR. Sexual functioning among breast cancer, gynecologic cancer, and healthy women. *J Consult Clin Psychol* 1985;53:25–32.
101. Bard M, Sutherland AM. Adaptation to radical mastectomy. *Cancer* 1952;8:656–671.
102. Cella DF, Tross S. Psychological adjustment to survival from Hodgkin's disease. *J Consult Clin Psychol* 1986;54:616–622.
103. Abend TA, Williamson GM. Feeling attractive in the wake of breat cancer: optimism matters, and so do interpersonal relationships. *Pers Soc Psychol Bull* 2002;28:427–436.
104. Taylor-Brown J, Kilpatrick M, Maunsell E, et al. Partner abandonment of women with breast cancer: myth or reality? *Cancer Pract* 2000;8:160–164.
105. Baider L, Cooper CL, De-Nour, AK, eds. *Cancer and the Family.* New York: John Wiley and Sons, 2000.
106. Sales E, Schulz R, Biegel D. Predictors of strain in families of cancer patients: a review of the literature. *J Psychosocial Oncology* 1992;10:1–26.
107. Vess JD, Moreland JR, Schwebel AI. A follow-up study of role functioning and the psychosocial environment of families of cancer patients. *J Psychosocial Oncology* 1985;3:1–14.
108. Ell K, Nishimoto R, Mantell J, Hamovitch M. Longitudinal analysis of psychological adaptation among family members of patients with cancer. *J Psychosom Res* 1988;32:429–438.
109. Ganz P, Coscarelli A, Fred C, et al. Breast cancer survivors: psychosocial concerns and quality of life. *Breast Cancer Res Treat* 1996;38:183–199.
110. Holzer B, Kemmler G, Kopp M, et al. Quality of life in breast cancer patients—not enough attention for long-term survivors? *Psychosomatics* 2001;42:117–123.
111. Ey S, Compas BE, Epping-Jordan JE, et al. Stress responses and psychological adjustment in patients with cancer and their spouses. *J Psychosocial Oncology* 1998;16:59–77.
112. Holzner B, Kemmler G, Kopp M, et al. Quality of life in breast cancer patients—not enough attention for long term survivors? *Psychosomatics* 2001;42:117–123.
113. Spencer S, Lehman J, Wynings C, et al. Concerns about breast cancer and relations to psychosocial well-being in a multiethnic sample of early-stage patients. *Health Psychol* 1999;18:159–168.
114. Steginga S, Occhipinti S, Dunn J, et al. The supportive care needs of men with prostate cancer. *Psychooncology* 2001;10:66–75.
115. Michael Y, Kawachi I, Berkman L, et al. The persistent impact of breast carcinoma on functional health status: prospective evidence from the Nurses' Health Study. *Cancer* 2000;89:2176–2186.

116. Broeckel J, Jacobsen P, Balducci L, et al. Quality of life after adjuvant chemotherapy for breast cancer. *Breast Cancer Res Treat* 2000;62:141–150.
117. Hewitt M, Breen N, Devesa, S. Cancer prevalence and survivorship issues: analyses of the 1992 National Health Interview Survey. *J Natl Cancer Inst* 1999;91:1480–1486.
118. Curran D, van Dongen JP, Aaronson NK, et al. Quality of life of early-stage breast cancer patients treated with radical mastectomy or breast-conserving procedures: results of the EORTC Trail 10801. *Eur J Cancer* 1998;34:307–314.
119. Rowland JH, Desmond KA, Meyerowitz BE, et al. Role of breast reconstructive surgery in physical and emotional outcomes among breast cancer survivors. *J Natl Cancer Inst* 2000;92:1422–1429.
120. Schover L, Yetman R, Tuason L, et al. Partial mastectomy and breast reconstruction. A comparison of their effects on psychosocial adjustment, body image, and sexuality. *Cancer* 1995; 75:54–64.
121. Taylor K, Lamdan R, Siegel J, et al. Treatment regimen, sexual attractiveness concerns and psychological adjustment among African American breast cancer patients. *Psychooncology* 2002;11:505–517.
122. Holly P, Kennedy P, Taylor A, et al. Immediate breast reconstruction and psychological adjustment in women who have undergone surgery for breast cancer: a preliminary study. *Psychol Health Medicine* 2003;8:441–452.
123. Al-Ghazal SK, Sully L, Fallowfield L, et al. The psychological impact of immediate rather than delayed breast reconstruction. *Eur J Surg Oncol* 2000;26:17–19.
124. Harcourt DM, Rumsey NJ, Ambler NR, et al. The psychological effect of mastectomy with or without breast reconstruction: a prospective, multicenter study. *Plast Reconstr Surg* 2003;111:1060–1068.
125. Wilkins EG, Cederna PS, Lowery JC, et al. Prospective analysis of psychosocial outcomes in breast reconstruction: one-year postoperative results from the Michigan Breast Reconstruction Outcome Study. *Plast Reconstr Surg* 2000;106:1014–1025.
126. Alderman A, Wilkins E, Lowery J, et al. Determinants of patient satisfaction in postmastectomy breast reconstruction. *Plast Reconstr Surg* 2000;106:769–776.
127. McNair DM, Lorr M, Droppleman LF. *EITS Manual of the Profile of Mood States.* San Diego, CA: Educational and Industrial Testing Services, 1971.
128. Radloff LS. The CES-D Scale: a self-report depression scale for research in the general population. *Appl Psychol Meas* 1977;1:385–401.
129. Beck AT, Epstein N, Brown G, et al. An inventory for measuring clinical anxiety: psychometric properties. *J Consult Clin Psychol* 1988;56:893–897.
130. Ware JE, Snow KK, Kosinski M. *SF-36 Health Survey: Manual and Interpretation Guide.* Lincoln, RI: Quality Metric Incorporated, 2000.

Chapter 12

Breast Reduction

V. Leroy Young, MD, and Marla E. Watson, MA

The American Society of Plastic Surgeons (ASPS) defines reconstructive surgery as being "performed on abnormal structures of the body, caused by congenital defects, developmental abnormalities, trauma, infection, tumors or disease. It is generally performed to improve function, but may also be done to approximate a normal appearance" (1). According to this definition, reduction mammoplasty is considered reconstructive in nature. Yet, aesthetic concerns play important roles in the motivations for surgery as well as postoperative satisfaction.

Women who suffer from breast hypertrophy—unusually large breast size in proportion to the rest of the body—fall into two broad categories: younger women and postmenopausal women (2). In younger women, enlarged breasts most often result from juvenile hypertrophy or obesity. Juvenile hypertrophy is relatively uncommon in the general population and the etiology is unknown. Nevertheless, these patients present to the plastic surgeon with some regularity. Some believe abnormally high levels of estrone or estradiol are responsible for the breast hypertrophy, but studies also have documented decreased levels of plasma progesterone (3). Others speculate that breast hypertrophy results from an exaggerated organ response to minimal concentrations of the estrogens and progesterone that regulate breast growth (2–3). Infrequently, reactions to drugs such as D-penicillamine may be responsible for the breast hypertrophy. Whatever the cause, the structure of the breast is essentially normal but there is a volume increase in its glandular and connective tissue components (4). In contrast, a hypertrophic breast associated with obesity usually contains more subcutaneous and interglandular fat deposits. For postmenopausal women, hypertrophic breasts are characterized by sagging and replacement of lobular tissue with fat (2).

Women who seek reduction mammoplasty (RM) are primarily interested in having average-sized breasts that are proportional to the rest of their bodies. As an additional benefit of the procedure, many women experience improved physical and psychosocial functioning that leads to an enhanced quality of life. In 2004, 105,592 breast reduction procedures were performed in the United States by board-certified plastic surgeons (1). This number represents a 25% increase since 2000 and will probably continue to rise as plastic surgery in general becomes more socially acceptable. Presently, the literature describes 72 different breast reduction techniques, many of which are variations of techniques first developed in the early 20th century (5). RM procedures have improved over the years as surgeons have developed technical innovations to reduce scarring and improve patient satisfaction.

This chapter will explore the reasons why women seek RM, including the pursuit of relief from the physical symptoms of breast hypertrophy that nonsurgical treatments do not offer. Relief of psychological distress caused by abnormal breast size is similarly important in the minds of many RM patients. The physical and psychological outcomes of breast reduction are then discussed, as are the high levels of patient satisfaction and reasons for dissatisfaction.

PREOPERATIVE MOTIVATIONS FOR BREAST REDUCTION

The primary preoperative motivations for breast reduction can be loosely classified as either physical or psychological in nature. One prospective study has identified six major areas of concern to women who seek breast reduction: (i) physical activity limitations; (ii) clothes fit and availability; (iii) physical problems and pain; (iv) embarrassment; (v) lack of confidence; and (vi) personal relationships and social life (6). In two large, retrospective studies, 98% to 100% of women endorsed one or more of these factors as the reason that they sought surgery (7–8). Relief of physical symptoms was reported by 91% and 78% of women in the two studies; self-consciousness about breast size was cited by 78% and 68%; and cosmetic concerns were named by 65%.

Physical Symptoms

One goal of RM is to reduce breast volume and weight, which can cause upper/lower back pain, neck and shoulder pain, breast pain, headaches, and ulnar nerve paresthesia (7,9–13). Although these symptoms are often trivialized by those who do not have large breasts, preoperative RM patients score higher on standardized pain indexes as compared to persons suffering from arthritis and chronic low back pain (13).

Common physical findings that contribute to discomfort include shoulder grooving from bra straps that support the breast weight (7,9–10,12–15), stooped posture (9,14,16), intertrigo beneath the breasts caused by sweating and irritation within the inframammary crease (7–10,12–16), and difficulty finding a comfortable sleeping position (8–9,16). Decreased sensation in the skin, nipple, and/or areola also occurs with some frequency (17–19). Although not completely understood, two theories are most often postulated as causes of decreased sensation: (i) chronic traction injury to the sensory nerves resulting from the pull of gravity on a heavy breast, and (ii) decreased density of sensory nerve receptors in the expanded nipple-areolar complex (17). Measurable preoperative respiratory difficulties—and their significant improvement after surgery—also have been reported (20–21).

For some women, the pain associated with breast hypertrophy may be severe enough to interfere with work. For example, 41% of reduction patients in one study had a working disability (on sick leave for some period of time) because of symptom severity (22). In addition, the pain and weight of very large breasts typically leads to reductions in exercise and engagement in everyday living activities, such as housework and playing with children. Studies have found that at least 83% of RM patients have difficulty taking part in physical activity most or all of the time prior to surgery (13,23).

The relationship between body mass and the physical symptoms associated with large breasts is equivocal. Several studies have suggested that the physical symptoms suffered by women who seek RM have been found to be independent of their body mass index (BMI) (9,24–25). Other studies, however, have found an association between overall body mass and physical symptoms. For example, in comparing obese and non-obese RM patients, Glatt et al. found that obese women were significantly more likely to have neck pain, breast pain, and intertrigo than non-obese patients (14). Netscher et al. compared the physical and psychosocial symptoms of 31 women seeking breast reduction, 21 seeking breast augmentation, and 88 student volunteers who had never thought about breast surgery (26). Not surprisingly, the breast reduction group had a significantly higher mean weight, larger bra cup size, and larger bra circumference size. When all subjects were categorized according to small, medium, or large body mass, bra circumference size, and bra cup size, the large body mass index group was significantly more likely to report only three conditions: back/neck pain, shoulder pain, and rashes. When the women were categorized by chest circumference, the large size group was significantly different on four conditions: back/neck pain, shoulder pain, rashes, and appearance concerns. When categorized according to bra cup, the large size group was significantly more likely to report back/neck pain, shoulder pain, rashes, breathing problems, tingling/numbness in upper extremities, activity limitations, and reduced exercise participation. Thus, a large bra cup size was associated with more of the physical symptoms of breast hypertrophy than either body mass or bra circumference.

The physical symptoms of macromastia appear to vary by age. Almost half (48%) of breast reduction patients are between the ages of 19 and 34 (1). Thirty-six percent are between 35 and 50 years old, 14% are 18 or younger, and 2% are 51 years old and older. Complaints about physical symptoms are more often voiced by women in their 30s and older, perhaps because of the accumulated years of carrying heavy and disproportionate weight on the chest, which can place unnatural loading on the upper body skeleton and musculature (27). However, studies that looked specifically at teenagers with breast hypertrophy found that large majorities of them—up to 100% in some studies—also reported back, neck, or shoulder pain (28–29).

Psychological Motivations

Breast hypertrophy may have a profound effect on women's lives by contributing to heightened self-consciousness, poor self-esteem, decreased confidence, and a negative body image (6,10,16,30–32). Large breasts can interfere with a woman's ability to have an active lifestyle and make it difficult to find clothing, swimsuits, or underwear that fit (6,10,16,30–32). Almost two-thirds of RM patients questioned before surgery "almost always" or "often" felt unattractive, and 40% felt their breast size adversely affected their sex lives (31).

Although younger patients suffer from physical problems, they may be more strongly motivated to have surgery because of psychosocial concerns (29,33). In addition to being the brunt of jokes and teasing comments related to their breast size during their formative years, teenagers may experience a great deal of unwanted attention from their male peers, who tend to pay more attention to their large breasts than see the person behind them (29). Adolescent girls with breast hypertrophy are often unable or embarrassed to wear bathing suits and fashionable clothing commonly worn by their peers (29). As a result, they may adopt strategies to camouflage their breasts, such as wearing baggy clothing, adopting a stooped posture, or intentionally gaining weight. If untreated, the emotional and social repercussions of abnormally large breasts in adolescence may resonate throughout adulthood.

Deliberate weight gain to hide macromastia is not uncommon among young women. Increased breast size also may inhibit a young woman's ability to engage in regular exercise or organized sports as a way to maintain a healthy lifestyle and normal body weight. While some teenagers choose to gain weight, others may develop eating disorders (34–35). One study reported on nine young women with bulimia nervosa who wore DD or DDD bra cup sizes by their mid-teens and began binge eating and purging as an inappropriate weight control strategy (35). After RM, eight of the nine had recovered from bulimia, and the one still recovering had reduced her binging and purging episodes by 80% (35).

Several studies have investigated the psychological motivations of RM using a variety of psychometric measures. In particular, quality of life, body image, depressive, and anxiety-related symptoms have received the greatest empirical attention.

Quality of life is a significant concern of women who seek breast reduction. The well-validated and standardized Medical Outcomes Survey Short Form–36 (SF-36) has been used most often to assess the health-related quality of life of breast reduction patients. The SF–36 has eight subscales: physical function, role limitation (physical), role limitation (mental), social function, mental function, vitality and energy, pain, and health perception. Several investigators have compared the preoperative scores of RM patients with normal controls from the general population and found that patients scored significantly lower than population controls on six (16,30) to all eight quality of life dimensions (11,13,31,36).

Other studies have examined additional psychological symptoms potentially related to breast hypertrophy. Using the Brief Symptom Inventory (BSI), Behmand et al. found that RM candidates had significantly higher ratings for depression, anxiety, interpersonal sensitivity, and hostility when compared to normal controls (36). Scores from preoperative RM patients on the Hospital Anxiety and Depression Scale (HADS) revealed significantly more symptoms of depression and anxiety when compared with an age-matched control group of large-breasted women who did not want surgery (30). The women who wanted surgery also had lower self-esteem and greater interpersonal difficulties than the large-breasted controls (30). Additionally, the surgical patients reported significantly more physical symptoms and limitations than the controls, which may have contributed to the pursuit of surgery.

Sarwer et al. compared the body image concerns of 30 breast reduction patients to 30 women who sought breast augmentation and found greater body image dissatisfaction among RM patients (32). The two groups of patients differed on seven of the ten subscales of the Multidimensional Body-Self Relations Questionnaire (MBSRQ), with preoperative breast reduction patients scoring significantly lower than preoperative augmentation patients on Appearance Evaluation, Body-Areas Satisfaction, Fitness Evaluation, Fitness Orientation, Health Evaluation, Health Orientation and Self-Classified Weight subscales. Using the Body Dysmorphic Disorder Examination–Self-Report (BDDE–SR) (adapted in this study for use as a measure of breast dissatisfaction), they also found that women who sought RM were significantly more dissatisfied with their breasts than women who sought augmentation (32). In addition, reduction patients were significantly more embarrassed about their breasts in public areas and in social settings and more likely to avoid physical activity because of self-consciousness about breast size. Furthermore, a significantly greater number of reduction patients believed their breast appearance was abnormal.

All plastic surgeons must be watchful for patients who may be suffering from psychological disturbances, especially body dysmorphic disorder (BDD) (see Chapters 14 and 16). However, clinical experience suggests that BDD is rarely encountered in women who seek breast reduction. Patients seeking RM have a real physical problem that is readily apparent, and they rarely, if ever, exaggerate its seriousness or its impact on their lives. When the obvious deformity is treated surgically, RM patients are unlikely to become fixated on another body area that they feel needs surgical correction.

The emotional pain and reduced quality of life suffered by women seeking breast reduction can be assessed with a variety of psychometric instruments. These measures can provide both patients and surgeons with a wealth of information about the specific psychosocial concerns experienced by patients prior to surgery. Specific questions in the initial consultation, as shown in Questionnaire 12-1 at the end of this chapter, can provide additional information on the extent of psychological distress resulting from breast hypertrophy. These questions easily can be worked into the surgeon's typical patient evaluation strategy to ascertain which specific concerns seem to have the greatest impact on prospective patients. They should also help surgeons determine whether a psychiatric consultation might be warranted, especially if a patient's psychological distress is excessive and inconsistent with the degree of breast hypertrophy observed.

NONSURGICAL TREATMENTS

Attempts to treat the physical symptoms of breast hypertrophy without surgery have historically included weight reduction, pain medications (over-the-counter, prescription, and narcotic), heat or cold treatments, hydrotherapy, postural training, relaxation training, exercise, physical therapy, chiropractic treatments, acupuncture, biofeedback, and the use of supportive bras or braces (10,13,15). In a multicenter prospective study, 179 women were asked to evaluate the extent to which these treatments were effective for alleviating their symptoms (13). Patients were compared with 88 women who also had breast hypertrophy but did not request surgery. Surgical patients were two to three times more likely than controls to have tried nonsurgical treatments with little or no improvement. For example, weight loss was tried by 85% of surgical patients, but no patient reported complete or permanent relief from their symptoms. Similarly, 77% of patients and 40% of controls reported analgesics use, but permanent relief was elusive for both groups. In contrast, surgery was very successful in relieving symptoms in the vast majority of patients (13). Other investigations reached similar conclusions (10,15). When considering the efficacy of nonsurgical treatments, surgeons should be aware that conservative treatments typically offer little, if any, symptom relief or psychological benefit. For most women, breast reduction is a last resort attempt at symptom relief, not the first.

CASE EXAMPLE

Case 1: M.O.

Patient M.O. is a 44-year-old woman with a weight of 182 lbs, height of 64 in., and BMI of 31 kg/m². She has a bra size of 40-DDD and presents for RM. She developed abnormally large breasts as an adolescent and further enlargement plus ptosis occurred with each of her three pregnancies. As she aged and gained weight, M.O. experienced escalating severity of pain in her back, neck, and shoulders, increasingly stooped posture, shoulder grooving, intertrigo, and bilateral numbness in her ring and little fingers. Although she had been working part-time in her family's restaurant for years, she planned to begin working full-time in a few months. She was to assume more managerial responsibilities that would include receiving shipments, shopping for perishables, supervising waitstaff, and some hostess duties. In addition to being worried about her ability to perform these physical tasks because of pain and fatigue that accompanied standing and walking, she was concerned about maneuvering through the crowded restaurant and bar, kitchen, and storage areas. At the same time, she wanted to dress in clothing that reflected well on the business. She had been self-conscious about her breast size since high school and now feared embarrassment in her more public role at the restaurant.

M.O. was an excellent breast reduction candidate. She had many of the typical physical symptoms associated with breast hypertrophy that would likely improve following RM. In addition, she was primarily motivated by the desire to reduce her physical discomfort, improve her stamina, look better in clothes, and feel less self-conscious in front of strangers.

POSTOPERATIVE CHANGES FOLLOWING BREAST REDUCTION

Patient Satisfaction

Patient satisfaction following breast reduction is typically high. Numerous studies have reported postoperative patient satisfaction rates between 84% to 99% (7,10,14,22,24,37–40). Between 92% and 100% of patients who have undergone surgery reported they would have surgery again or recommend RM to others (7,10,14,16,23–24,28,37,41–43). Many plastic surgeons find RM one of the most satisfying procedures they perform because patients report so many positive changes in their lives. Because of these benefits, some women seem to accept less-than-optimal aesthetic results. In a study designed to examine cosmetic outcomes, 34 patients were asked to evaluate the appearance of their breasts 19 months after surgery (41). Four surgeons, blinded to the identity of the patients and operating surgeon, also evaluated the patients' photographs. Patients' ratings of their aesthetic results were significantly higher than the surgeons' ratings on dimensions including overall body harmony, appearance out of clothes, overall breast and nipple–areolar complex symmetry, and breast shape.

Physical Changes

Numerous studies have documented the decrease in physical pain and increase in physical activity patients typically experience following RM. In addition, patients often experience changes in body weight and psychosocial status.

Pain

Macromastia has long been viewed as a condition based on anatomic size of the breasts in relation to the rest of the body. However, more than size seems to be involved in motivating patients to seek surgery. As discussed earlier, not all women with large breasts report the pain and discomfort that lead them to a surgeon's office. Gonzalez et al. have proposed that the definition of breast hypertrophy include a complex of chronic pain symptoms affecting at least three anatomic upper body areas, such as back, neck, or shoulder pain as well as pain resulting from brassiere strap grooves (9). When compared to a group of small-breasted women, preoperative reduction patients reported pain that was three standard deviations higher for all pain variables. Postoperatively, the RM patients' pain levels were statistically indistinguishable from controls. All patients reported improvement in their symptoms, with 25% experiencing a total elimination of pain. Numerous other studies have found that RM improves or completely relieves pain symptoms in the great majority of patients (6–7,10–11,14,16,22,24–25,37,44–47).

Blomqvist et al. have produced the longest prospective study to evaluate pain and quality of life in breast reduction patients (11,46). They followed 39 of the original 49 participants for at least 3 years postoperatively. Patients reported significant improvements at the 6-month, 12-month, and 36-month postoperative time-points for the six pain locations studied: neck pain, shoulder pain, lower back pain, breast pain, shoulder grooving, and headache. The majority of patients said they had complete elimination of their preoperative pain in these areas. In addition, significant improvements were found in patients' body posture, choice of clothing, sexual relations, and working capacity at all time points. Although sleeping improved after surgery, the change was not significant.

In another prospective study, Chao et al. investigated pain, posture, and muscle strength in women who sought breast reduction (48). Preoperatively and again 6 months postoperatively, 55 women completed muscle strength testing using a standardized muscle grading scale, as well as assessments of head and shoulder postural measurements. At the postoperative assessment, patients experienced significant strength improvements in the rhomboideus, middle trapezius, and lower trapezius muscles. Strength of the pectoralis major and minor muscles also improved, but the changes were not significant. In addition, the values for the postural measurements of head translation and cranial rotation improved significantly. These patients also experienced highly significant decreases in pain and disability ratings after breast reduction, regardless of preoperative BMI.

Chadbourne et al. performed a meta-analysis of prospective and observational investigations published between 1986 and 1999 that investigated the physical symptoms of breast hypertrophy (12). Data from 29 studies, consisting of 4,173 patients, were pooled to compare preoperative and postoperative reported frequencies of

▶ **TABLE 12-1** Mean Percentage (and Range) of Women Reporting Symptoms of Breast Hypertrophy in 29 Studies of RM

Symptom	% of Women Reporting Symptom Preoperatively	% of Women Reporting Symptom Postoperatively
Shoulder grooving	84.1 (20–96)	7.6 (0–24)
Shoulder pain	79.7 (48–99)	6.0 (2–24)
Upper/lower back pain	72.9 (46–92)	13.0 (3–33)
Neck pain	65.4 (31–94)	9.7 (2–27)
Intertrigo	50.3 (22–77)	4.4 (1–17)
Breast pain	50.1 (6–90)	13.0 (1–46)
Headache	33.7 (2–89)	8.8 (0–27)
Pain/numbness in hands	18.6 (11–23)	6.5 (3–9)

Adapted from Chadbourne EB, Zhang S, Gordon MJ, et al. Clinical outcomes in reduction mammaplasty: a systematic review and meta-analysis of published studies. *Mayo Clin Proc* 2001;76:503–510.

several physical symptoms. As shown in Table 12-1, there was a significant decrease in the percentage of women reporting these symptoms following RM.

Physical Activity

Most women who undergo RM report greater involvement in physical activities after surgery, likely as a function of the reduced physical discomfort associated with large breasts. Two studies observed that 90% of patients had difficulty participating in sports or exercise before surgery; the percentages dropped to 5% (13) or 17% (16) after RM. In another investigation, 63% of RM patients had a marked increase in activity level after surgery. An additional 12% of patients reported a moderate increase and 9% reported a mild increase (25). Makki et al. reported that 61% of their RM patients exercised more and 74% became more physically active postreduction (8). Several other investigators also found increases in participation in daily life tasks and exercise programs, as well as an increase in social activity levels, postoperatively (10,29,42,44,47). As one example, McMahan et al. found that the ability of teenagers to participate in athletic activities and exercise improved by at least 87% after RM (29). As noted above, of the 41% of reduction patients who had a working disability (on sick leave at least some of the time) because of preoperative symptom severity, approximately three quarters of these women returned to work after surgery without further absences (22).

Body Weight

The physical pain and limited ability to engage in active lifestyles likely contributes to weight problems in women with breast hypertrophy. RM in overweight and obese women often requires removal of large amounts of breast tissue. Several studies (9,24–25,48), but not all (23), have found no correlation between the amount of breast tissue removed and postoperative symptom relief. Thus, both obese and non-obese women are likely to experience improvements in physical symptoms following RM, regardless of the amount of breast tissue removed. However, there appears to be a relationship between larger tissue resections and higher complication frequencies (10,22,24,38). Because patients with large resections are more likely to be obese, they also may suffer from more weight-related comorbid conditions that influence wound healing. During preoperative consultations the greater risk for complications in obese patients must be thoroughly explained.

Several investigators have examined the relationship between obesity and breast reduction outcomes. Glatt et al. found that obese RM patients were more likely to report significantly more preoperative neck and breast pain than were non-obese patients (14). The non-obese women, in contrast, were significantly more likely to suffer personal embarrassment because of their breast size. There were no significant differences when obese and non-obese patients were asked about back pain, shoulder pain, shoulder grooving, skin irritation, poor posture, or trouble finding clothes that fit. After surgery, there were few differences between the obese and non-obese patients: both groups experienced similar relief of physical symptoms and improved body image satisfaction.

Other studies have similarly found that patients with a higher BMI benefit from RM just as much as women with a lower BMI (6,13,24). In the study by Collins et al., 179 patients from multiple surgeon practices were compared to a control group of large-breasted women who did not want surgery (13). Eighty-five percent of reduction patients had tried weight loss before proceeding to surgery. More than half of them found it completely ineffective at relieving breast-related symptoms and no patient found permanent and complete symptom relief from losing weight. In the large-breasted control group, 40% had tried weight loss, but only 9% found that it produced full and permanent symptom relief.

As of 2002, approximately one third of the U.S. population was overweight, defined as a BMI >25 kg/m^2, and an additional one third were obese, as judged by a BMI >30 kg/m^2 (49). Among women, 6.4% now suffer from extreme obesity, defined as a BMI >40 kg/m^2. In response to the growing obesity epidemic, and the rise in extreme obesity, an increasing number of Americans have turned to bariatric surgery to lose weight. We can assume that some percentage of women who have lost large amounts of weight from bariatric surgery or more conservative weight loss treatments also suffer from breast hypertrophy and may seek breast reduction following significant weight loss. In our experience, the major problem in this group of women is breast sagging due to excessive amounts of skin rather than breast tissue. It may be that patients who have undergone a massive weight loss are more likely to need a mastopexy to reduce the skin envelope rather than a tissue reduction. If additional body contouring is requested, procedures must be carefully staged to reduce the risk of complications.

Psychological Changes

Table 12-2 summarizes major results from studies that have examined psychosocial changes following RM. These investigations have evaluated a variety of psychological domains using a wide range of psychometric measures such as the SF-36, MB-SRQ, Body Image Questionnaire (BIQ), and Body Satisfaction Scale (BSS). Most studies used a prospective design to compare preoperative and postoperative data from the same group of patients. Several included a control group of women, typically recruited from the local population, who did not seek surgery. Other studies compared patients to the normative values provided with the measures. Despite these methodological differences, the results consistently demonstrate that women experience psychological benefits following RM.

▶ **TABLE 12-2 Summary of Findings from Studies that Assessed Changes in Psychosocial Functioning Following Breast Reduction[a]**

Authors, Year	# Patients/ Controls	Avg FU time	Measures Used	Major Findings
Hollyman et al., 1986 (50)	11/19	6 mo	1, 2	Patients were significantly more anxious and depressed, had more somatic anxiety, and scored higher on hysteria scale both before and after surgery. Postoperatively, patients had significant improvements in self-confidence, femininity, and sexual attractiveness scores.
Klassen et al., 1996 (31)	128 preoperative and 58 postoperative/ norms of the measures	6 mo	3, 4, 5	Preoperative patients scored significantly lower than controls on all quality of life dimensions. Postoperative patients reported significant improvement in self-esteem. After surgery, patients reported significant improvements on all quality of life dimensions; patients scored significantly better than controls on all dimensions. Proportion of cases that scored high enough to have possible psychiatric disturbance fell from 41% before surgery to 11% after surgery.
Shakespeare and Cole, 1997 (16) Shakespeare and Postle, 1999 (6)	110 preoperative, 90 at postoperative month 6, and 60 at postoperative month 24/norms of the measures	6 mo	3, 5	Preoperative patients scored significantly lower than controls on physical function, role limitation-physical, social function, pain, mental health, and energy. Postoperative patients reported significant improvement in self-esteem. After surgery, patients reported significant improvements in physical function, social function, pain, mental health, and energy; no differences as compared to controls.
Guthrie et al., 1998 (30) and Faria et al., 1999 (40)	33 preoperative and 19 postoperative	4 mo	3, 5–8	Preoperative patients reported greater symptoms of anxiety and depression, greater body image dissatisfaction, and lower quality of life in 6 areas (physical function, role limitation-physical, social function, mental health, energy, and pain). After surgery, patients reported significant improvement in quality of life, self-esteem, and body image, as well as significant reduction in anxiety and depressive symptoms.

(continued)

▶ **TABLE 12-2 Summary of Findings from Studies that Assessed Changes in Psychosocial Functioning Following Breast Reduction[a]** *(Continued)*

Authors, Year	# Patients/ Controls	Avg FU time	Measures Used	Major Findings
Glatt et al., 1999 (14)	61 postoperative patients/30 preoperative patients and norms of the measure	5 yr	9	Postoperative patients reported significant improvements in body image.
Blomqvist et al., 2000 (11), 2004 (46)	39/normal controls	6, 12, 36 mo	5	Preoperative patients scored significantly lower than controls in all 8 quality of life domains. After surgery, patients had significant improvement in all 8 quality of life domains; scores comparable to controls.
Behmand et al., 2000 (36)	69/normal controls	9 mo	5, 10	Preoperative patients in ≤24 and 35–44 age groups scored significantly lower than controls on 7 of 8 subscales/patients in 24–34 age group scored significantly lower for all 8 measures/patients in ≥45 age group scored significantly lower on 3 of 8 subscales (physical function, pain, and energy). After surgery, patients had significant improvements on all subscales for all age groups. Preoperative patients had significantly higher levels of interpersonal sensitivity, depression, anxiety, and hostility than controls; patients had significantly lower levels of all 4 symptoms after surgery and were comparable to controls.
Collins et al., 2002 (13)	179/88 women with breast hypertrophy not seeking surgery and 96 normal controls	8 mo	5, 11–14	Preoperative patients scored significantly lower than controls on all quality of life dimensions. Postoperatively, patients had significant improvements in overall health, quality of life, and body image as well as reductions in pain and other breast related symptoms.

[a]Measures Key
1 = Crown-Crisp Experimental Index
2 = Visual analog scales measuring anxiety, depression, anger, femininity, self-confidence, and sexual attractiveness
3 = Rosenberg Self-Esteem Scale (RSE)
4 = General Health Questionnaire (GHQ-28)
5 = Short Form–36 (SF–36, with 8 subscales: physical function, role limitation-physical, role limitation-mental, social function, mental health, energy/vitality, pain, general health perception)
6 = Hospital Anxiety and Depression Scale (HADS)
7 = Body Image Questionnaire (BIQ)
8 = Body Satisfaction Scale (BSS)
9 = Body Dysmorphic Disorder Examination–Self Report (BDDE–SR)
10 = Brief Symptom Inventory (BSI)
11 = EuroQol
12 = McGill Pain Questionnaire (MPQ)
13 = Multidimensional Body–Self-Relations Questionnaire—Appearance (MBSRQ Appearance)
14 = Breast-Related Symptoms (BRS)

Hollyman et al. completed the first psychometric investigation of breast reduction patients in 1986 (50). Eleven RM patients completed the Crown-Crisp Experimental Index (CCEI) and were compared to 19 controls similar in age. The breast reduction group—both before and after surgery—was found to be significantly different from controls on 4 of 6 subscales: they were more anxious, more depressed, had more somatic anxiety, and scored higher on the hysteria scale. Based on these results, the authors concluded that women requesting breast reduction have "abnormal psychoneurotic profiles" that surgery does not address.

This interpretation of the findings presents a rather psychopathological picture of RM patients. Methodological limitations of the study, however, call into question the validity of the conclusion. While the study clearly suggested an elevation in these symptoms, it is unclear if these scores are truly representative of formal diagnosable conditions such as major depression or anxiety disorders. In addition, the sample size of 11 women is very small. Finally, the CCEI is a somewhat obscure psychometric measure that has not been used in any subsequent investigations of breast reduction patients. Most contemporary studies have not focused on preoperative psychopathology, in part because this approach is inconsistent with the experiences of present-day surgeons. Results of these studies indicate that most patients who present for plastic surgery do not display formal psychopathology, at least not at a rate greater than that found in the general population. (See Chapters 14 and 15 for a more detailed discussion of these issues.)

The next major prospective controlled study to evaluate psychosocial functioning in breast reduction patients did not appear for 10 years, when Klassen et al. used several measures to assess RM patients (31). Based on a comparison of preoperative and postoperative scores, patients demonstrated significant improvements in quality of life (as assessed by all eight subscales of the SF-36) and self-esteem (as assessed by the Rosenberg Self-Esteem Scale). Furthermore, the postoperative scores on all eight subscales of the SF-36 were significantly higher than those for controls. When patients were questioned about their satisfaction with the procedure, 98% said their change in appearance was what they wanted, 86% thought the result of surgery was either excellent or very good, and 74% were very pleased with the impact surgery had on their lives.

Shakespeare and Cole confirmed the significant self-esteem improvements after surgery and also found that preoperative patients were not preoccupied with self-image problems or aesthetic considerations (16). Only four of 110 women evaluated preoperatively reported being "depressed" about appearance concerns. Shakespeare and Postle subsequently evaluated the same group of patients 2 years after surgery (6). As compared to patient's RSE scores 6 months after surgery, 52% had higher self-esteem scores, 30% had similar scores, and 18% had lower scores. Of the 11 women with lower scores, eight were nevertheless happy with their surgical outcome but had other problems, including severe scarring or weight gain.

Shakespeare and Postle also found that improvements on the SF–36 scores were comparable at 6-month and 24-month time points, suggesting long-term positive changes in quality of life after surgery. Postoperative scores also were comparable to—or higher than—controls on all eight subscales. In a series of open-ended questions, study participants were asked to provide additional information about their experiences with RM. Seventy-two percent of patients reported having no pain or very little discomfort after surgery. These physical improvements may have been related to other positive changes. For example, these women reported an increased ability to engage in more physical activities and a more active family life. Seventy percent mentioned that breast reduction made them feel better about themselves. Seventy-two percent said their improved appearance gave them greater self-confidence in many areas of life, and others noted a positive change in other people's attitudes toward them, including observations that they were viewed more as colleagues by coworkers and thought their chances of job advancement were improved after surgery.

These comments vividly illustrate how breast reduction may be associated with improvements in the physical and psychological health of patients. For many women, the reduction in pain and discomfort of large breasts is associated with greater physical activity and enjoyment of daily life activities. Postoperatively, many women either lose weight or feel more physically fit, and the great majority is able to dress in more stylish clothes. Because they look more "normal" after surgery, they believe that they are treated differently by others, which, in turn, may lead to an enhanced self-image.

Improvements in quality of life have been found in other studies (11,13,32,44,46). For example, Blomqvist et al. found significant improvements on all eight subscales of the SF-36 one year postoperatively (11). Scores remained stable 3 years after surgery, although scores on the "role limitations due to physical health" subscale were no longer significant as compared to the preoperative scores (46). This study, as well as the study by Boschert et al. (44), further suggests that quality of life benefits occur independently from the patient's age or body mass. A few studies have found that RM is associated with improvements in other psychosocial domains. Behmand et al. found significant improvements in depressive symptoms, anxiety, interpersonal sensitivity, and hostility following breast reduction (36). In another study, RM was followed by significant decreases in depression and anxiety as measured by the HADS (40).

Glatt et al. specifically investigated the body image concerns of post-RM patients (14). They found the reduction patients' postoperative scores on the BDDE-SR (again adapted for use as an index of breast dissatisfaction) were significantly lower than those reported by women awaiting breast reduction surgery, as well as those who sought other forms of cosmetic surgery. Post-RM patients also completed the Breast Chest Rating Scale (BCRS) to evaluate how women perceived their current breast size, and what they believed to be the ideal size, female size preference, and male size preference. The postreduction patients were significantly different from the female norms on the BCRS for all scales except the breast size preferred by men. Even after surgery, RM patients perceived their own breast size to be significantly larger than did controls. Moreover, they believed the ideal breast size and the size preferred by most women to be significantly smaller than did controls. The BCRS results seem to suggest that breast reduction patients would prefer to have even smaller breasts, although the vast majority was satisfied with their postoperative breast size. These findings may reflect that women who underwent breast reduction still recall the self-consciousness and social embarrassment their breast size caused them before surgery.

POSTOPERATIVE DISSATISFACTION

As noted above, the vast majority of women report high levels of postoperative satisfaction following RM. The most common reason for dissatisfaction with reduction mammoplasty is scarring (7–8,23,25,37,38). One prospective study found that 22% of patients believed their scars were worse or much worse than expected (16). Thirteen percent of patients judged their scars to be poor and 12% rated them as unacceptable (41). All with "unacceptable" scars had experienced a postoperative complication such as infection, wound breakdown, or hypertrophic scar formation. It should be noted, however, that 94% of patients in this study said they would have breast reduction again or recommend it to friends. Thus, dissatisfaction with scars did not necessarily equate to dissatisfaction with the surgery as a whole.

Complications following breast reduction are not uncommon. Several authors have reported complication rates between 33% and 53% (7–8,24–25,37,39). Most were described as minor problems with wound healing or scars that were addressed with office procedures. Complications that are more serious—such as changes in nipple sensation, fat necrosis, infection, marked asymmetry, and hypertrophic scars—do not typically lead to a need or request for additional surgery. Reported revision rates for these complications range from 0% to 9% (7,10,24–25,37,39). The tolerance for less-than-desirable aesthetic results among breast reduction patients is impressive. For example, 45% of patients in one study had a major or minor complication, yet only 9% required or requested revision; in addition, 95% reported being "happy" or "very happy" with their results (24). As with scars, complications do not seem to be associated with high rates of dissatisfaction among RM patients. When revision procedures are needed, surgical fees are not typically charged, though operating room charges may accrue if the procedure cannot be done in the surgeon's office.

Efforts to reduce scarring have led many surgeons to use procedures that result in only one vertical scar (which runs between the areola and inframammary crease) rather than the classic approach that creates an inverted "T" scar (which adds an additional scar along, often beyond, the inframammary crease). The latter approach is still recommended by many for larger volume breast reductions, but the vertical short-scar technique can produce excellent results for most large volume reductions. In the study of women who underwent the inverted T procedure as adolescents, the majority (60%) complained about their prominent scars, yet none requested scar revision and 94% would have the surgery again (29). In a follow-up study of 15 patients who underwent RM between the ages of 14 to 20, Evans and Ryan found that all 15 were satisfied with their surgical results (28).

Unfortunately, no matter how good the postoperative size and shape, scars will form, and some individuals are prone to develop wide and/or raised scars. If RM serves as patients' first surgical procedure, their scarring tendency may be unknown until months later, when patients may feel they have been disfigured by a new problem. This explains why litigation following RM is more often prompted by hypertrophic scars than complications such as nipple loss or asymmetry (51).

Problems with asymmetry can involve the size, shape, or position of the breasts or nipple–areolar complexes. Few studies have reported on dissatisfaction with breast symmetry but frequencies seem to range from 2% to 10% (8,23,25,42). Breast size or shape asymmetry is relatively easy to correct with touch-up liposuction, though few patients request revision unless there is a cup size or more difference between the breasts.

The most important way to reduce postoperative dissatisfaction is to conduct detailed preoperative discussions and carefully prepare patients for scarring and other complications that may develop. The likely postoperative appearance of the breasts must be thoroughly explained before surgery and is best illustrated by photographs of other patients. There appears to be a relationship between those who felt that preoperative discussions were inadequate and those dissatisfied with the final result (37). Nevertheless, 94% of women in this study were either satisfied or very satisfied with the surgery, and 92% would have it again or recommend it to others. In another study, one third of patients said more extensive preoperative discussions would have been helpful in preparing them for what to expect after surgery (i.e., extent of scarring, breast appearance, etc.) (39). In addition to explaining what postoperative scars might look like, surgeons should stress that few women have symmetrical breasts before surgery, and the amount of tissue removed can only be estimated. Consequently, some degree of postoperative asymmetry would not be unusual. Good preoperative photographs are important for documenting pre-existing asymmetry. As with all plastic surgery procedures, thorough informed consent is the best way to reduce postoperative dissatisfaction. (See Chapters 18 and 19 for a more detailed discussion of issues of informed consent.)

Breast reduction produces a major body change. A woman who goes into surgery with a DDD bra cup size and comes out a C cup will be at least somewhat shocked, no matter how much she hated the size of her breasts before. Goin et al. have pointed out that some patients feel euphoric about their new breasts, while others may "mourn the loss" of their old breasts (52). Still others have used their breasts, and accompanying excess body weight, as a buffer to unwanted social interactions and suddenly feel vulnerable. Patients need to be told that it may take some time before their new breast size is incorporated into their self-image. Cognitive-behavioral psychotherapeutic interventions, as discussed in Chapter 4, may be particularly helpful with these issues.

CASE EXAMPLE

Case 2: C.B.

C.B. was almost 18 years old when she sought reduction mammoplasty. She was 63 inches tall, weighed 118 lbs, giving her a BMI of 21 kg/m^2. She wore a 34-DDD bra. She suffered from back and neck pain, as well as shoulder grooving. Throughout high school, she had been teased about her breast size, become the brunt of jokes, and was self-conscious, especially around boys. She rarely dated and avoided school social activities. Throughout grade school and middle school, C.B. had been an avid soccer player, but she quit during 9th grade because she was so embarrassed by the way her breasts bounced when she ran. Her posture was stooped and she wore baggy clothing during her preoperative consultations. She wanted to have breast reduction surgery before starting college and looked forward to beginning another chapter of her life in a new place where she would not feel abnormal or "deformed." Though she was concerned about potential scarring, she seemed mature enough to accept it in exchange for greater psychological comfort with herself and others. In fact, she feared she would never be the person she was capable of being because her breasts were "in the way."

She underwent reduction mammoplasty with the vertical short-scar technique and removal of approximately 500 grams of tissue from each breast. At her last postoperative visit, C.B. had completed her freshman year at college. She was wearing a 32-C bra and was satisfied with her result. For the first time since early adolescence, she enjoyed shopping for clothes. She had built a large circle of new friends, was involved in the social life of the campus and dated regularly. Her self-confidence had markedly improved, she was much more outgoing than before surgery, and she commented on how much better she felt about herself and her life. Her scarring was minimal, she was pleased with the shape of her breasts, and she did not fear undressing in front of others in the dorm.

CONCLUSIONS

Women with breast hypertrophy frequently suffer with a significant, quantifiable health burden. The majority of these women pursue breast reduction to relieve the physical symptoms that nonsurgical treatments did not effectively alleviate. The most common physical symptoms of breast hypertrophy often interfere with the ability to keep up with everyday living activities at home, at work, and in social settings. Simple ambulation and more intense physical activity can seem a chore. The psychological distress caused by abnormal breast size is an equally important reason for seeking breast reduction, particularly for younger women. Viewing themselves as "abnormal," patients report they are socially embarrassed and self-conscious, cannot wear the same types of clothing as their peers, and lack self-confidence.

Following surgery, patients report high levels of postoperative satisfaction and the vast majority report that they would undergo the procedure again or recommend it to others, even with the experience of minor complications. The vast majority of women report either a significant reduction or elimination of many of the physical symptoms that motivated the desire for surgery in the first place. These changes frequently occur regardless of age or body mass. Studies that have measured psychosocial variables with objective instruments consistently indicate that breast reduction leads to significant improvements in physical symptoms, activity levels, self-esteem, body image, and overall quality of life. Such positive changes might be expected when comparing patients preoperatively and postoperatively. The similarities between postreduction women and age-matched controls in these domains, however, are especially striking and suggest that RM typically has the effect of "normalizing" patients as compared to their peers with normal sized breasts. Thus, from both a physical and psychological perspective, RM is judged to be a successful treatment for the vast majority of women who seek it.

Preoperative Questions to Assess Psychological Issues in Patients Seeking Breast Reduction

Three suggested response choices are: Frequently, Occasionally, Almost Never

■ Are you embarrassed by your breast size?

■ Does your breast size make you reluctant to participate in social activities with family, friends, or co-workers?

■ Do you feel self-conscious or uncomfortable around men you don't know well because of your breast size?

■ Do you feel your breast size detracts from your overall appearance?

■ Does your breast size interfere with these kinds of everyday activities?

    ☐   Routine household tasks
    ☐   Job duties
    ☐   Family activities

■ Do you feel uncomfortable in intimate situations?

■ Do you receive (or overhear) inappropriate comments about your breast size?

■ Do you feel your breasts make you unattractive?

■ Do you feel depressed or anxious about your breast size?

■ Do you think you'd feel better about yourself if your breasts were smaller?

■ Are there other areas of your body you are unhappy with? _____

■ Have you had any other plastic surgery procedure(s)? _____

REFERENCES

1. American Society of Plastic Surgeons. 2004. Procedural Statistics [American Society of Plastic Surgeons Web site]. Available at: http://www.plasticsurgery.org. Accessed June 1, 2005.
2. Spira M. Pathology of the hypertrophic breast. In: Goldwyn RM, ed. *Reduction Mammoplasty*. Boston: Little, Brown and Company, 1990:25–27.
3. Bland KI, Romrell LJ. Congenital and acquired disturbances of breast development and growth. In: Bland KI, Copeland EM III, eds. *The Breast: Comprehensive Management of Benign and Malignant Diseases*. Vol. 1. 2nd ed. Philadelphia: WB Saunders, 1998:214–232.
4. Goldwyn RM. Comments on Chapter 3. In: Goldwyn RM, ed. *Reduction Mammoplasty*. Boston: Little, Brown and Company, 1990:28.
5. de Souze A, Saltz R. The common principles of effective breast reduction techniques. *Aesthetic Surg J* 2000;20:213–217.
6. Shakespeare V, Postle K. A qualitative study of patients' views on the effects of breast-reduction surgery: a 2-year follow-up survey. *Br J Plast Surg* 1999;52:198–204.
7. Davis GM, Ringler SL, Short K, et al. Reduction mammaplasty: long-term efficacy, morbidity, and patient satisfaction. *Plast Reconstr Surg* 1995;96:1106–1110.
8. Makki AS, Ghanem AA. Long-term results and patient satisfaction with reduction mammaplasty. *Ann Plast Surg* 1998;41:370–377.
9. Gonzalez F, Walton RL, Shafer B, et al. Reduction mammaplasty improves symptoms of macromastia. *Plast Reconstr Surg* 1993;91:1270–1276.
10. Schnur PL, Schnur DP, Petty PM, et al. Reduction mammaplasty: an outcome study. *Plast Reconstr Surg* 1997;100:875–883.
11. Blomqvist L, Eriksson A, Brandberg Y. Reduction mammaplasty provides long-term improvement in health status and quality of life. *Plast Reconstr Surg* 2000;106:991–997.
12. Chadbourne EB, Zhang S, Gordon MJ, et al. Clinical outcomes in reduction mammaplasty: a systematic review and meta-analysis of published studies. *Mayo Clin Proc* 2001;76:503–510.
13. Collins ED, Kerrigan CL, Kim M, et al. The effectiveness of surgical and nonsurgical interventions in relieving the symptoms of macromastia. *Plast Reconstr Surg* 2002;109:1556–1566.
14. Glatt BS, Sarwer DB, O'Hara DE, et al. A retrospective study of changes in physical symptoms and body image after reduction mammaplasty. *Plast Reconstr Surg* 1999;103:76–82.
15. Chalekson CP, Neumeister MW, Zook EG, Russell RC. Outcome analysis of reduction mammaplasty using the modified Robertson technique. *Plast Reconstr Surg* 2002;110:71–79.
16. Shakespeare V, Cole RP. Measuring patient-based outcomes in a plastic surgery service: breast reduction surgical patients. *Br J Plast Surg* 1997;50:242–248.
17. Godwin Y, Valassiadou K, Lewis S, Denley H. Investigation into the possible cause of subjective decreased sensory perception in the nipple-areola complex of women with macromastia. *Plast Reconstr Surg* 2004;113:1598–1606.
18. Temple CLF, Hurst LN. Reduction mammaplasty improves breast sensibility. *Plast Reconstr Surg* 1999;104:72–76.
19. Harbo SO, Jørum E, Roald HE. Reduction mammaplasty: a prospective study of symptom relief and alterations of skin sensibility. *Plast Reconstr Surg* 2003;111:103–110.
20. Starley IF, Bryden DC, Tagari S, et al. An investigation into changes in lung function and the subjective medical benefits from breast reduction surgery. *Br J Plast Surg* 1998;51:531–534.
21. Sood R, Mount DL, Coleman JJ III, et al. Effects of reduction mammaplasty on pulmonary function and symptoms of macromastia. *Plast Reconstr Surg* 2003;111:688–694.
22. Atterhem H, Holmner S, Janson P-E. Reduction mammaplasty: symptoms, complications, and late results. *Scand J Plast Reconstr Hand Surg* 1998;32:281–286.
23. Brühlmann Y, Tschopp H. Breast reduction improves symptoms of macromastia and has a long-lasting effect. *Ann Plast Surg* 1998;41:240–245.
24. Dabbah A, Lehman JA Jr, Parker MG, et al. Reduction mammaplasty: an outcome analysis. *Ann Plast Surg* 1995;35:337–341.
25. Miller AP, Zacher JB, Berggren RB, et al. Breast reduction for symptomatic macromastia: can objective predictors for operative success be identified? *Plast Reconstr Surg* 1995;95:77–83.
26. Netscher DT, Meade RA, Goodman CM, et al. Physical and psychosocial symptoms among 88 volunteer subjects compared with patients seeking plastic surgery procedures to the breast. *Plast Reconstr Surg* 2000;105:2366–2373.
27. Letterman G, Schurter M. The effects of mammary hypertrophy on the skeletal system. *Ann Plast Surg* 1980;5:425–431.
28. Evans GRD, Ryan JJ. Reduction mammaplasty for the teenage patient: a critical analysis. *Aesthetic Plast Surg* 1994;18:291–297.
29. McMahan JD, Wolfe JA, Cromer BA, et al. Lasting success in teenage reduction mammaplasty. *Ann Plast Surg* 1995;35:227–231.
30. Guthrie E, Bradbury E, Davenport P, et al. Psychosocial status of women requesting breast reduction surgery as compared with a control group of large-breasted women. *J Psychosom Res* 1998;45:331–339.
31. Klassen A, Fitzpatrick R, Jenkinson C, et al. Should breast reduction surgery be rationed? A comparison of the health status of patients before and after treatment: postal questionnaire survey. *BMJ* 1996;313:454–457.
32. Sarwer DB, Bartlett SP, Bucky LP, et al. Bigger is not always better: body image dissatisfaction in breast reduction and breast augmentation patients. *Plast Reconstr Surg* 1998;101:1956–1961.
33. Birtchnell S, Whitfield P, Lacey JH. Motivational factors in women requesting augmentation and reduction mammoplasty. *J Psychol Res* 1990;34:509–514.
34. Losee JE, Jiang S, Long DE, et al. Macromastia as an etiologic factor in bulimia nervosa: 10-year follow up after treatment with reduction mammaplasty. *Ann Plast Surg* 2004;52:452–457.

35. Kreipe RE, Lewand AG, Dukarm CP, et al. Outcome for patients with bulimia and breast hypertrophy after reduction mammaplasty. *Arch Pediatr Adolesc Med* 1997;151:176–180.
36. Behmand RA, Tang DH, Smith DJ Jr. Outcomes in breast reduction surgery. *Ann Plast Surg* 2000;45:575–580.
37. Brown AP, Hill C, Khan K. Outcome of reduction mammaplasty—a patients' perspective. *Br J Plast Surg* 2000;53:584–587.
38. Brown DM, Young VL. Reduction mammoplasty for macromastia. *Aesthetic Plast Surg* 1993;17:211–223.
39. Hughes LA, Mahoney JL. Patient satisfaction with reduction mammaplasty: an early survey. *Aesthetic Plast Surg* 1993;17:345–349.
40. Faria FS, Guthrie E, Bradbury E, et al. Psychosocial outcome and patient satisfaction following breast reduction surgery. *Br J Plast Surg* 1999;52:448–452.
41. Godwin Y, Wood SH, O'Neill TJ. A comparison of the patient and surgeon opinion on the long-term aesthetic outcome of reduction mammaplasty. *Br J Plast Surg* 1998;51:444–449.
42. Raispis T, Zehring RD, Downey DL. Long-term functional results after reduction mammaplasty. *Ann Plast Surg* 1995;34:113–116.
43. Serletti JM, Reading G, Caldwell E. Long-term patient satisfaction following reduction mammoplasty. *Ann Plast Surg* 1992;28:363–365.
44. Boschert MT, Barone CM, Puckett CL. Outcome analysis of reduction mammaplasty. *Plast Reconstr Surg* 1996;98:451–454.
45. Jones SA, Bain JR. Review of data describing outcomes that are used to assess changes in quality of life after reduction mammaplasty. *Plast Reconstr Surg* 2001;108:62–67.
46. Blomqvist L, Brandberg Y. Three-year follow-up on clinical symptoms and health-related quality of life after reduction mammaplasty. *Plast Reconstr Surg* 2004;114:49–54.
47. Mizgala CL, MacKenzie KM. Breast reduction outcome study. *Ann Plast Surg* 2000;44:125–133.
48. Chao JD, Memmel HC, Redding JF, et al. Reduction mammaplasty is a functional operation, improving quality of life in symptomatic women: a prospective, single-center breast reduction outcome study. *Plast Reconstr Surg* 2002;110:1644–1652.
49. Hedley AA, Ogden CL, Johnson CL, et al. Prevalence of overweight and obesity among U.S. children, adolescents and adults, 1999–2002. *JAMA* 2004;291:2847–2850.
50. Hollyman JA, Lacey JH, Whitfield PJ, et al. Surgery for the psyche: a longitudinal study of women undergoing reduction mammaplasty. *Br J Plast Surg* 1986;39:222–224.
51. Daane SP, Rockwell WB. Breast reduction techniques and outcomes: a meta-analysis. *Aesthetic Surg J* 1999;19:293–303.
52. Goin MK, Goin JM, Gianini MH. The psychic consequences of a reduction mammaplasty. *Plast Reconstr Surg* 1977;59:530–534.

Chapter 13

Genital Reconstruction and Gender Identity Disorders

Walter O. Bockting, PhD, and Leo C. T. Fung, MD

This chapter introduces plastic surgeons and other health professionals to the psychological aspects of reconstructive surgery to alter primary and secondary sex characteristics. These surgical procedures are most commonly performed to feminize or masculinize the appearance of children born with ambiguous genitalia (referred to as *intersex* patients) and of adult transgender/transsexual patients. These procedures are also used in rare cases of genital trauma, such as circumcision accidents or genital mutilation (1–2). The discussion here will be limited to the psychological aspects of genital reconstruction in the context of sex (re)assignment in childhood or adulthood.

Few health providers are knowledgeable about, or have experience with, transgender or intersex patients. After reading this chapter, surgeons and other health professionals should have a better understanding of the psychosocial context in which these patients request surgical treatment and, therefore, be better equipped to coordinate care with an interdisciplinary team of professionals. In many parts of the United States, specialists can be found through the Harry Benjamin International Gender Dysphoria Association. It is an organization of professionals in the fields of psychology, psychiatry, social work, endocrinology, surgery, and the law dedicated to the understanding and treatment of both gender identity disorders and intersexuality.

This chapter is divided into two main parts addressing genital reconstruction in the treatment of (i) intersex conditions and (ii) gender identity disorders. Case vignettes taken from the first author's clinical practice illustrate the therapeutic issues and interventions. The chapter concludes with a Questionnaire 13-1, a list of questions to ask patients who request genital reconstructive surgery.

GENITAL RECONSTRUCTION IN THE TREATMENT OF INTERSEX CONDITIONS

Intersex is an umbrella term used to refer to individuals born with a discrepancy between their genetic, gonadal, hormonal, or genital sex (3–5). A variety of intersex conditions exist, including chromosomal/gonadal conditions (e.g., Klinefelter Syndrome, Turner Syndrome), female pseudohermaphroditism (e.g., Congenital Adrenal Hyperplasia [CAH]), and male pseudohermaphroditism (e.g., Androgen Insensitivity Syndrome, 5-alpha-Reductase Deficiency). The incidence of children with ambiguous genitalia is estimated at 1 to 2 per every 2,000 births (4).

Guidelines for genital reconstructive surgery in children born with ambiguous genitalia are highly controversial. Initial guidelines were based on the hypothesis of psychosexual neutrality at birth (6). The implication was that early genital surgery would facilitate unambiguous gender-appropriate rearing and development of the expected "optimal" gender identity (5). Hence, children with ambiguous genitalia were traditionally assigned the gender that the external genitalia, after reconstruction, could best support. These assignments appeared to have worked for many patients; however, some developed significant gender dysphoria and were reassigned to the other gender later in life (6).

Since the establishment of these initial guidelines, research has pointed to the potential role of sexual differentiation of the brain in the development of gender identity and role. This work suggests that biology plays a larger role in gender identity development than initially assumed (7). Along with this new knowledge came greater awareness of the potential negative consequences of early genital surgery. The concerns raised by adult intersex individuals centered on the lack of knowledge and information provided to patients and their families and the performance of sometimes unnecessary surgery that later proved to be detrimental to sexual functioning (8). Recently, proposed guidelines for the management of intersexuality reflect this awareness and illustrate a shift toward greater caution in surgical intervention (9). We agree with Cohen-Kettenis and Pfaefflin (3) that decisions regarding sex assignment and genital surgery are best made on a case-by-case basis after careful review of the available empirical evidence, the specific condition, and psychosocial context of the patient and his or her family.

Surgical procedures performed as part of the management of congenital intersex conditions should be directed toward establishing the necessary anatomy for sexual function and cosmesis, in keeping with the gender identity desired by the patient. Ideally, the patient would first reach a decision regarding the desired gender identity. Then, the necessary surgical procedures would be performed. This ideal is often not possible or, at best, is only partly feasible. On the one hand, early surgery is preferable, because it takes advantage of the superior healing and tissue remodeling potential of children as compared to adults. On the other hand, allowing the patient to reach a sufficiently mature age to determine the desired gender identity could circumvent future gender identity disorder. Health care providers take both factors into account when counseling intersex patients and families about surgical treatment.

It is beyond the scope of this chapter to cover, in depth, the wide range of surgical procedures available to intersex patients. We will explore the principles behind some of these procedures in the context of optimizing the integration of surgery into the psychological development and overall well-being of the patient, while optimizing surgical outcome.

Healing and Tissue Considerations

Infants and children have superior healing and regenerative capabilities as compared to adults. This difference is especially pronounced in the early postnatal period. Surgeries performed before a child is full-grown usually result in cosmetically superior results. The benefits of these properties are well recognized in hypospadias repair. When surgical intervention is desirable to an undervirilized male, it is standard practice to perform the surgery when the child is roughly between 1 and 2 years of age (10).

The tissue of the young child has a greater degree of elasticity. For genital reconstruction, this can produce a superior cosmetic result and be the critical determinant in whether or not a certain surgical procedure can be used successfully to bridge a gap in tissue. This principle is well understood in the repair of undescended testes. In a young infant, the mobilized intact spermatic cord allows the testis to reach a relatively long distance. This minimizes the degree of surgical dissection necessary to bring the undescended testis into intra-scrotal position. Should the repair be done at an older age in a child with the same degree of testicular undescent, it becomes exponentially more difficult to bring the testis into position.

In conditions where there is minimal deficiency in vaginal tissue, such as in patients with CAH associated with minimal virilization, early versus late surgery probably makes little difference. It is in the highly virilized 46, XX patients—with a long distance between the internalized vaginal cavity and the perineum—that the timing of surgery can have a critical impact on physical outcome. In an infant or young child, relatively large gaps between the high internalized vagina and the perineum can generally be bridged simply by surgical mobilization and the use of adjacent perineal tissue (11–12). At an older age, however, these gaps can no longer be bridged using only locally available tissue. Alternative methods, including the use of skin grafts from a separate donor site (13) or a piece of intestine interposing between the internal vaginal tissue and the perineal skin (14–15) become necessary. Such procedures are more invasive and inferior in anatomical outcome. In the case of the skin graft procedures, they usually require long-term self-dilation of the vagina (13).

Vaginal Dilation

In the adult or adolescent female, vaginal dilation can be performed with little or no difficulties. Although vaginal dilation is not particularly painful, it can be traumatic for a prepubertal child (16). Thus, reconstructive procedures expected to require vaginal dilation should generally be avoided in these children (17). Other procedures that do not require dilation can be used, or the surgery can be delayed until the patient is old enough to participate in postoperative management. Vaginal plasties which do not require long-term dilation during childhood, include primary vaginal reconstruction using vaginal mobilization (12) and local perineal skin flaps (18–19). The vaginal cavity typically remains patent throughout childhood. Although some degree of outlet stenosis is likely, this can be easily addressed with vaginal self-dilation at, or after, puberty and prior to sexual activity. Neo-vaginas created with an interposed intestinal segment do not require long-term dilation during the prepubertal period (14–15).

Vaginal plasties which use skin grafts from a distant donor site are prone to significant contractures and, therefore, need to be maintained by long-term dilation (13). This is generally true even for full-thickness skin grafts, though partial-thickness skin grafts are especially prone to contracture. In another technique, pressure is applied to a perineal dimple progressively via a dilator or a probe. This stretches the perineal skin internally to become a vagina suitable for intercourse, but requires long-term dilation for maintenance (20). These techniques can produce satisfactory results, but are less desirable for the prepubertal child.

For patients who have a functional uterus, but a deficient or obstructed vagina, vaginal reconstruction is often a matter of necessity to provide suitable menstrual outflow, prevent infections, and optimize potential fertility. If a patient has a female gender identity but lacks a functional uterus and female genitalia, the need for vaginal reconstruction depends on whether or not the patient desires a reconstructed vagina for functional, psychological, or aesthetic reasons.

Hormonal Brain Imprinting and Limitations in Reconstructive Procedures

It was once thought that a newborn could be successfully reared into a well-adjusted male or female, regardless of the infant's chromosomal sex, if given the appropriate postnatal hormonal, surgical, and environmental interventions. Unfortunately, this is not always the case. There are examples of 46, XY male infants raised as girls who developed into happy and well-adjusted adult women; but there are also examples of patients who later chose to change to a male gender identity. Before birth, the imprinting effects of androgen exposure in utero appears to have a significant and lasting influence on a person's gender identity.

Adding to the complexity is the reality that genital reconstruction techniques are by no means perfect. A reasonable outcome can generally be achieved for female external genitalia, even if tissue availability is limited. The same cannot be said for male external genitalia. Unless there is already sufficient usable penile tissue present, penile reconstruction by other means (e.g., forearm pedicled flaps) remains suboptimal both cosmetically and functionally (21–22).

Given these two considerations, intersex patients who would ultimately desire female genitalia can generally be expected to achieve a satisfactory surgical outcome. The situation is more challenging when a patient has been subjected to significant imprinting of the brain under the exposure of androgen and when there is insufficient penile tissue for satisfactory male external genitalia. Such a situation is often encountered in 46, XY patients with cloacal exstrophy. Rearing this patient as a male will result in external genitalia that will continue to appear ambiguous, yet rearing as a female could result in serious future dissatisfaction and a change in gender identity to male. There is no obvious solution to this dilemma.

The Timing of Gonadal Surgery

The timing of gonadal surgery is critical and can significantly impact both the physical and psychological outcomes. Consider the case of a 46, XY patient with testes and male-typical androgen function being considered for a female sex due to not having sufficient penile tissue to allow for effective construction of male genitalia. If the child is to be reared as female, it would be desirable to remove any further androgen influence as soon as possible, necessitating the removal of all functional testicular tissue. In contrast, the patient may ultimately wish to have a male gender identity, and the irreversible nature of removing the testes would not only alter the developmental process as a male, but also destroy any potential for fertility. Once again, a decision regarding the management of the gonads must be made long before the child is mature enough to participate in the decision-making process. Unfortunately, there is no perfect solution.

Psychological Impact of Growing Up with Ambiguous Genitalia

In some situations, intersexuality can be managed by waiting until the patient becomes sufficiently mature to decide upon the desired gender identity. However, foregoing early surgery requires the patient to go through a significant portion of childhood with ambiguous genitalia. Some parents are more likely to accept their child's ambiguous genitalia than others. Once the child becomes aware of having genitalia that are quite different from his or her peers, the child may develop a sense of shame. If other children become aware of this difference, the child may be teased or ridiculed. Nevertheless, the impact of growing up with ambiguous genitalia may be less traumatic than previously assumed, especially when adequate social support is available. In the absence of empirical research, however, we cannot conclude that foregoing surgery does not result in psychological harm.

Considerations Specific to Different Groups of Intersex Conditions

Intersex conditions often are classified either by the genetic makeup or anatomical characteristics of the patient. Neither approach serves the present discussion well. In considering surgical procedures for intersex conditions, the major categories are more appropriately divided into three groups (see Table 13-1).

Group I

Group I conditions do not require genital reconstruction; the external sexual characteristics are in keeping with the expected gender identity. These conditions are predominantly genetic in nature and may affect reproductive potential. Examples

▶ **TABLE 13-1 Grouping of Intersex Conditions by Need and Possibilities of Genital Reconstruction**

	Desired Sexual Identity	*Physical Anatomy*	*Genital Surgical Reconstruction*
I a	Male	Typical male	None needed
b	Female	Typical female	None needed
II a	Male	Ambiguous	Anatomically functional; reconstruction possible
b	Female	Ambiguous	Anatomically functional; reconstruction possible
III a	Male	Ambiguous	Anatomically functional; reconstruction not possible
b	Female	Ambiguous	Anatomically functional; reconstruction not possible

include 46, XY patients with CAH (precocious puberty with a male phenotype), and females with gonadal dysgenesis (XO karyotype, Turner's Syndrome, female phenotype). They also include disorders that may require surgery for other, nonreconstructive concerns such as gonadal malignancy. Although the exact risk of dysgenetic gonads undergoing malignant transformation is unknown, dysgenetic gonads containing all or part of a Y chromosome are considered at risk for gonadoblastoma (23) and are generally recommended to be excised (24).

Group II

Group II conditions are characterized by two features: (i) ambiguity of the external genitalia and (ii) physical anatomy that can be expected to yield satisfactory reconstruction of the external genitalia. With successful reconstruction, these patients can be expected to have a good cosmetic result and achieve satisfactory sexual function. However, many of these conditions are associated with infertility. Conditions in Group II include most 46, XX patients with CAH and male pseudohermaphrodites where the hypospadiac penis and/or undescended testes are amenable to surgical reconstruction. The group also includes true hermaphrodites, where an appropriate sex of rearing can be determined with relative certainty and where the corresponding external genitalia can be achieved surgically.

For these patients, early surgery can be performed in view of the superior healing potential of young children. This approach seems reasonable in male reconstructions. Even if the patient later develops a female gender identity, a subsequent surgical reversal from male to female would be feasible. The best management approach is not as clear in treating the severely virilized female. In most instances, feminizing surgery yields satisfactory long-term results both physically and psychologically. But what would happen if the patient has had such a degree of androgen brain imprinting that a male gender identity develops? The feminizing surgery would have removed the possibility that the severely androgenized external genitalia be modified into satisfactory male genitalia. This situation argues that at least some 46, XX patients with CAH may not fit the Group II categorization, but fall into Group III.

Group III

This group constitutes conditions where the management issues are unresolved. This may occur when male genitalia are desired, but unable to be successfully reconstructed. This group also includes the severely virilized 46, XX patient with CAH and true hermaphrodites for whom the optimal sex of rearing is unclear and where significant limitations in the anticipated outcome of genital surgery exist. In these challenging situations, the difficult task of selecting the sex of rearing and deciding upon additional surgery is relegated to the child's parents or legal guardian. The health professionals' role should be limited to providing unbiased information regarding the pros and cons of the full range of treatment options. Because there are no perfect solutions, each decision will necessarily lead to some desired benefits, while foregoing other desirable potentials.

Psychological Support

Psychological support and counseling should be provided for children born with ambiguous genitalia and their families. Parents may experience a range of emotions when learning about their child's condition, from initial shock and confusion, shame and anxiety, to anger and sadness. Addressing these feelings will facilitate the acceptance necessary to act in the child's best interest. Parents will have questions about their child's future, including issues of sexual orientation as well as sexual and reproductive functioning. At birth, parents should be informed completely about their child's condition and counseled in order to make a fully informed decision regarding sex assignment and the available medical interventions. Such counseling is best provided by a mental health professional who is part of a multidisciplinary team that specializes in the clinical management of intersexuality. These teams are not always readily available and parents are not always amenable to seeing a psychologist or psychiatrist (25). The treating physician can help by explaining that counseling is a regular part of the assessment and treatment process. Peer support organizations are another potential resource.

Affected patients are best served by accurate information about their condition and prognosis. However, information needs to be paced and provided in a sensitive, age-appropriate manner (26) and preferably by the parents (3). This is easier said than done. Many parents have great difficulty talking about gender and sexuality, especially to children. Above all, parents, counselors, and treating physicians should agree on what information to provide and when. Information and emotional support will help most children and adolescents to accept and adapt to their intersexuality. Children and adolescents who are ridiculed by their peers for being different may need additional assistance in the form of psychological and school-based interventions. Teasing by peers appears to be an important contributor to mental health problems of intersex patients (27).

All intersex patients are likely, at one time or another, to struggle with shame as a result of the stigma associated with their condition. In an analysis of the life histories of intersex adults, their adaptation to being different was likened to the "coming out" process for gay and lesbian individuals, in which shame and secrecy transformed into pride (28–29). Contact with similar others enabled participants to "own" their intersexuality, create greater visibility to combat isolation, and shape their treatment. Intersex patients may encounter challenges associated with their condition at any point in their lives. These may stem from gender identity or body image concerns (30), sexual functioning or fertility concerns (8), academic performance issues (e.g., as a result of cognitive deficits associated with Klinefelter's Syndrome) (3), or socialization difficulties (e.g., associated with Turner's Syndrome) (31).

GENITAL RECONSTRUCTION IN THE TREATMENT OF GENDER IDENTITY DISORDERS

Transgender is an umbrella term used to refer to a diverse group of individuals who cross or transcend culturally defined categories of gender (32). Transgender individuals include transsexuals (who desire or have had hormone therapy and/or genital reconstructive surgery), transgenderists (who live full-time in the cross-gender role and may take sex hormones, but do not desire genital reconstructive surgery), cross-dressers or transvestites (who wear clothing associated with another sex for emotional or sexual gratification), drag queens or drag kings (who adopt a hyperfeminine or hypermasculine presentation), and individuals identifying as bigender or "two-spirit" (both woman and man). A transgender patient might report having an intersex condition, as illustrated in the first vignette at the end of this chapter. Often, however, a physical examination of the transgender patient does not confirm intersexuality. Data on the prevalence and incidence of transsexualism are scarce. Prevalence is estimated at one in 11,900 for male-to-females (MtF) and one in 30,400 for female-to-males (FtM) (33). Incidence estimates range from .15 to 1.58 per 100,000 persons annually (34).

Transgender individuals may meet criteria for gender identity disorders (see Table 13-2) as described in the *Diagnostic Statistical Manual of Mental Disorders* (DSM) (35) or the International Classification of Diseases (36). A key criterion of the DSM definition is that "the disturbance causes clinically significant distress or impairment in social, occupational, or other important areas of functioning" (p. 581). For individuals who experience such distress, sex reassignment surgery may alleviate significant impairment in interpersonal and/or vocational functioning. For these reasons, the surgery is almost always medically necessary, not elective or cosmetic.

Since the 1970s, the Benjamin Association has set forth standards of care for the treatment of gender identity disorders (37). The standards delineate eligibility and readiness criteria for cross-gender hormone therapy and sex reassignment surgery. In addition, the standards offer guidelines for competency and practice for surgeons and other professionals (see Table 13-3). To ensure quality of care, the standards require that two mental health professionals independently evaluate and recommend sex reassignment surgery before the surgeon makes the final determination whether or not to operate on a transsexual patient.

Although these standards are widely used, not everyone who takes feminizing or masculinizing hormones or requests sex reassignment surgery, has been prepared in accordance with them. Needs assessment studies in transgender communities across the U.S. have found rates of illicit hormone use ranging from 29% to 71% (38–40). This is especially common among the more marginalized and impoverished, including those who work in the sex industry (41). In light of the psychological and social issues that applicants for sex reassignment may face (as described below), it is essential for every surgeon working with transgender patients to familiarize themselves with the standards of care and adhere to their guidelines.

Sex Reassignment and Identity: From Gender Dichotomy to Gender Diversity

The meaning and associated clinical approach to sex reassignment has gone through an important paradigm shift since the first surgery in the United States (42). In the 1960s and 1970s, treatment was guided by a dichotomous view of gender (male versus female, man versus woman, masculine versus feminine); the focus of sex reassignment was to assist males to become women and women to become men (43–44). Indeed, the effectiveness of sex reassignment was evaluated on the basis of how well transsexuals were able to "pass" as members of the "opposite" sex (45). A change in one's genitalia signified the ultimate change in sex.

This paradigm began to shift in the 1980s when Prince coined the term "transgenderist" to refer to males who live full-time as women without undergoing genital reconstructive surgery (46). A growing number of transgenderists and a generation of postoperative transsexuals began to question the dichotomous understanding of gender. Stone (47), a postoperative MtF transsexual, was one of the first to call for transsexuals to come out and affirm their unique identity and experience. Rather than starting a new life as a member of the other sex, individuals began to claim a transgender or transsexual identity that continues beyond the transition or sex reassignment phase.

▶ **TABLE 13-2 Diagnostic Criteria that May Include an Indication for Sex Reassignment Surgery**

DSM IV-TR (American Psychiatric Association, 2000)		ICD-10 (World Health Organization, 1992)	
302.85	*Gender Identity Disorder in Adolescents or Adults*	*F(64.0)*	*Transsexualism*
A.	A strong and persistent cross-gender identification (not merely a desire for any perceived cultural advantages of being the other sex), . . . manifested by symptoms such as a stated desire to be the other sex, frequent passing as the other sex, desire to live or be treated as the other sex, or the conviction that he or she has the typical feelings and reactions of the other sex	1.	The desire to live and be accepted as a member of the opposite sex, usually accompanied by the wish to make his or her body as congruent as possible with the preferred sex through surgery and hormone treatment
B.	Persistent discomfort with his or her sex or sense of inappropriateness in the gender role of that sex, . . . manifested by symptoms such as preoccupation with getting rid of primary and secondary sex characteristics (e.g., request for hormones, surgery, or other procedures to physically alter sexual characteristics to simulate the other sex) or belief that he or she was born the wrong sex	2.	The transsexual identity has been present persistently for at least 2 years
C.	The disturbance is not concurrent with a physical intersex condition	3.	The disorder is not a symptom of another mental disorder or a chromosomal abnormality
D.	The disturbance causes clinically significant distress or impairment in social, occupational, or other important areas of functioning		
302.6	*Gender Identity Disorder Not Otherwise Specified*	*F(64.9)*	*Gender Identity Disorder, Unspecified*
	This category is included for coding disorders in gender identity that are not classifiable as a specific Gender Identity Disorder. Examples include:		No specific criteria, yet could be used for gender dysphoria among patients with an intersex condition
1.	Intersex conditions (e.g., partial androgen insensitivity syndrome or congenital adrenal hyperplasia) and accompanying gender dysphoria		
2.	Transient, stress-related cross-dressing behavior		
3.	Persistent preoccupation with castration or penectomy without a desire to acquire the sex characteristics of the other sex		

Adapted from the World Health Organization. *International Statistical Classification of Diseases and Related Health Problems.* 10 rev. Geneva, Switzerland: World Health Organization, 1992.

▶ **TABLE 13-3 Standards of Care for the Treatment of Gender Identity Disorders**[a]

Guidelines for Providers	Mental Health Professional	Physician Prescribing Hormones	Surgeon Performing Sex Reassignment Surgery
Competence	• Master or doctoral degree • Documented supervised training in psychotherapy • Specialized training in the treatment of sexual disorders • Continuing education in the treatment of gender identity disorders	• Board-certified physician • Well-versed in the relevant medical and psychological aspects of treating patients with gender identity disorders	• Board-certified urologist, gynecologist, plastic or general surgeon competent in urological diagnosis • Documented supervised training in sex reassignment surgery • Continuing education in reassignment surgery

Guidelines for Applicants	Eligibility Criteria		Readiness Criteria
Hormone therapy	• At least 3 months of psychotherapy *or* real life experience[b] • Demonstrable knowledge of the effects and side effects, social benefits, and risks of hormones and documented informed consent • One letter from a competent mental health professional recommending hormone therapy		• Further consolidation of gender identity during psychotherapy or the real life experience • Progress in mastering other identified problems leading to stable mental health • The patient is likely to take hormones in a responsible manner
Female-to-male chest surgery	• At least 3 months of psychotherapy *or* real life experience • Demonstrable knowledge of the potential risks and benefits of chest surgery and documented informed consent • One letter from a competent mental health professional recommending chest surgery		• Further consolidation of gender identity during psychotherapy or the real life experience • Progress in mastering other identified problems leading to stable mental health
Male-to-female breast surgery	• At least 3 months of psychotherapy *or* real life experience • At least 18 months of hormone therapy[c] • Demonstrable knowledge of the potential risks and benefits of breast surgery and documented informed consent • One letter from a competent mental health professional recommending breast surgery		• Further consolidation of gender identity during psychotherapy or the real life experience • Progress in mastering other identified problems leading to stable mental health
Genital reconstructive surgery	• Legal age of majority • At least 12 months of continuous hormone therapy[c] • At least 12 months of continuous full-time real life experience • Demonstrable knowledge of the cost, required lengths of hospitalizations, likely complications, and postsurgical rehabilitation requirements of the various surgical approaches and documented informed consent • Awareness of different competent surgeons • Two letters from competent mental health professionals recommending genital surgery. At least one of these professionals needs to have a doctoral degree		• Demonstrable progress in consolidating one's gender identity • Demonstrable progress in dealing with work, family, and interpersonal issues resulting in a significantly better state of mental health

[a]The guidelines summarized here pertain to adults. Guidelines for children and adolescents are somewhat different and can be found at www.hbigda.org.
[b]The real life experience is a period of living continuously and full-time in the preferred gender role.
[c]Exceptions can be made (e.g., in case of medical contraindications to hormone therapy).

This paradigm shift gave birth to an increasingly visible transgender community that offers peer support and empowerment for transgender persons and their families. For example, in coalition with the gay, lesbian, and bisexual community, the transgender community has been able to counteract the social stigma associated with gender nonconformity through the adoption of human rights legislation that protects against discrimination. Today, being transsexual means having a distinct identity, and the focus of treatment is to facilitate a transgender coming out process. This process may or may not include hormone therapy and/or sex reassignment surgery. Hormone therapy is no longer necessarily followed by genital surgery (42,48) and has become a valid treatment option in and of itself. Conversely, patients who do not want or need hormone therapy still might undergo surgery (e.g., orchiectomy, mastectomy/chest surgery). Evaluation by a mental health professional specialized in the treatment of gender identity disorder is, in these cases, even more important to ensure that the patient is adequately prepared for the psychosocial consequences of the various expressions of transgender identity.

The task of the mental health professional is to prepare the applicant for sex reassignment and for living life as a transsexual person. Some patients have already begun to embrace a transgender identity when they present for hormones or surgery. Others struggle to accept their transgender identity as a consequence of the social stigma attached to their gender nonconformity and, as a result, may suffer from internalized transphobia (i.e., discomfort with one's own transgenderism stemming from internalized normative gender expectations).

Growing up with transgender feelings poses a significant challenge to psychosocial development (49). When a child learns that his or her inner feelings do not match the expectations associated with the sex assigned at birth based on the external genitalia, these inner feelings are kept private or are suppressed. Instead, a false self that is congruent with society's expectations is presented and affirmed. This "splitting" of identity into a private and public self—polarized in terms of gender—is a source of distress that can contribute to the development of such mental health concerns as anxiety, depression, and substance abuse, as well as personality disorders related to one's sense of autonomy and capacity for intimacy. When life in the gender associated with the public self eventually fails (50), the "woman trapped in a male body" (or "man trapped in a female body") may present with a request for sex reassignment aimed at eradicating everything associated with their sex assigned at birth in an effort to start a new life as a member of the "opposite" sex. Hence, despite the paradigm shift described above, some individuals may still present with a request to "change sex" and undergo extensive plastic surgery of the face and body to be able to pass as a nontransgender woman or man. Treatment in accordance with the Benjamin Standards of Care and exposure to peers in the transgender community can alleviate this internalized transphobia and start the process of self-acceptance and identity integration (51). This may help the patient to make a fully informed decision about sex reassignment surgery.

The fact that MtF transgender persons are increasingly able to live as women without genital surgery does not mean that such surgery is becoming obsolete. Rather, the motivation for obtaining a vagina has shifted from being the ultimate change in sex to a change in genitals for itself. Whereas in the past, MtF transsexuals may have been satisfied with genital surgery despite functional limitations (e.g., lack of depth of the neo-vagina, absence of a clitoris) (52), today, sexual function, along with aesthetic appearance, has become even more important in patient satisfaction. For FtMs, removal of the breasts and the creation of a male-appearing chest remain important to live successfully as a transgender or transsexual man. Most, however, do not opt for phalloplasty and instead live as transsexual men without a penis, because the surgical outcome is aesthetically and functionally less than satisfactory (53). This does not mean that female-to-male genital reconstructive surgery is not important. Rather, it means that surgical techniques in this area need to be advanced. Moreover, even if social change toward greater acceptance of gender diversity continues, there will be individuals who experience a strong, visceral aversion to their primary sex characteristics and who can benefit greatly from genital reconstructive surgery.

Surgical Procedures

Sex reassignment surgery includes mastectomy for FtMs, breast augmentation for MtFs, and genital reconstructive surgery. The most common technique for vaginoplasty is the penile-inversion technique (54). With this technique, the outer skin of the penis becomes the inner lining of the vagina, the labia are created from the scrotum, and the glans of the penis is reduced to form a clitoris. The most common complication of the penile inversion technique is stenosis (narrowing) of the vagina. An alternative technique not as likely to result in stenosis is the recto-sigmoid technique, in which colon tissue is used for the inner lining of the vagina. The most common technique for phalloplasty is the radial forearm flap technique (55). A flap of skin and subcutaneous tissue is taken from the forearm to create the penis, and the labia become the scrotum in which testicle implants are inserted. The vagina is closed and the urethra extended. A penile implant is needed for the penis to become erect. Following the procedure, penile sensation is limited and loss of some of the transplanted tissue is a possible complication. An alternative is metoidioplasty (clitoral release), which does not require a skin graft and maximizes sexual sensitivity (56). Most common are hysterectomy and oopherectomy, the latter being particularly important to prevent ovarian cancer for patients who take masculinizing hormones.

For MtFs, a number of other feminizing surgeries may be performed. Options include reduction thyroid chrondroplasty, suction-assisted lipoplasty of the waist, rhinoplasty, facial bone reduction, rhytidectomy, and blepharoplasty. For FtMs, other surgeries include liposuction to reduce fat in hips, thighs, and buttocks. In contrast to breast/chest and genital surgery, these procedures do not require written recommendation from mental health professionals (37).

Surgery Prevalence

Table 13-4 shows the prevalence of these surgeries among a sample of 538 transsexuals surveyed via the Internet (57). These data confirm clinical observations that female-to-male chest surgery and male-to-female vaginoplasty are the most commonly requested procedures. Thirty-two percent reported having had any type of sex reassignment surgery, and 59% reported wanting to have sex reassignment surgery in the future. Furthermore, nine participants (2%) reported having had silicone injections in their breasts, hips, lips, cheeks, and buttocks. Only half of these silicone injections were performed by medical providers. Illicit use of silicone can have disastrous consequences such as distortion of the body part being injected, granuloma formation, and chronic draining wounds (58).

Outcome of Surgery

Studies have shown that the vast majority of transsexuals are satisfied with sex reassignment surgery. Satisfaction rates range from 87% for MtFs to 97% for FtMs (59). Dissatisfaction and postoperative psychopathology have been associated with inadequate surgical results (60–61). Making a gender role transition has been shown to improve mood and other psychological symptoms (62). Regrets and reversal to the original gender role are rare (63) and have been associated with poor differential psychiatric diagnosis, failure to carry out the real life experience, and unsatisfactory surgical results (64). Socioeconomic status, relationships, and sexual satisfaction have been shown to improve with sex reassignment (65).

▶ TABLE 13-4 Sex Reassignment Surgery among 538 Transsexuals in the U.S.

Type of Surgery	Male-to-Females (N=278)	Female-to-Males (N=260)	Total (N=538)
Breast/chest	29 (10%)	91 (35%)	120 (22%)
Vaginoplasty/vaginectomy and metoidioplasty	53 (19%)	7 (3%)	60 (11%)
Labiaplasty/scrotoplasty	43 (15%)	6 (2%)	49 (9%)
Orchiectomy (removal of testicles)/oophorectomy (removal of ovaries)	51 (18%)	34 (13%)	85 (16%)
Hysterectomy	n/a	36 (14%)	36 (7%)
Adam's apple reduction (tracheal shave)	15 (5%)	N/A	15 (3%)
Facial surgery	14 (5%)		14 (3%)
Hair transplant	2 (.7%)	1 (.4%)	3 (.5%)
Rib removal	1 (.3%)	N/A	1 (.2%)
Hip enlargement/reduction		1 (.4%)	1 (.2%)
TOTAL	67 (24%)	105 (61%)	172 (32%)

Note: N/A=not applicable. None of the female-to-males reported having had a phalloplasty.

Assessment of the Applicant for Sex Reassignment

Applicants for sex reassignment surgery should receive a psychological evaluation by mental health professionals competent in the diagnosis and treatment of sexual and gender identity disorders (37). The task of the mental health professional is to accurately diagnose the patient's condition and any coexisting psychopathology. Depression and anxiety, as well as features of schizotypal, narcissistic, and antisocial personality disorder, are common (35). The professional should ascertain the eligibility and readiness of the patient for sex reassignment surgery as outlined in the Benjamin Standards of Care (Table 13-3). In addition to standard topics covered in any psychological evaluation, assessment should include a history of gender dysphoria and cross-dressing. An assessment of sexual fantasy and behavior is also necessary to illuminate the relationship between identity and sexuality and to identify any compulsive sexual behavior.

Sexual identity is assessed using a descriptive model with the following four components: sex assigned at birth, gender identity, social sex role, and sexual orientation (66). At birth, sex is usually assigned based on the external genitalia as male or female. When the external genitalia are ambiguous, other markers of sex, such as internal genitalia, chromosomal sex, and hormones are considered before a sex assignment is made. Although the vast majority of applicants for sex reassignment were not born with ambiguous genitalia, it is not uncommon for patients to wonder or believe that they were born intersex in an effort to validate their gender identity.

The second component, gender identity, refers to the basic conviction of being a man, woman, or other gender (e.g., transgender). The clinical interview remains the best way to assess gender identity. The patient is asked to describe his or her experience of gender, and a detailed biopsychosocial developmental history is obtained. Gender identity is the most important of the four components in the decision whether or not reassignment surgery might be indicated (48).

The third and fourth components, social sex role and sexual orientation, are integral parts of the patient's identity. Social sex role is defined as characteristics in personality, appearance, and behavior culturally defined as masculine or feminine. Sexual orientation includes sexual behavior, fantasy, and emotional attachment to men and/or women, and is best defined on the basis of gender identity rather than sex assigned at birth. For example, the sexual orientation of a patient assigned female at birth who is convinced that his gender identity is that of a man and who is attracted to men is best described as homosexual or gay, rather than heterosexual (67–68). The relevance of sexual orientation and social sex role in the decision for sex reassignment is limited. For example, a patient assigned male at birth who is convinced that his gender identity is that of a woman may be quite masculine and attracted to women. Her masculinity does not make her feelings of being a woman any less valid. The goal of treatment is to assist this patient in being as authentic as she can be and to integrate her womanhood, masculinity, and sexual orientation toward women into an integrated transgender identity. Like many nontransgender women, this may mean living life as a lesbian, masculine woman.

Social sex role can be assessed using standardized instruments such as the Bem Sex Role Inventory (69) and Personal Attributes Questionnaire (70). Sexual orientation can be assessed using the Assessment of Sexual Orientation form (67). Transsexuals may identify as straight, lesbian, gay, or bisexual. Among the 278 MtF transsexuals described above (Table 13-4), 32% reported being attracted to men, 31% to women, and 37% to both men and women. Among the 260 FtMs, 57% reported being attracted to women, 13% to men, and 28% to both genders.

Standardized psychological tests and paper-and-pencil questionnaires should be used to compare the patient's psychosexual adjustment to established norms as well as to cross-validate information gathered during the clinical interview. Examples of useful tests for assessing coexisting psychological and sexual disorders are the Minnesota Multiphasic Personality Inventory-2 (71), the Tennessee Self-Concept Scale (72), and the Derogatis Sexual Functioning Inventory (73). Other useful questionnaires include the Transgender Identity Survey (74) to assess dimensions of internalized transphobia, the Cross-Gender Questionnaire (75) to assess cross-gender identification and experience, and the Compulsive Sexual Behavior Inventory (76).

A physical examination is recommended for patients who are taking hormones. Patients may have taken hormones without medical supervision. Transgender patients may have avoided regular medical care due to anticipated or actual negative experiences with health providers (77). A physical exam might therefore be indicated to screen for any untreated medical conditions and to promote prevention of common diseases such as cancer, cardiovascular disease, or diabetes (78). A psychiatric evaluation is recommended for patients who might benefit from psychotropic medications to alleviate symptoms of anxiety, depression, or other mental disorders. Finally, a chemical dependency evaluation is recommended for patients presenting with substance use. Taken together, these examinations will allow for the request for sex reassignment to be evaluated in the context of the patient's overall mental, physical, and sexual health.

Psychological Treatment

After the assessment is complete, an individualized treatment plan is negotiated with each patient. A comprehensive treatment model of gender dysphoria (51,79) comprises the following four tasks: (i) management of coexisting psychological problems; (ii) facilitating identity formation; (iii) identity management (including possible surgery); and (iv) aftercare.

Management of Coexisting Psychological Problems

Patients may present with a range of psychological difficulties. For example, 52% of MtF and 44% of FtM transsexuals reported clinical levels of depression (57). These conditions may coexist with or be exacerbated by their gender dysphoria. Addressing these problems first serves to stabilize the patient and facilitate the development of a therapeutic relationship for exploring and resolving gender identity conflict. If treatment is effective, these disorders do not necessarily contraindicate sex reassignment. Rather, the potential of sex reassignment in improving the overall health and well-being of the patient is carefully considered.

Facilitating Identity Formation

After coexisting psychological problems have been addressed, the focus of treatment shifts to clarifying gender identity conflict and understanding the request for sex reassignment in light of the patient's psychosocial development. One way to accomplish this is for the patient to write his or her autobiography up to the present time and share it with the therapist. In addition, the patient may wish to explore how he or she sees life after sex reassignment surgery. The personal history can be analyzed using a symbolic-interactionist approach (80–82). That analysis focuses on the meaning the patient assigns to past, present, and future life experiences. These meanings can be further explored and restructured as a result of journal writing and discussion of the relevant history in individual, group, or family therapy. Patients are encouraged to verbalize gender feelings and conflicts. Feelings are re-examined, and barriers to identity development are identified and resolved (51).

The impact of growing up with transgender feelings in a society with few positive transgender role models is a common theme in this phase of therapy. Transgender feelings usually date back to childhood and, when initially expressed, are met with a lack of understanding, disapproval, and sometimes abuse. As a result, many transgender people attempt to conform to what is expected of them on the basis of their sex assigned at birth, and hide or suppress their transgender feelings. The shame that ensues is long lasting and undermines the development of a sense of autonomy as well as the capacity for intimacy. Revisiting some of these experiences and releasing the associated grief can empower patients to begin to accept their transgender experience and acknowledge it to peers, family, and friends.

Identity Management

Many transsexual patients have already decided that they want sex reassignment before they consult with a mental health professional. However, in accordance with the Benjamin Standards of Care, the professional needs at least 3 months to begin to understand and support the patient's decision for hormone therapy or sex reassignment surgery. The fact that sex reassignment can only be accessed with a referral from a specialized mental health professional has been criticized by some members of the transgender community as unnecessarily pathologizing (83–84). The "gatekeeper" role poses a challenge for therapists and patients in establishing and maintaining a trusting therapeutic relationship (85). Nonetheless, the standards of care may be at least in part responsible for the lack of regret among patients who have completed sex reassignment. Indeed, patients' choices among the available medical interventions can change during the course of therapy. For example, acceptance of a transgender identity that transcends the gender dichotomy may alleviate a patient's quest to have extensive facial surgery in an effort to pass as a nontransgender woman. Moreover, a trusting therapeutic relationship can be a real asset for patients going through a social gender role transition as they come out to friends, family, co-workers, and community.

In addition to the referral of a mental health professional, the Benjamin Standards of Care call for a real life experience of at least 12 months of living continuously and full-time in the preferred gender role prior to surgery. The real life experience ensures that patients have a realistic understanding of what it is like to live as a transsexual before having irreversible surgeries. The real life experience is described as "the act of fully adopting a new or evolving gender role or gender presentation in everyday life" (37, p. 17). This does not mean that the patient needs to adopt a stereotypical cross-gender role and pass as a member of the other sex. Rather, it means that patients need to continuously express their authentic transgender identity. Some patients, however, may be reluctant and avoid expressing their preferred gender identity in interpersonal settings where they feel particularly vulnerable to rejection. The real life experience requires, however, that the patient transitions full-time to the preferred gender role when ready. Living part-time in the preferred gender role is a necessary step for many, but does not count toward the requirement of one year of full-time expression.

In preparing for the real life experience, patients are encouraged to take calculated risks by first coming out to those most likely to accept them. The therapist can help patients plan for or facilitate disclosure to friends and family. An important principle for patients to understand is that family and friends need to go through their own coming out process. They may experience grief over the loss of their relative or friend as they know him or her, a process mirroring Kübler-Ross's stages of grief characterized by denial, anger, bargaining, depression, and eventual acceptance (86–87). Immediate acceptance, therefore, is not a realistic expectation. While family and friends proceed through these stages, the patient is in particular need of support from peers and the therapist who can help put into perspective the reactions of family and friends.

Another critical issue is coming out in the workplace. Most human resource departments have little experience with employees who change gender on the job. Consequently, the transgender employee often has to assume a dual role: that of the employee making the transition and the only "expert" on whom the company relies in planning for this transition. For both the transsexual employee and the workplace, it is much better for a third party to come in to hear all concerns, develop and negotiate a plan, and provide the necessary education. A qualified and experienced mental health professional could fulfill this role in a consulting capacity.

This transition toward living full-time in the preferred gender role usually is a tumultuous time for the transsexual patient. Relationships may change or end and jobs might be lost. New relationships and support systems often replace these losses. In time, most patients manage to recover and develop resilience in coping with the challenges of living life as a transsexual—challenges related to social stigma that they will likely continue to face for the rest of their lives.

Aftercare

The mental health professional plays an important role in preparing the patient for surgery, but also providing aftercare. Sex reassignment surgery can be an intense emotional experience for the transsexual patient. Patients usually have worked hard for many years to overcome multiple personal and social challenges and may experience considerable feelings of grief, as well as relief, when the goal of surgery is finally realized. Surgery is often performed far away from home due to the scarcity of specialized surgeons; thus, it is important to plan for available support from family, friends, peers, or health providers. If at all possible, at least one member of the patient's support system should be available in person for emotional support. Others, including the patient's therapist, should be available via phone or e-mail. Upon the patient's return home, both medical and psychological follow-up care should be available.

Hormone therapy and sex reassignment surgery can affect the patient's sexual functioning. Feminizing hormones tend to reduce sexual desire. Erections may become more difficult to obtain, or maintain, and are sometimes painful. Masculinizing hormones tend to increase sexual desire and, as such, can have an impact (positive or negative) on primary relationships. Hormones are discontinued prior to surgery to reduce the risk of complications. They are resumed, with an adjusted regimen, after the testicles or ovaries have been removed. Regular dilation of the neo-vagina after surgery is critical to prevent stenosis, especially if the patient is interested in receptive vaginal intercourse. Although many MtF transsexuals maintain their ability to reach orgasm after surgery, some do not (88). Moreover, many transsexuals will want to experiment sexually with their changed anatomy. Such sexual experimentation may include sex with men for both MtFs and FtMs, even if they are predominantly attracted to women. For some FtMs, once they have established their identity as men, sex with other men may serve to explore male sexuality, nurture their masculinity, and satisfy their curiosity and longing for a functioning penis (89). Sexual health, including HIV/STD prevention education, is an important topic to address before, and after, sex reassignment surgery.

The prevalence of HIV and other STDs among certain subgroups of the transgender population is high. In a sample of 392 MtF transgender persons in San Francisco, 35% tested positive for HIV and 53% were diagnosed with an STD (38). The Benjamin Association issued a resolution that it is unethical to deny availability or eligibility for sex reassignment surgery solely on the basis of blood-seropositivity for conditions such as HIV or hepatitis B (37). This resolution was necessary, because some surgeons had denied surgery on the basis of HIV status alone. Guidelines for surgery on HIV-positive transsexuals include coordination with the physician treating the patient's HIV, evaluation of the patient's medical history and lab data, and discussion of the most recent treatment regimen (90). When these guidelines and the proper precautions against infection of health care workers are followed, the outcome of sex reassignment surgery for HIV-positive transsexuals is satisfactory (91).

CASE EXAMPLES

The following case vignettes, taken from the first author's clinical practice, illustrate many of the psychological aspects of sex (re)assignment discussed in this chapter. Although most intersex patients appear satisfied with their sex assigned at birth, some are not. Gender dysphoria is more common among prenatally androgenized individuals who were raised as females (3). An example is the experience of Alex, detailed in the first vignette, whose treatment for gender dysphoria was guided by the Benjamin Standards of Care (37). This case illustrates the importance of counseling in assisting intersex patients and their families to cope with the implications of early genital reconstruction in light of later gender identity and sexuality.

The second vignette of Carole, a MtF transsexual, illustrates the impact of social stigma and shame associated with gender nonconformity. Carole's request for extensive feminizing surgery can be interpreted as overcompensation to alleviate her shame. Psychotherapy helped her to achieve a greater level of acceptance of her transsexual identity, allowing her to make a more fully informed decision regarding surgery.

The last vignette shares the story of Tim, a FtM transsexual, who experienced the physical changes of puberty as traumatic. This, along with his struggle to find a peer group he could identify with, resulted in depression. Once Tim identified his transsexuality, masculinized his body, and connected with the transgender community, he blossomed. Tim's story illustrates the importance of evaluating the request for genital reconstruction in the overall context of the patient's life and mental health.

Case 1: Alex: Intersexuality

Alex was referred to our clinic at age 22 by his endocrinologist for evaluation and treatment of gender dysphoria. At the time of referral, he was living in the female role. He was born with 46, XX CAH, salt-losing type, and as a result of androgen exposure, he was virilized, his clitoris was the size of a small penis, and no vaginal opening was present. He was raised female. Within the first three years of life, his clitoris was surgically reduced. In early adolescence, a vaginal opening was created. Since birth, cortisone and salt-replacements were prescribed, but Alex had been intermittently noncompliant in taking these medications, especially after he became increasingly unhappy with his female sex assignment. To cope with his gender dysphoria and other stressors in his life, Alex began abusing alcohol and drugs at age 12, which developed into chemical dependency. A psychological evaluation at age 14 concluded: Alex "may feel deformed or damaged in some way, and he might be quite angry about the physical anomalies and medical interventions." Presently he has been sober for 1 year and stated as his goal: "I would like to proceed with surgery to be a full-fledged man instead of being an 'it'."

According to Alex, his family dealt with his intersexuality by not talking about it. This was confirmed by a family therapy session with his mother who had great difficulty talking about her son's condition. Yet, at the end of the session, Alex's mother was able to acknowledge that she felt guilty about having chosen the "wrong sex" for her child after birth. Alex was the youngest of four children, having two sisters and one brother. Alex never knew his birth father. Alex's mother raised the four children as a single parent. One of his sisters revealed: "I feel like I failed as an older sister, because I did not explain to you how great being a girl could be." After counseling, she ended up respecting Alex's decision to live as a man.

Alex reported a history of childhood sexual abuse. This was extensively addressed in therapy prior to supporting Alex's request for reassignment to the male sex. Alex began living full-time in the male gender role and changed his name legally. A physical exam in preparation for masculinizing hormone therapy revealed a split-type clitoris with the urethral opening and another area of erectile tissue below that which, upon urination or stimulation, would hypertrophy under the skin. In accordance with the Benjamin Standards of Care, initial hormone therapy was followed by chest surgery and phalloplasty (using the radial forearm flap technique). He insisted on the latter surgery despite knowing its limitations.

Alex phoned his therapist shortly after one of his main genital reconstructive surgeries. Alone in a hotel room, he experienced a panic attack with fears of not healing and death. He developed postoperative depression, a recurrence of a lifelong depression compounded by grief over lost time and missed opportunities. This depression was successfully treated with antidepressant medications. Subsequent sex therapy helped Alex with his long-standing difficulty reaching orgasm. Participation in an aftercare group for patients who completed sex reassignment surgery was recommended.

Case 2: Carole: Male-to-Female Transsexualism

Carole is a 31-year-old African-American MtF transsexual who presented with a request for sex reassignment. Specifically, she requested feminizing hormone therapy, extensive facial surgery (of nose, cheeks, chin, brow ridge, and Adam's apple), breast augmentation, and vaginoplasty. Her history of gender dysphoria dated back to early childhood. She had been a feminine boy, teased for her mannerisms and behavior. She recalled feeling ashamed, because she was considered a disgrace to her family. In her early teenage years, Carole suffered abuse from peers in school and the neighborhood. At age 15 she ran away to a shelter. When she returned home, she began to live in the female gender role. Her parents tolerated this until Carole was caught visiting a gay bar. Shortly thereafter, she moved in with her boyfriend. She took feminizing hormones on and off, first obtained through friends and later prescribed by a doctor. Carole felt ready for surgery to "finally become a woman."

Carole met criteria for gender identity disorder. She also reported a history of experimenting with crystal meth and cocaine as well as more regular use of marijuana. A no-use contract was established for these substances. In addition, Carole met criteria for diagnoses of dysthymia and histrionic personality disorder. The personality disorder affected her in many ways, particularly in relationships with men. Carole recognized that she took care of her partner at the expense of her own needs.

Carole's symptoms of depression were treated with pharmacotherapy. She agreed to discontinue regular marijuana use and quit smoking cigarettes to lower the risks associated with hormone therapy and to improve her physical health. In psychotherapy, Carole reviewed her history and confronted the grief associated with the rejection and ridicule she received from her family and peers. The relationship with her mother improved considerably after Carole included her in family therapy. Carole's mother revealed that she blamed herself for Carole's transgender identity, a "lifestyle" not approved of by her church. Carole shared with her mother a faith in God and was able to put her mother's struggle into perspective. Carole also brought her male partner to therapy, but was not able to change her pattern of codependency in this relationship. Eventually, she left him for another man.

Carole joined a therapy group with other transgender individuals in various stages of coming out. In this group, Carole confronted her feelings of shame. This process led to a deeper acceptance of her transgender identity. She developed a friendship with another transsexual. She recognized that even if she could pass with the help of extensive plastic surgery, she would always be different from non-transgender women. She was able to feel proud of being transsexual. Her desire for facial plastic surgery waned.

Feminizing hormones had resulted in modest breast growth; however, considering Carole's broad shoulders and chest, she felt the breast growth was insufficient. More than a year after the initial intake had passed when Carole requested support for breast augmentation and genital reconstructive surgery. She consulted with a plastic surgeon who specialized in transgender surgery. After Carole's therapist submitted the required paperwork, her health insurance company agreed to cover the cost of the procedure. Within days after the surgery, Carole called her therapist and reported that the surgery had gone well and that she felt great relief. She then cried. Follow-up care was provided by a physician in Carole's hometown whose nurses helped her to continue dilation to preserve adequate depth and width of the vagina. Months later, Carole joined a brief psycho-educational group for transsexuals exploring their sexual health. She participated in homework exercises designed to increase comfort with her body and genitals. Eventually she was able to achieve orgasm.

Case 3: Tim: Female-to-Male Transsexualism

Tim was 40 years old when he was referred to our clinic by a therapist who had been treating him for depression. He disclosed to this therapist that he felt he could no longer go on living as a woman. A tomboy as a child, he thought he was a lesbian and got involved in the lesbian community as a young adult. All his life, people had frequently commented on his masculinity ("you are too butch"), which, according to Tim, made relationships with lesbian women difficult. He felt he belonged neither in the gay community nor in the straight community. Tim was interested in learning about the possibility of sex reassignment.

In reviewing Tim's sexual history, it became clear that the gender dysphoria was long-standing and persistent. He felt bothered by "anything womanly" in puberty and did not like the changes his body went through. He took showers in the dark. He felt he belonged with the guys. He did not talk about these feelings with his parents, because they "had their own problems" (referring to his mother's drinking). After falling in love with a woman, Tim explored the lesbian community and thought he had found his home. However, he gradually came to the conclusion that he is also different from them, which after several failed lesbian relationships caused him to become depressed.

Tim met criteria for diagnoses of major depression and gender identity disorder. As he began to accept his transgender identity, the depression lifted. He participated in individual and group psychotherapy. He came out to his parents and sister. What helped them to accept Tim's transsexuality was the improvement they observed in his mood and happiness. Tim connected with other FtM transsexuals in the community and initiated a monthly social at his house. He finally felt he belonged. Eight months into therapy, he received support for masculinizing hormone therapy and mastectomy. One year later, he had a hysterectomy and oophorectomy. The affirmation of his gender identity greatly improved Tim's self-esteem. He liked himself and, as a result, took better care of his health. He worked out regularly, and he developed a crush on a female personal trainer who worked at his gym.

Unfortunately, the personal trainer did not reciprocate Tim's efforts to get to know her. Tim struggled with fear of rejection, and also with the fact that he did not have a penis. Tim eventually met a woman via the Internet with whom he connected well. She was a heterosexually identified woman with two children from a previous marriage. They fell in love and became sexual. Tim learned that he could have a satisfying sexual relationship without the presence of a penis. He no longer brought up the option of metoidioplasty or phalloplasty. The couple wanted to get married and, in order to do so, Tim sought to amend his birth certificate to reflect his male gender identity. The state initially refused, because Tim had not had genital reconstructive surgery. Letters from Tim's therapist and physician explaining that Tim had lived many years as a man sufficed to change the state's decision. Tim is now happily married, and his depression is in full remission.

CONCLUSIONS

Genital reconstructive surgery may be needed or desired for individuals born with ambiguous genitalia or following genital trauma or mutilation. However, genital reconstructive surgery is a medically necessary intervention shown to be effective for patients with gender identity disorder who are selected and prepared for such surgery in accordance with the Benjamin Standards of Care. In addition, not all patients with an intersex condition or with gender identity disorder need or want genital surgery. Surgery is simply one of the options available to actualize and affirm gender identity. In the case of intersexuality, the long-term impact of early surgery on identity development and sexual functioning needs to be carefully considered. In the case of transsexuality, the pros and cons of genital surgery need to be evaluated in the context of the transgender coming out process, which is first and foremost a psychosocial process. Consultation with a mental health professional and living at least one year full-time in the preferred gender role, as required by the Benjamin Standards of Care, can help in this process. Surgeons working with these populations should be sensitive to the psychological aspects of having an intersex condition or transgender identity, coordinate care with other providers in the patient's care system, and participate in continuing education in this specialized area of sexual medicine.

Greater visibility of intersexuality and transgenderism will increase our awareness that not only gender, but also sex, is less binary than often assumed. Within a binary paradigm, transsexualism illustrates the psychological pain associated with a conflict between one's genital anatomy and sex assignment versus one's gender identity. Genital surgery is among the options that can bring considerable relief; but, when performed in infancy, genital surgery may for some become a source of psychological pain, especially when the sole purpose of the surgery was cosmetic and when surgery negatively affected sexual functioning (29). An acknowledgment of the diversity in sex and gender has great potential to lessen the discomfort and shame associated with genital nonconformity.

Patient Assessment

- How do you identify in terms of your gender? Please describe what this means for you.
- What sex were you assigned at birth? How comfortable are you with this sex assignment?
- To your knowledge, were you born with ambiguous genitalia? If so, what do you know about the cause of this ambiguity and what was the response of your family? Did you or your family consult with a health provider regarding your situation, and if so, what happened?
- What surgery are you requesting?
- Please explain how you expect the surgery to help you.

Are you aware of the Benjamin Standards of Care? Specifically:

- Have you consulted with mental health professionals with special expertise in the area of intersexuality, transgenderism, or transsexuality? If yes, who, when (for how long)? Are these professionals supportive of the surgery you are requesting? If no, would you be willing to consult with a mental health professional? (Make referral.)
- Are you living full-time in your preferred gender role? If yes, for how long have you lived full-time in this role?
- Have you received feminizing or masculinizing hormone therapy? If yes, for how long, and who prescribes your hormones?
- What is your understanding of the nature and the potential risks and benefits of the surgery?
- How do you think this surgery might affect your sexual functioning?
- What plan do you have in place for your recovery? Who will be there to assist and support you?
- Who in your circle of family and friends is aware of your plans to undergo this surgery? How supportive are they?
- Who is your primary care physician, and is this physician aware of your plans to have surgery?

REFERENCES

1. Bradley SJ, Oliver GD, Chernick AB, Zucker KJ. Experiment of nature: Ablatio penis at 2 months, sex reassignment at 7 months, and a psychosexual follow-up in young adulthood. *Pediatrics* 1998;102(1):9.
2. Money J. Ablatio penis: normal male infant sex-reassigned as a girl. *Arch Sex Behav* 1975;4:65–71.
3. Cohen-Kettenis PT, Pfaefflin F. *Transgenderism and Intersexuality in Childhood and Adolescence: Making Choices.* Developmental clinical psychology and psychiatry, 46. Thousand Oaks, CA: Sage Publications, Inc., 2003.
4. Blackless M, Charuvastra A, Derryck A, et al. How sexually dimorphic are we? *Am J Hum Biol* 2000;12(2): 151–166.
5. Money J, Ehrhardt AA. *Man and Woman, Boy and Girl: The Differentiation and Dimorphism of Gender Identity from Conception to Maturity.* Baltimore, MD: The Johns Hopkins University Press, 1972.
6. Diamond M. Sexual identity and sexual orientation in children with traumatized or ambiguous genitalia. *J Sex Res* 1997;34:199–211.
7. Meyer-Bahlburg HFL. Gender assignment and reassignment in 46, XY pseudohermaphroditism and related conditions. *J Clin Endocrinol Metab* 1999;84(10):3455–3458.
8. Minto CL, Liao LM, Woodhouse CR, et al. The effect of clitoral surgery on sexual outcome in individuals who have intersex conditions with ambiguous genitalia: a cross-sectional study. *Lancet* 2003;361(9365):1252–1257.
9. Diamond M, Sigmundson HK. Management of intersexuality: guidelines for dealing with person with ambiguous genitalia. *Arch Pediatr Adolesc Med* 1997;151:1046–1050.
10. American Academy of Pediatrics. Timing of elective surgery on the genitalia of male children with particular reference to the risks, benefits, and psychological effects of surgery and anesthesia. *Pediatrics* 1996; 97:590.
11. Ludwikowski B, Hayward O, Gonzalez R. Total urogenital sinus mobilization: expanded applications. *Br J Urol Int* 1998;83:820.
12. Pena A. Total urogenital sinus mobilization: an easier way to repair cloacas. *J Pediatr Surg* 1997;30:2.
13. Buss J, Lee R. McIndoe procedure for vaginal agenesis: results and complications. *Mayo Clin Proc* 1989;64:758.
14. Hendren W, Atala A. Use of bowel for vaginal reconstruction. *J Urol* 1994;152:752.
15. Hitchcock R, Malone P. Colovaginoplasty in infants and children. *Br J Urol* 1994;73:196.
16. Slijper FME, Drop SLS, Molenaar JC, de Muinck Keizer-Schrama MSMPF. Long-term psychological evaluation of intersex children. *Arch Sex Behav* 1998;27(2):125–144.
17. Husmann D. Intersex. In: Gillenwater J, Grayhack J, Howards S, Mitchell M, eds. *Adult and Pediatric Urology.* 4th ed. Philadelphia: Lippincott Williams & Wilkins, 2001:2558.
18. Belloli G, Campobasso P, Musi L. Labial skin flap vaginoplasty using tissue expanders. *Pediatr Surg Int* 1997;12:168.
19. Passerinai-Glazel G. A new one-stage procedure for clitorovaginoplasty in severely masculinized female pseudohermaphrodites. *J Urol* 1989;142:565.
20. Frank R. The formation of an artificial vagina without an operation. *Am J Obstet Gynecol* 1938;35:1053.
21. Chang T, Huang W. Forearm flap in one stage reconstruction of the penis. *Plast Reconstr Surg* 1984;74:251.
22. Gilbert D, Jordan G, Devine C, et al. Phallic construction in prepubertal and adolescent boys. *J Urol* 1993; 149:1521.
23. Hall JG, Gilchrist DM. Turner syndrome and its variants. *Pediatr Clin North Am* 1990;37:1421–1441.
24. Diamond DA. Sexual differentiation: normal and abnormal. In: Walsh P, Retick A, Vaughan D, Wein A, eds. *Campbell's Urology.* 8th ed. Philadelphia: WB Saunders, 2003:2405.
25. Eugster EA. Reality vs. recommendations in the care of infants with intersex conditions. *Arch Pediatr Adolesc Med* 2004;158(5):426–428.
26. Alderson J, Madill A, Balen A. Fear of devaluation: understanding the experience of intersexed women with androgen insensitivity syndrome. *Br J Health Psychol* 2004;9(1):81–100.
27. Rickert VI, Hassed SJ, Hendon AE, Cunniff C. The effects of peer ridicule on depression and self-image among adolescent females with Turner syndrome. *J Adolesc Health* 1996;19(1):34–38.
28. Preves SE. For the sake of the children: destigmatizing intersexuality. *J Clin Ethics* 1998;9(4):411–420.
29. Preves SE. *Intersex and Identity: The Contested Self.* New Brunswick, NJ: Rutgers University Press, 2003.
30. Krege S, Walz KH, Hauffa BP, et al. Long-term follow-up of female patients with congenital adrenal hyperplasia form 21-hydroxylase deficiency, with special emphasis on the results of vaginoplasty. *BJU Int.* 2000;86(3):253–258.
31. McCauley E, Feuillan P, Kushner H, Ross JL. Psychosocial development in adolescents with Turner syndrome. *J Dev Behav Pediatr* 2001;22(6):360–365.
32. Bockting WO, Robinson BE, Rosser BRS. Transgender HIV prevention: a qualitative needs assessment. *AIDS Care* 1998;10(4):505–526.
33. Bakker A, Kesteren PJM, van Gooren LJG, Bezemer PD. The prevalence of transsexualism in the Netherlands. *Acta Psychiatr Scand* 1993;87:237–238.
34. Olsson S, Moeller AR. On the incidence and sex ratio of transsexualism in Sweden, 1972–2002. *Arch Sex Behav* 2003;32(4):381–386.
35. American Psychiatric Association. *Diagnostic and Statistical Manual of Mental Disorders.* 4th ed. Text revision. Washington, DC: American Psychiatric Association, 2000.
36. World Health Organization. *International Statistical Classification of Diseases and Related Health Problems.* 10 rev. Geneva, Switzerland: World Health Organization, 1992.
37. Meyer W III, Bockting W, Cohen-Kettenis P, et al. The standards of care for gender identity disorders, sixth version. *J Psychol Human Sex* 2001;13(1):1–30.
38. Clements K, Katz M, Marx R. *The Transgender Community Health Project: Descriptive Results.* San Francisco: San Francisco Department of Public Health, 1999.

39. Nemoto T, Operario D, Keatley J. Health and social services for male-to-female transgenders of color in San Francisco. *International Journal of Transgenderism* 2005;8(2/3).
40. Xavier JM, Bobbin M, Singer B. A needs assessment of transgendered people of color living in Washington, DC. *International Journal of Transgenderism*. In press.
41. Reback CJ, Lombardi E, Simon PA, Frye DM. HIV seroprevalence and risk behaviors among transgendered women who exchange sex in comparison with those who do not. *J Psychol Human Sex* 2005;17(1/2).
42. Bockting WO. Transgender coming out: implications for the clinical management of gender dysphoria. In: Bullough B, Bullough VL, Elias J, eds. *Gender Blending*. Amherst, NY: Prometheus Books, 1997:48–52.
43. Hastings DW. Inauguration of a research project on transsexualism in a university medical center. In: Green R, Money J, eds. *Transsexualism and Sex Reassignment*. Baltimore, MD: Johns Hopkins University Press, 1969: 243–251.
44. Hastings DW. Postsurgical adjustment of male transsexual patients. *Clin Plast Surg* 1974;1(2):335–344.
45. Hastings D, Markland C. Post-surgical adjustment of twenty-five transsexuals (male-to-female) in the University of Minnesota study. *Arch Sex Behav* 1978;7(4):327–336.
46. Feinberg L. *Transgender Warriors: Making History from Joan of Arc to RuPaul*. Boston: Beacon Press, 1996.
47. Stone S. The empire strikes back: a posttranssexual manifesto. In: Epstein J, Straub K, eds. *Body Guards: The Cultural Politics of Gender Ambiguity*. New York: Routledge, 1991:280–304.
48. Bockting WO. From construction to context: gender through the eyes of the transgendered. *SIECUS Report.* 1999;28(1):3–7.
49. Fraser L. *Psychodynamic viewpoint: a Jungian perspective*. Plenary address at: 18th Harry Benjamin International Symposium on Gender Dysphoria; September 11, 2003; Gent, Belgium.
50. Diamond M. Self-testing among transsexuals: a check on sexual identity. *J Psychol Human Sex* 1996;8(3): 61–82.
51. Bockting WO. The assessment and treatment of gender dysphoria. *Directions in Clinical and Counseling Psychology* 1997;7(11):1–23.
52. Turner I, Edlich RF, Edgerton MT. Male transsexualism—a review of genital surgical reconstruction. *Journal of Personality Deviation* 1978;43:385–387.
53. Rachlin K. Factors which influence individual's decisions when considering female-to-male genital reconstructive surgery. *International Journal of Transgenderism* [serial online]. 1999;3(3). Available at www.symposion.com/ijt.
54. Karim RB, Hage JJ, Mulder JW. Neovaginoplasty in male transsexuals: review of surgical techniques and recommendations regarding eligibility. *Ann Plast Surg* 1996;37:669–675.
55. Hage JJ, Bouman GG, de Graaf FH, Bloem JJ. Construction of the neophallus in female-to-male transsexuals: the Amsterdam experience. *J Urol* 1993;149(6):1463–1468.
56. Hage JJ. Metaidoioplasty: an alternative phalloplasty technique in transsexuals. *Plast Reconstr Surg* 1996; 97:161–167.
57. Bockting WO, Miner MH, Robinson BE, et al. *Identity and sexuality of transgender people in the U.S.: Findings from an Internet-based survey*. Manuscript in preparation.
58. Hage JJ, Kanhai RC, Oen AL, et al. The devastating outcome of massive subcutaneous injection of highly viscous fluids in male-to-female transsexuals. *Plast Reconstr Surg* 2001;107(3):738–741.
59. Green R, Fleming D. Transsexual surgery follow-up: status in the 1990s. *Annu Rev Sex Res* 1990;1:163–174.
60. Lawrence AA. Factors associated with satisfaction or regret following male-to-female sex reassignment surgery. *Arch Sexu Behav* 2003;32(4):299–315.
61. Ross MW, Need JA. Effects of adequacy of gender reassignment surgery on psychological adjustment: a follow-up of fourteen male-to-female patients. *Arch Sex Behav* 1989;18(2):145–153.
62. Blanchard R, Steiner BW. *Clinical Management of Gender Identity Disorders in Children and Adults*. Washington, DC: American Psychiatric Press, 1990.
63. Kuiper AJ, Cohen-Kettenis PT. Gender role reversal among postoperative transsexuals. *International Journal of Transgenderism* [serial online] Month, 1998;2(3). Available at www.symposion.com/ijt.
64. Pfaefflin F. Regrets after sex reassignment surgery. *J Psych Human Sex* 1992; 5(4):69–85.
65. Pfaefflin F, Junge A. Thirty years of international follow-up studies of sex reassignment surgery: a comprehensive review, 1961–1991. *International Journal of Transgenderism* [serial online]. Available at www.symposion.com/ijt.
66. Shively M, DeCecco J. Components of sexual identity. *J Homosex* 1977;3:41–48.
67. Coleman E. Assessment of sexual orientation. *J Homosex* 1987;14(1/2):9–24.
68. Coleman E, Bockting WO, Gooren LJG. Homosexual and bisexual identity in sex-reassigned female-to-male transsexuals. *Arch Sex Behav* 1993;22(1):37–50.
69. Bem SL. The measurement of psychological androgyny. *J Consult Clin Psychol* 1974;42(2):155–162.
70. Spence JT, Helmreich RL. *Masculinity and Femininity: Their Psychological Dimensions, Correlates, and Antecedents*. Austin: University of Texas Press, 1978.
71. Hathaway SA, McKinley JC. *Minnesota Multiphasic Personality Inventory*. Minneapolis: The University of Minnesota Press, 1989.
72. Fitts WH. *Tennessee Self Concept Scale*. Los Angeles: Western Psychological Services, 1964.
73. Derogatis LR, Melisaratos N. The DSFI: a multidimensional measure of sexual functioning. *J Sex Marital Ther* 1979;5:244–281.
74. Bockting WO. Transgender identity, sexuality, and coming out: implications for HIV risk and prevention. Proceedings of the NIDA-sponsored satellite sessions in association with the XIV International AIDS Conference, Barcelona, Spain, July 2002. Bethesda, MD: U.S. Department of Health and Human Services, 2003.
75. Doctor RF, Fleming JS. Dimensions of transvestism and transsexualism: the validation and factorial structure of the Cross-Gender Questionnaire. *J Psych Human Sex* 1992;5(4):15–38.
76. Coleman E, Miner M, Ohlerking F, Raymond N. Compulsive sexual behavior inventory: a preliminary study of reliability and validity. *J Sex Marital Ther* 2001;27:325–332.
77. Feldman J, Bockting W. Transgender health. *Minn Med* 2003;86(7):25–32.

78. Feldman J. New onset of type 2 diabetes mellitus with feminizing hormone therapy: case series. *International Journal of Transgenderism* [serial online] 2002;6(2). Available at www.symposion.com/ijt.

79. Bockting WO, Coleman E. A comprehensive approach to the treatment of gender dysphoria. *J Psych Human Sex* 1992;5(4):131–155.

80. Minton HL, McDonald GJ. Homosexual identity formation as a developmental process. *J Homosex* 1984;9(2/3):91–104.

81. Plummer K. *Sexual Stigma: An Interactionist Account*. London, England: Routledge Kegan Paul, 1975.

82. Plummer K. *Beyond Childhood: Organizing "Gayness" in Adult Life*. Workshop at the international conference, Homosexuality Beyond Disease. Amsterdam, The Netherlands.

83. Pollack R. What is to be done? A commentary on the recommended guidelines. In: Israel GE, Tarver DE II. *Transgender Care*. Philadelphia: Temple University Press, 1997:229–235.

84. Stryker S. Over and out of academe: transgender studies come of age. In: Israel GE, Tarver DE II. *Transgender Care*. Philadelphia: Temple University Press, 1997:241–247.

85. Bockting W, Robinson B, Benner A, Scheltema K. Patient satisfaction with transgender health services. *J Sex Marital Ther* 2004;30(4):277–294.

86. Kübler-Ross E. *On Death and Dying*. London, England: The Macmillan Company, 1996.

87. Emerson S, Rosenfeld C. Stages of adjustment in family members of transgender individuals. *J Fam Psychother* 1996;7(3):1–12.

88. Lief HI, Hubschman L. Orgasm in the post-operative transsexual. *Arch Sex Behav* 1993;22(2):145–155.

89. Hein D, Kirk M. Education and soul-searching: the Enterprise HIV prevention group. *International Journal of Transgenderism* [serial online]. 1999;3(1/2). Available at www.symposion.com/ijt. Accessed on June 1, 2005.

90. Kirk S. Guidelines for selecting HIV positive patients for genital reconstructive surgery. *International Journal of Transgenderism* [serial online]. 1999;3(1/2). Available at www.symposion.com/ijt. Accessed on June 6, 2005.

91. Wilson AN. Sex reassignment surgery in HIV positive transsexuals. *International Journal of Transgenderism* [serial online]. 1999;3(1/2). Available at www.symposion.com/ijt. Accessed on May 27, 2005.

SECTION III

Psychological Perspectives on Cosmetic Surgery

Chapter 14

Cosmetic Surgery of the Face

Canice E. Crerand, PhD, Thomas F. Cash, PhD, and Linton A. Whitaker, MD

In 2004, over 9.2 million cosmetic surgical and nonsurgical procedures were performed in the United States (1). Rhinoplasty, blepharoplasty, and rhytidectomy (facelift) were among the most popular surgical procedures, as they typically are. Nonsurgical or minimally invasive procedures, such as botulinum toxin (Botox®) injections, are becoming even more popular than these surgical procedures. Of the 9.2 million cosmetic procedures performed in 2004, over 7.5 million were minimally invasive procedures (1). The popularity of these and other facial procedures is not surprising, given that the face is often an individual's most prominent and defining physical feature (2).

As the number of individuals who seek cosmetic facial procedures increases, so does the need to understand the psychological characteristics of the patients who seek them. Plastic surgeons and mental health professionals have long been interested in this issue, even before the recent rise in popularity. Understanding the psychological characteristics of patients who desire and undergo cosmetic procedures is important for practical reasons. Cosmetic procedures are often considered "psychological interventions," as many patients report postoperative improvements in their self-esteem and satisfaction with their appearance (3). However, these procedures may not be appropriate for all individuals, particularly those with certain psychiatric disorders. Thus, an understanding of the psychological functioning of cosmetic surgery patients is important as it relates not only to who desires these procedures but potentially to their outcome.

This chapter will review studies of the psychological characteristics of patients seeking facial cosmetic treatments. Particular attention will be paid to studies of patients seeking rhinoplasty, anti-aging treatments, and facial skeletal procedures. The chapter will also discuss the psychological characteristics of patients who seek hair replacement and/or transplantation. The relationship between two psychiatric disorders (body dysmorphic disorder and social anxiety disorder) and facial cosmetic surgery will be reviewed. The chapter concludes with suggestions for future research and implications for clinical practice.

RHINOPLASTY

Historically, rhinoplasty has been one of the most popular cosmetic procedures. In 1992, rhinoplasty was the second most commonly performed cosmetic procedure with 50,175 procedures performed in the United States (4). Its popularity has endured, as evinced by the fact that 305,475 rhinoplasties were performed in 2004, again making it the second most commonly performed cosmetic surgical procedure (1). Over the past 50 years, the psychological characteristics of rhinoplasty patients have received as much attention as any cosmetic procedure. As observed by Sarwer et al. (2,5), these studies, as well as studies of patients who have undergone other procedures, can be grouped into three generations of research.

First Generation Studies

Early reports of the psychological characteristics of rhinoplasty patients date back to 1940s and 1950s. Many of these investigations, as well as studies conducted into the 1960s, relied heavily on clinical interviews and observations of patients. The results of these studies suggested that rhinoplasty patients were highly psychopathological (6–7). One set of investigators went so far as to state that *all* patients desiring rhinoplasty were mentally ill (6). They described their sample of patients as suffering from a variety of psychiatric issues, ranging from feelings of inferiority to psychosis (6). In another study, 53% of patients received preoperative diagnoses of personality disorders (8). Following surgery, 10 patients were reported to have had "significant postoperative disturbances," such as symptoms of anxiety, depression, and psychosis.

Many early investigators conceptualized the desire for rhinoplasty from a psychodynamic perspective, the prevailing theoretical orientation in psychiatry at the time. The nose was often thought to symbolize the penis, and the desire for rhinoplasty was conceptualized as the patient's unconscious displacement of sexual conflicts onto his or her nose (9). For adolescent females, the desire for rhinoplasty was interpreted as an attempt to remove elements of her father's personality from her own (10). In another investigation, female rhinoplasty patients were described as over-identifying with their fathers because of an ambivalent relationship with an inadequate mother, which led to conflicts about femininity (11). Rhinoplasty was thought to provide resolution to these conflicts.

These early reports suggested that the majority of rhinoplasty patients were psychologically disturbed. In some cases, surgery exacerbated, rather than eliminated, this psychopathology. These findings, however, must be viewed in light of several methodological limitations. The reliance upon unstructured, psychodynamically oriented interviews suggests that the observations may have been biased, particularly since, from a psychodynamic perspective, appearance concerns are thought to be symptoms of underlying psychopathology. The lack of description provided for the clinical interviews prohibits replication of these findings. The majority of studies had relatively small sample sizes and failed to incorporate appropriate control groups. Finally, at the time these early reports were published, cosmetic surgery was clearly not as socially acceptable or readily available as it is today. In light of this social context, it is possible that surgery patients from this generation were, in fact, more psychopathological than the patients who seek rhinoplasty today (3).

Second Generation Studies

During the 1970s and 1980s, "second generation studies" of rhinoplasty patients began to include valid and reliable psychometric measures (2,5). Many studies incorporated control groups as well as preoperative and postoperative assessments. In contrast to previous studies, the majority found less evidence of preoperative psychopathology (12–15), and several noted postoperative benefits (13–14,16–17).

For example, Hay (12) investigated preoperative psychological characteristics in 45 patients seeking rhinoplasty using psychiatric interviews and several personality measures, including the Eysenck Personality Inventory. Compared to a control group, rhinoplasty patients reported higher levels of hostility, neuroticism, and obsessiveness. According to the psychiatric interviews, 26 of the 45 patients were considered to be "normal" or suffering from only mild personality reactions stemming from their appearance concerns. Postoperatively, 17 patients were asked to complete some of the same psychometric measures (16). The majority reported satisfaction with their surgery as well as reductions in levels of hysteria (16).

A subsequent study that administered clinical interviews and several psychometric tests, including the General Health Questionnaire, also found increased levels of anxiety, obsessiveness, and paranoia preoperatively compared to age- and gender-matched controls (13). Following surgery, patients reported decreases in all of these symptoms, and there were no significant differences between the rhinoplasty and control patients (13). Another study similarly reported improvements in symptoms of depression and anxiety postoperatively in 25 patients (17). Studies incorporating the use of the Minnesota Multiphasic Personality Inventory (MMPI) reported that the personality profiles of rhinoplasty patients were essentially normal preoperatively (14–15), and no changes in personality were noted postoperatively (14). Improvements in self-concept were reported (14).

Collectively, studies from the second generation of research suggest that rhinoplasty patients exhibited less psychopathology compared to earlier studies. Furthermore, postoperative assessments largely suggested that surgery produced improvements in psychological symptoms such as depression and anxiety. Nonetheless, many of these studies suffered from methodological problems, such as small sample sizes and the lack of appropriate control groups, which limit the generalizability of their findings.

Third Generation Studies

More recent studies (e.g., 1990 to present) of rhinoplasty patients have utilized improved methodologies, including reliable and valid self-report questionnaires and clinical interviews with established diagnostic criteria. Most studies have also included preoperative and postoperative assessments and appropriate control groups.

One study assessed 72 rhinoplasty patients preoperatively and postoperatively using two self-report instruments, the Maudsley Personality Inventory (MPI) scales for Extroversion and Neuroticism and the Inventory for Personality and Anxiety Testing (IPAT) scale for Anxiety (18). Anxiety and neuroticism scores decreased postoperatively, and patients also reported increases in extraversion. In a subsequent study, 79 rhinoplasty patients were assessed preoperatively and postoperatively with the MPI and IPAT (19). Decreases in neuroticism and anxiety were found postoperatively at the 6-month and 5-year follow-up assessments. However, increases in extraversion were present at the 6-month follow-up only.

Interestingly, 34% of the sample had higher than normal scores on the MPI and IPAT preoperatively and showed symptoms of mild to moderate dysmorphophobia (more commonly referred to as body dysmorphic disorder), somatization disorders, social phobia, and personality "abnormalities" (19). For the majority of these patients, psychological symptoms were still apparent at both follow-up assessments. Overall, these results suggest that some psychological changes may be short-lived, as in the case of extraversion. Furthermore, surgery may not improve more significant psychological symptoms.

Other third generation studies suggested that rhinoplasty patients did not experience inordinate levels of psychiatric symptoms. Goin and Rees (20) administered the Brief Symptom Inventory, a measure of psychological symptoms, to a sample of 121 rhinoplasty patients. Preoperatively, patient responses fell within the normal range. Postoperatively, patients reported reductions in anxiety, depression, and obsessiveness.

Hern et al. (21) evaluated 27 rhinoplasty or septorhinoplasty patients and a group of patients seeking septoplasty using the CORE questionnaire, a standardized measure designed to assess dimensions of psychological status, including well-being, symptoms or problems, and life/social functioning. No differences between groups were reported for the well-being and symptoms/problems dimensions, although rhinoplasty patients reported more problems with life functioning. A related study found that rhinoplasty patients were no more likely to report problems with interpersonal relationships compared to septoplasty patients (22).

Another recent study investigated psychopathology among 25 patients presenting for septorhinoplasty compared to two control groups: outpatients from an otolaryngology practice seeking nonsurgical treatment and outpatients awaiting noncosmetic nasal surgery. Pre- and postoperative psychiatric interviews and standardized psychological measures (e.g., Beck Depression Inventory, Symptom Checklist-90) were administered (23). No preoperative differences were found between septorhinoplasty patients and both control groups on the psychometric tests. Psychiatric interviews suggested that patients were "psychologically normal" although a few patients had mild adjustment disorders. Postoperatively, patients reported satisfaction with their surgical results and improvements in social desirability. Half of the patients with adjustment disorders reported symptom reductions following surgery.

Rankin and Borah (24) assessed quality of life in a sample of 105 patients, 21 of whom sought rhinoplasty. Preoperatively, rhinoplasty patients reported high levels of appearance dissatisfaction on a measure of quality of life. Significant improvements in appearance satisfaction and reductions in appearance-related embarrassment were noted postoperatively.

Within this third generation of research, the psychological construct of body image has received increased attention (2,5). Although, intuitively, body image is often thought to refer to the body as a whole, facial appearance clearly influences an individual's body image. Sarwer et al. (3) proposed a model of the relationship between body image dissatisfaction and cosmetic surgery. Briefly, the model contends that physical and psychological factors influence attitudes toward the body and, therefore, interest in changing the body through cosmetic surgery. These attitudes are thought to consist of two parts: (i) valence, or the importance of body image to an individual's self-esteem, and (ii) value, defined as the degree of body dissatisfaction (2–3,5). These two dimensions are comparable to what Cash, in Chapter 4 of this volume, terms body image investment and body image evaluation, respectively. It is theorized that persons who derive much of their self-esteem from their appearance (high valence or investment) and who also report high levels of body image dissatisfaction (high value or negative body image evaluation) may be more likely to seek cosmetic surgery (2–3,5).

To date, only one study has specifically examined the body image concerns of rhinoplasty patients. Preoperatively, the body image concerns of 32 female rhinoplasty patients were compared to those of 97 women who sought rhytidectomy and/or blepharoplasty (25). Patients completed two standardized self-report measures of body image: the Multidimensional Body-Self Relations Questionnaire (MBSRQ) (26–27) and the Body Dysmorphic Disorder Examination, Self-Report (BDDE-SR) (28). Rhinoplasty patients reported greater dissatisfaction with their noses, as assessed by the BDDE-SR, compared to the degree of concern with facial appearance reported by the rhytidectomy and/or blepharoplasty patients.

Conclusions

It is difficult to reconcile the findings from the three generations of research, largely because of methodological differences. First generation studies, which relied heavily on psychodynamically oriented interviews, suggested that the majority of rhinoplasty patients were psychologically disturbed and that surgery may exacerbate psychopathology. Studies from the second generation of research incorporated standardized assessments of psychological symptoms. These studies mostly indicated that rhinoplasty patients were less psychopathological and that surgery could produce improvements in psychological symptoms.

Third generation studies, which have addressed some of the methodological weaknesses of earlier studies, found that most rhinoplasty patients are psychologically healthy individuals. The one investigation of body image in rhinoplasty patients provides preliminary evidence that these patients experience heightened body image dissatisfaction specifically focused on their noses. While earlier generations of studies suggested that the desire for rhinoplasty was a symptom of psychopathology, this study offers a more plausible explanation, namely that patients seek rhinoplasty as a means of improving specific body image dissatisfaction (2). These results are also more consistent with the clinical experiences of most present-day cosmetic surgeons.

ANTI-AGING PROCEDURES

Rhytidectomy and Blepharoplasty

Rhytidectomy and blepharoplasty are two of the most popular cosmetic surgical procedures for those interested in restoring or maintaining a youthful appearance. In 2004, 114,279 facelifts and 233,334 blepharoplasty procedures were performed in the United States (1). Because these procedures are often performed concurrently, studies of patients who seek these anti-aging procedures will be reviewed together.

Early reports suggested that facelift patients were highly psychopathological. Patients were frequently characterized as dependent and depressed (29). For example, one study reported that nearly 70% of patients received a preoperative psychiatric diagnosis, most commonly neurotic depressive reactions or chronic personality disturbances (29). However, the majority of patients reported postoperative improvements in well-being and did not experience any postoperative "emotional disturbances" (29).

Like studies of rhinoplasty patients, studies of aging face patients that incorporated standardized self-report measures found lower rates of psychopathology. In one study, postoperative psychometric assessments revealed decreases in psychological symptoms such as depression (30). Another study assessed preoperative and postoperative quality of life and depression using standardized measures in a sample of 105 patients seeking a variety of cosmetic procedures, including rhytidectomy (24). These patients rated dissatisfaction with appearance and loss of self-confidence as the most important factors contributing to their current quality of life. Following surgery, they reported significant increases in appearance satisfaction and confidence. Overall, they did not report preoperative depression, with scores falling significantly below the population norms.

Recent studies examined the body image concerns of patients seeking anti-aging procedures. In an investigation of the preoperative body image concerns of 100 women seeking cosmetic surgery, nearly half (n = 46) sought facelift or blepharoplasty procedures (31). Patients reported higher levels of dissatisfaction for the feature for which they sought surgery, but they did not report increased dissatisfaction with overall body image (31). Postoperatively, patients reported decreases in body image dissatisfaction for the feature that was treated, but no changes in overall body image (32). Rhytidectomy and/or blepharoplasty patients have reported greater investment in appearance as well as greater satisfaction with overall body image as compared to women who sought rhinoplasty (25).

Dunofsky (33) investigated body image, narcissism, self-esteem, and anxiety among women who had facial cosmetic surgery. Women who underwent cosmetic surgery had significantly higher levels of narcissism and less body image dissatisfaction compared to a control group. No differences were found between groups on measures of self-esteem and anxiety. Because preoperative assessments were not obtained in this study, the significance of this finding is unclear.

In summary, recent studies of rhytidectomy and blepharoplasty patients indicate that these patients are not as psychopathological as earlier studies suggested. Body image studies indicate that patients seeking anti-aging procedures may place greater emphasis on their appearance and report less dissatisfaction with their overall body image as compared to patients who seek other procedures. However, these patients may seek surgery to decrease body image dissatisfaction specifically associated with aging facial features.

Minimally Invasive Anti-aging Procedures

In 2004, over 7 million minimally invasive procedures were performed in the United States (1). These treatments have surpassed the popularity of the more traditional anti-aging surgical procedures in part because they offer subtle appearance improvements without the associated cost and risks of surgery.

Nearly 2.3 million Botox® injections were performed in the United States in 2004, making this procedure the most popular of all cosmetic treatments (1). The toxin is typically injected into areas of the face (i.e., forehead creases, crow's feet) in order to reduce the appearance of wrinkling. It is also effective at treating excessive sweating. Other popular minimally invasive procedures include fat injections, collagen injections, chemical peels, dermabrasion, and laser resurfacing. Like Botox® injections, these procedures can improve the appearance of wrinkled, scarred, or sun-damaged skin. In 2004, the Food and Drug Administration approved a new product specifically designed to improve lipoatrophy in persons with HIV disease. In addition, new generations of customized facial implants are being used to treat this condition (34). It is quite possible that these products will also be used for cosmetic purposes in persons without HIV disease in the near future.

Despite their popularity, little is known about the psychological characteristics or body image concerns of the patients who seek these and other minimally invasive procedures. A German study of 30 patients who received Botox® injections for facial lines examined posttreatment social outcomes and attitudes toward appearance using two self-report measures (35). Nearly 50% of the sample reported greater confidence in their appearance, and over half reported increases in attractiveness (35).

Recently, a report described the phenomenon of "botulinophilia," a term used to describe a potential subtype of body dysmorphic disorder (BDD) characterized by persistent demands for Botox® injections to treat excessive sweating (hyperhidrosis), despite any clinical evidence of a physical problem (36). Thirteen patients requesting Botox® for assumed hyperhidrosis were evaluated for BDD with a semistructured interview utilizing DSM-IV criteria. Twenty-three percent met formal diagnostic criteria for BDD (36).

Few studies have investigated the psychological characteristics of patients who sought other minimally invasive facial procedures. A recent study of 178 patients seeking laser skin resurfacing reported that 18% received prior treatment for depression (37). Another study evaluated the psychosocial benefits associated with alpha hydroxy acid, a topical treatment that is used to reduce roughness and fine wrinkling. Patients noted significant improvements in appearance and relationship satisfaction following treatment (38). Given their popularity, studies of the psychological concerns of patients who seek these treatments are needed.

OTHER FACIAL PROCEDURES

Facial Skeletal Procedures

Requests for "atypical" facial cosmetic procedures have also been reported in the literature. These procedures involved bone contouring, bone grafting, or the insertion of cheek, chin, or other facial implants. Edgerton, Langmann, and Pruzinsky (39) described 15 patients who sought extensive symmetrical facial skeletal recontouring procedures in order to address discontent with facial width. These "facial width deformity" patients reported concerns with minor, largely unnoticeable anatomic deviations, such as their heads being too wide or too thin.

Preoperative psychiatric interviews revealed that the majority of these patients experienced significant impairment in psychosocial functioning. Only three patients received a formal psychiatric diagnosis. However, the clinical descriptions of these patients suggest that some may have been suffering from BDD. Postoperatively, patients reported improvements in body image and psychosocial functioning although psychometric measures were not utilized to assess these changes (39).

While requests for facial skeletal cosmetic procedures may be atypical, more patients are requesting procedures such as cheek and chin implants in order to change the structural appearance of their faces. In 2004, over 25,000 chin or cheek implantation procedures were performed (1). Comparatively, only 1,741 cheek implant and 4,115 chin augmentation procedures were performed in 1992 (4). The increase in popularity of these procedures underscores the need for more research regarding the psychological characteristics and body image concerns of patients who seek these procedures.

Acne Treatment

Patients with facial skin conditions have had a long-standing interest in improving their appearance. Many complain of active acne or acne-related scarring. This is not surprising, considering that acne affects at least 80% of adolescents (40). The prevalence of acne typically decreases with age; however, it may persist through adulthood, affecting at least 8% of adults aged 25 years to 34 years, and 3% of adults aged 35 years to 44 years (41).

In the past, the psychosocial effects of acne were often dismissed, largely because acne has long been considered a non-life-threatening, age-related, cosmetic condition (42). However, more health professionals now recognize the impact acne may have on the psychological and social well-being of its sufferers. Studies suggest that 30% to 50% of adolescents experience psychological difficulties associated with acne, including body image concerns, embarrassment, social impairment, anxiety, frustration, anger, depression, and poor self-esteem (43). Several studies evaluated the psychological characteristics of patients seeking treatment for acne. These studies indicate that depression, social anxiety, low self-esteem, and body image dissatisfaction commonly occur among these patients (42,44–46). Suicidal ideation and suicide attempts also have been documented (45,47).

Patients presenting with facial acne appear to be particularly vulnerable to the psychological effects of the disease. Compared to patients with truncal acne, facial acne patients reported lower self-esteem and greater body image dissatisfaction (46). At least one study (48) has pointed to a focused dissatisfaction with facial appearance (rather than overall appearance dissatisfaction), the magnitude of which is related to self-perceived (not objective) severity of the acne and, in turn, to the experience of social inhibition and distress. This is consistent with studies of cosmetic surgery patients, which have typically found increased dissatisfaction with the specific feature considered for surgery, rather than the more global body image (2,5).

Acne patients experience similar degrees of impairment in quality of life as compared to patients with other chronic medical conditions, including epilepsy and diabetes (49). As suggested above and consistent with theories of body image dissatisfaction, the patient's perception of acne severity (rather than the objective severity) appears to be closely related to the degree of psychosocial distress (50).

Acne treatment appears to result in improvements in psychosocial functioning (51–52). Kellett and Gawkrodger (44) reported significant reductions in anxiety and depression following treatment with isotretinoin. However, among measures of general emotional distress, they did not find a significant change from pretreatment to posttreatment. The authors conclude that some of the psychological effects of acne may remain despite successful treatment. This finding makes intuitive sense, given that acne can result in permanent scarring. Extended duration of acne and acne excoriee (skin picking) are associated with greater likelihood of scarring (53).

Facial acne may leave emotional scars, even if there are no residual cutaneous scars. Cash and Santos (54) studied 193 young adults with various histories of facial acne during adolescence, none of whom had current acne or scarring from previous acne. Former acne sufferers, especially women and those recalling more subjectively severe acne, reported less current facial satisfaction and more body image dysphoria, than peers who had not had facial acne as teenagers.

Available evidence suggests that some acne patients experience significant distress and impairment in quality of life that may last longer than the physical manifestations of this disorder. The psychosocial distress associated with acne has implications for providers who perform aesthetic treatments such as dermabrasion and laser treatment to improve the appearance of acne-related scars. These providers may be able to assess for the psychological effects of this disorder and provide appropriate mental health treatment referrals when appropriate.

Vitiligo

Vitiligo is a progressive condition characterized by loss of pigmentation in the skin, resulting in irregular hypopigmented patches on the skin's surface (55). Generalized vitiligo, the most common form, is characterized by bilateral, symmetric depigmentation of the face (particularly periorificial area), the neck, torso, wrists, and legs (56). Vitiligo can result in depigmentation across the entire body (56). The prevalence of this condition is estimated to be about 1% to 2% of the world population (57). Age of onset is typically childhood or young adulthood (56), a time when appearance plays a critical role in social development. Medical treatments include topical cosmetics, PUVA (a combination of psoralens and UVA light to stimulate repigmentation), corticosteroids, and surgical skin grafting (56). However, there is no cure for the disease (57).

As with acne, the psychological distress associated with vitiligo is often underestimated, namely because it is considered a cosmetic condition (55). Nevertheless, it appears to have a negative impact on the social and emotional well-being of its sufferers (58). A controlled study of cognitive-behavioral therapy (CBT) in a small sample of vitiligo patients found that, at baseline, patients reported difficulties with body image, self-esteem, and quality of life (55). Following treatment, those in the CBT group reported significant improvements in these areas compared to the control group (55). Although additional studies are needed, treatment providers should be aware of the potential for emotional distress in these patients.

Similar psychological sequelae have been reported among patients with other chronic skin conditions, including eczema and psoriasis (45,59–60). A thorough review of the psychological characteristics of patients who seek dermatological treatment is beyond the scope of this chapter. Interested readers are directed to those reviews and books on the topic (61–63).

Micropigmentation

Micropigmentation (also known as "permanent makeup" or "dermagraphics") is a permanent cosmetic procedure in which pigment is implanted into the epidermis in order to enhance or define features, including the eyebrows, eyelashes, and lips. No exact statistics are available on the number of procedures performed each year. Dissatisfaction with results is considered to be one of the most common complications, and unrealistic patient expectations and psychopathology are thought to increase the likelihood of treatment dissatisfaction (64). Patients with schizophrenia, depression or anxiety, personality disorders, and those desiring a "perfect self-image" may be poor candidates (65). However, these issues have yet to be empirically studied.

HAIR LOSS AND HAIR TRANSPLANTATION

The human face is crowned and sometimes framed by scalp and/or face hair. Hair is an adorning feature that possesses considerable cultural, social, and personal significance (66–67). It may be cut, colored, curled, and coiffed. Hair is a part of the body that is readily malleable by individuals as they construct their social identity or attempt to "look their best." Indeed, a walk down the hair-care products aisle of most supermarkets or drugstores (in Western societies) can be a form of exercise. So what happens when people begin to lose their hair?

Psychosocial Impact of Androgenetic Hair Loss

There are a number of hair-loss conditions. The most prevalent is *androgenetic alopecia* (AGA), or common genetically predisposed hair loss. The condition is mediated by androgenic metabolism (especially dihydrotestosterone) and progresses with age. It is visibly evident in the majority of men over their life span. AGA also occurs in a significant minority of women, although the pattern of alopecia is one of diffuse thinning rather than the more conspicuous receding frontal hairline and vertex balding that occurs among men.

In recent years, researchers have begun to investigate the psychosocial effects of AGA for both sexes. Collectively, the extant studies indicate that this can be a very distressing condition for both genders, albeit more troubling for women (68–69). The stress and distress associated with AGA among men is greater the earlier the onset of the hair loss, for younger men not involved in an intimate relationship, and for men who are more psychologically invested in their appearance (70–71). The impact on men is more on body image than other aspects of psychosocial adjustment, whereas the effects of AGA on women may be more extensive, including lower self-esteem (71). As with other appearance-altering conditions, the subjective severity of AGA is more related to its psychosocial impact than are objective or clinical indices of severity (68).

AGA Medical Treatment Outcomes

Most outcome data for AGA treatment comes from large-scale, controlled clinical trials of minoxidil and finasteride (68,72–73). The psychological outcome measures in these studies have largely focused on patients' perceptions of and satisfaction with resultant hair growth. The results generally support efficacy on these limited dimensions. There is a dearth of outcomes research using more psychologically sophisticated, scientific measures. One uncontrolled, "usual care" study of 144 men treated with topical minoxidil confirmed moderate hair growth and improvements on hair-specific quality of life measures (e.g., hair-loss distress and perceived social noticeability of the hair loss), but not on more global measures such as anxiety, depression, self-esteem, or social confidence (74). However, the research did observe better hair-specific and global outcomes among those men whose initial hair growth expectations were realistic, whereas men who expected extensive regrowth had less satisfying outcomes.

Hair Transplants

In recent years, there have been major advances in surgical methods of hair replacement, including micrografting and flap techniques, especially for men with AGA. Unlike the medical treatments, which do not produce substantial hair regrowth for most patients, hair transplantation is a more certain and permanent method of hair replacement in less time. According to the American Society for Aesthetic Plastic Surgery (ASAPS), 22,890 hair transplants were performed in the United States in 2004, with 85.2% of these performed on men (75). By contrast, the ASPS reported

48,925 hair transplants in 2004 (88% on men) (1). Perhaps due to the availability of prescription and other over-the-counter medical treatments for AGA, there has been a 62% decline in the number of transplants performed since 1997 (75). Surprisingly, there exists no systematic research on the psychosocial outcomes of hair transplantation. Given the clear adverse impact of AGA on body image, such research is certainly needed. Of course, relative to a medical treatment that might produce gradual regrowth, a hair transplant will produce visible changes that may be more immediately discernible to others. Perhaps some men are unwilling to exchange the self-consciousness from their hair loss for the self-consciousness from revelation that they have had a hair transplant. Needed are investigations of the psychological characteristics of persons who seek hair transplants and outcome studies to discern what changes and benefits result from these procedures.

PSYCHIATRIC DISORDERS AND FACIAL COSMETIC PROCEDURES

No large-scale studies on the rate of psychopathology among cosmetic surgery patients have been conducted to date. Thus, it is unknown if certain psychiatric disorders occur more frequently among patients who seek facial cosmetic procedures. One psychiatric disorder, body dysmorphic disorder (BDD), may be more common among cosmetic surgery patients and particularly among those who seek facial procedures. Another disorder of potential relevance to patients who seek facial cosmetic procedures is social anxiety disorder (social phobia).

Body Dysmorphic Disorder

BDD is defined by the *Diagnostic and Statistical Manual,* Fourth Edition, Text Revision (DSM-IV-TR) by the following three criteria: (i) a preoccupation with an imagined defect in appearance, or if a slight physical defect is present, the person's concern is exaggerated; (ii) the appearance preoccupation must result in significant emotional distress or impairment in functioning; and (iii) the preoccupation with appearance is not due to another mental disorder (76).

Reports of BDD date back to 1886, when Morselli (77) described it as "dysmorphophobia." Although not recognized as a distinct psychiatric disorder in the United States until the publication of *DSM-III-R* in 1987 (78), descriptions of BDD first appeared in the American dermatology and plastic surgery literatures much earlier. Reports in the dermatology literature described patients presenting with "dermatological nondisease" (79), whereas those in the plastic surgery literature detailed "minimal deformity" and "insatiable" patients (80–81). Similar to current clinical descriptions, these patients presented with excessive concerns about slight or nonexistent appearance flaws and reported dissatisfaction with their postoperative results (82).

Prevalence

BDD is estimated to occur in 1% to 2% of the general population (76). This rate has yet to be definitively confirmed with an epidemiological study, although two large studies of BDD in community samples reported prevalence rates of 0.7% (83–84). Rates of 2.5% to 5% have been reported in university samples (85–88). BDD, however, appears to be far more common among patients presenting for cosmetic treatments. In the United States, one study found that 7% of female cosmetic surgery patients met criteria for BDD (31). A recent study of patients seeking only facial cosmetic procedures found that 8% met diagnostic criteria (89).

Among international samples, rates of BDD among cosmetic surgery patients range from 9% to 53% (90–93). In most of these studies, the majority of patients sought facial cosmetic procedures (91–93). Methodological differences (e.g., the use of different measures to assess for BDD) and limitations (e.g., lack of control groups) are likely responsible for the wide range of rates of BDD reported in these studies.

Rates of 9% to 15% have been reported in patients seeking dermatological treatment, most commonly for acne (94–96). Among patients seeking reconstructive procedures, 7% to 16% report distress and appearance preoccupation consistent with BDD (89,97). Patients with BDD also request treatment from orthodontists, maxillofacial surgeons, and paraprofessionals (98–100). The rate of BDD in these and other medical settings has not been studied.

Clinical Features

Age of onset for BDD is typically late adolescence. The condition is thought to occur with equal frequency among men and women, and most clinical and demographic features appear to be similar between genders (101–102). Any body part can be a source of preoccupation, however, patients typically report concerns with the skin, face, nose, and hair (98,101). Women frequently report preoccupation with their hips, legs, breasts, and weight, while men report concerns about their height, genitals, hair, and body build (101–102). Preoccupation with more than one feature is common (98). The course of BDD tends to be chronic; symptom severity, areas of concern, and insight may vary over time (101,103).

Patients often experience intrusive thoughts about their "defects." Some may hold beliefs about perceived appearance flaws with delusional intensity. Others may recognize that their concerns are exaggerated (104–105). Patients with BDD often engage in compulsive behaviors, such as mirror checking, camouflaging, and reassurance seeking often as a means of decreasing their distress (106). Skin picking is common (107–108). Engaging in compulsive appearance-related behaviors for more than one hour per day is considered a diagnostic indicator of BDD (103,109–110).

BDD frequently results in significant emotional distress, impairment in social and occupational functioning, and decreased quality of life (110–111). In some instances, patients may become housebound (101). Self-harm and suicidal tendencies are also common. Veale (112) described several patients who attempted "do-it-yourself" cosmetic procedures. Studies suggest that up to 40% of BDD sufferers experience suicidal ideation (103). Rates of attempted suicide range from 17% to 33% (101,103,113). Case reports of completed and attempted suicides among dermatology patients suggest that many of these patients suffered from BDD (47,79).

Comorbidity

BDD typically co-occurs with other psychiatric disorders, most frequently with depression (114). Anxiety disorders, particularly obsessive–compulsive disorder and social phobia, as well as substance use, personality, and eating disorders also commonly co-occur with BDD (101,103,113–117). The high comorbidity rate associated with BDD and the reluctance of patients to reveal their concerns to providers often results in misdiagnosis (110,113).

Nonpsychiatric Treatment

Individuals with BDD often seek cosmetic and dermatological treatments as a means of decreasing their appearance concerns (98,101,112–113). In the largest study of the use of aesthetic treatments among BDD patients (n = 250), 76% sought and 66% received treatment, with dermatological procedures and cosmetic surgery being the most popular treatments (98). Although providers often refuse to treat BDD patients, patients may "doctor shop" until they find a physician who will perform the desired procedure (98,118).

Studies suggest that nonpsychiatric treatments are often ineffective. One study found that the majority (72%) of nonpsychiatric treatments received by patients with BDD resulted in either no change or a worsening in BDD symptoms (98). Another study found that 81% of BDD patients were dissatisfied with the results of cosmetic treatments (113). After surgery, some patients report no change in their symptoms, whereas others may develop new appearance preoccupations (98,101). Furthermore, patients with BDD may be more likely to threaten or enact legal action and/or violence against their surgeons (118–120). Because of these issues, the presence of BDD is often considered a contraindication for cosmetic procedures (121–123).

Pharmacological and Psychotherapeutic Treatment

Studies suggest that selective serotonin reuptake inhibitor (SSRI) antidepressant medications and cognitive-behavioral therapy are effective strategies for treating BDD (124–136). Treatment research, however, is still in its early stages. Future studies of the effectiveness of psychiatric and psychological treatments are needed (136–137).

Summary

A significant minority of facial cosmetic surgery patients may present with BDD. Persons with BDD seek cosmetic treatments to address their appearance-related distress, although such treatments appear to be largely ineffective. These studies underscore the need for treatment providers to be aware of the potential for BDD in their patients (see Chapter 16) and to provide appropriate mental health referrals when necessary (5,138).

Social Anxiety Disorder

Patients with facial appearance concerns frequently report self-consciousness and feelings of anxiety in social settings (32,89,97). For some persons, this anxiety may manifest itself in the form of social anxiety disorder. According to DSM-IV-TR (76), social anxiety disorder is characterized by an excessive or persistent fear of social situations that involves exposure to unfamiliar people or to possible scrutiny by others. Exposure to feared situations may result in significant anxiety. Social situations may be avoided or endured with distress. Additionally, the anxiety or avoidance must result in distress or impairment in functioning.

The presentation and prevalence of social anxiety among patients seeking facial cosmetic procedures has received little empirical attention. Two studies suggest that 8%–10% of cosmetic surgery patients meet criteria for anxiety disorders (92,139). However, no studies have specifically examined the rate of social anxiety disorder in cosmetic populations.

Diagnostically, it can be difficult to differentiate social anxiety disorder from more commonplace body image concerns. Both positive and negative thoughts and feelings about one's body are influenced by feedback received from others. An individual's beliefs, perceptions, and feelings about his or her appearance may influence his or her thoughts about how others view his or her appearance as well (140). Thus, negative attitudes toward one's body may, in fact, result in social anxiety, as the individual assumes that others will also dislike his or her appearance.

Social anxiety and severe body image concerns likely overlap. As noted above, social anxiety disorder is a common BDD comorbidity, and most patients with comorbid BDD and social phobia report that the onset of social phobia predated their BDD symptoms (103,114,141). It has been suggested that the core feature of social phobia, namely the negative evaluation of the self in relation to others, might predispose those with early onset social phobia to develop the distorted self-evaluations characteristic of BDD (141). These findings illustrate the need for research regarding the rates of social anxiety disorder among patients seeking cosmetic surgery. Patients presenting with significant social anxiety should also be evaluated for the presence of BDD.

CONCLUSIONS

Facial cosmetic procedures, particularly minimally invasive treatments, continue to increase in popularity. Studies suggest that patients seeking facial procedures experience a wide variety of psychological symptoms. Most investigations indicate that patients experience postoperative psychosocial benefits. However, the duration of these benefits is largely unknown. Early studies conceptualized the desire for aesthetic treatments as being indicative of psychopathology. Recent investigations suggest that body image may provide a more reasonable explanation as to why individuals seek to change their facial appearance.

Many of the studies reviewed in this chapter examined the psychological characteristics of women. Men are increasingly presenting for cosmetic treatments, particularly to address concerns such as hair loss. Empirical evaluations of gender differences in body image and other psychological characteristics among those who seek facial procedures are necessary. Future studies also should address the motivations of patients who seek facial procedures and the relationship of body image and preoperative psychopathology to treatment outcome. Needed are studies that incorporate appropriate control groups and standardized pre- and postoperative assessments (including structured clinical interviews and self-report measures). Particular attention should be paid to the duration of postoperative effects.

The findings of the available studies have implications for clinical practice. Although the majority of patients presenting for cosmetic surgery are likely to be psychologically appropriate for treatment, it is not uncommon for patients requesting facial procedures to experience psychosocial distress and impairment in quality of life, particularly those seeking treatments for chronic skin conditions. As discussed in Chapter 16, patients complaining of minimal facial flaws should be evaluated for BDD, given that persons with BDD seek cosmetic treatments with great frequency. Additionally, patients presenting with symptoms of social anxiety or depression should be assessed for BDD because of the comorbidity associated with this disorder. Treatment providers are in a unique position to identify patients experiencing distress and to provide appropriate referrals.

REFERENCES

1. *2005 Report of the 2004 National Clearinghouse of Plastic Surgery Statistics*. Arlington Heights, IL: American Society of Plastic Surgeons, 2005.
2. Sarwer DB, Crerand CE. Body image and cosmetic medical treatments. *Body Image: An International Journal of Research*. 2004;1:99–111.
3. Sarwer DB, Wadden TA, Pertschuk MJ, Whitaker LA. The psychology of cosmetic surgery: a review and reconceptualization. *Clin Psychol Rev* 1998;18:1–22.
4. *2005 Report of the 2004 National Clearinghouse of Plastic Surgery Statistics*. Arlington Heights, IL: American Society of Plastic Surgeons, 2005.
5. Sarwer DB, Magee L, Crerand CE. Cosmetic surgery and cosmetic medical treatments. In: Thompson JK, ed. *Handbook of Eating Disorders and Obesity*. Hoboken, NJ: John Wiley and Sons, 2004:718–737.
6. Linn L, Goldman IB. Psychiatric observations concerning rhinoplasty. *Psychosom Med* 1949;11:307–315.
7. Hill G, Silver AG. Psychodynamic and esthetic motivations for plastic surgery. *Psychosom Med* 1950; 12:345–352.
8. Meyer E, Jacobson WE, Edgerton MT, Canter A. Motivational patterns in patients seeking elective plastic surgery. *Psychosom Med* 1960;22(3):193–202.
9. Book HE. Sexual implications of the nose. *Compr Psychiatry* 1971;12(5):450–455.
10. Gifford S. Cosmetic surgery and personality change: a review and some clinical observations. In: Goldwyn RM, ed. *The Unfavorable Result in Plastic Surgery: Avoidance and Treatment*. Boston: Little, Brown and Company, 1973:11–33.

11. Jacobson WE, Meyer E, Edgerton MT, et al. Screening of rhinoplasty patients from the psychologic point of view. *Plast Reconstr Surg* 1961;28(3):279–281.
12. Hay GG. Psychiatric aspects of cosmetic nasal operations. *Br J Psychiatry* 1970;116:85–97.
13. Robin AA, Copas JB, Jack AB, et al. Reshaping the psyche: the concurrent improvement in appearance and mental state after rhinoplasty. *Br J Psychiatry* 1988;152:539–543.
14. Wright MR, Wright WK. A psychological study of patients undergoing cosmetic surgery. *Arch Otolaryngol* 1975;101:145–151.
15. Micheli-Pellegrini V, Manfrida GM. Rhinoplasty and its psychological implications: Applied psychology observations in aesthetic surgery. *Aesthetic Plast Surg* 1979;3:299–319.
16. Hay GG, Heather BB. Changes in psychometric test results following cosmetic nasal operations. *Br J Psychiatry* 1973;122:89–90.
17. Marcus P. Psychological aspects of cosmetic rhinoplasty. *Br J Plast Surg* 1984;37:313–318.
18. Ercolani M, Baldaro B, Rossi N, et al. Short-term outcome of rhinoplasty for medical or cosmetic indication. *J Psychosom Res* 1999;47(3):277–281.
19. Ercolani M, Baldaro B, Rossi N, Trombini G. Five year follow-up of cosmetic rhinoplasty. *J Psychosom Res* 1999;47(3):283–286.
20. Goin MK, Rees TD. A prospective study of patients' psychological reactions to rhinoplasty. *Ann Plast Surg* 1991;27:210–215.
21. Hern J, Hamann J, Tostevin P, et al. Assessing psychological morbidity in patients with nasal deformity using the CORE questionnaire. *Clin Otolaryngol* 2002;27:359–364.
22. Hern J, Rowe-Jones J, Hinton A. Nasal deformity and interpersonal problems. *Clin Otolaryngol* 2003; 28:121–124.
23. Borges-Dinis P, Dinis M, Gomes A. Psychosocial consequences of nasal aesthetic and functional surgery: a controlled prospective study in an ENT setting. *Rhinology* 1998:36:32–36.
24. Rankin M, Borah GL, Perry AW, Wey PD. Quality-of-life outcomes after cosmetic surgery. *Plast Reconstr Surg* 1998;102(6):2139–2145.
25. Sarwer DB, Whitaker LA, Wadden TA, Pertschuk MJ. Body image dissatisfaction in women seeking rhytidectomy or blepharoplasty. *Aesthetic Surgery Journal* 1997;17:230–234.
26. Brown TA, Cash TF, Mikulka PJ. Attitudinal body-image assessment: factor analysis of the Body-Self Relations Questionnaire. *J Pers Assess* 1990;55(1):135–144.
27. Cash TF. *Body image assessments*. Available at www.body-images.com. Accessed December 19, 2004.
28. Rosen JC, Reiter J. Development of the body dysmorphic disorder examination. *Behav Res Ther* 1996; 34(9):755–766.
29. Webb WL, Slaughter R, Meyer E, Edgerton M. Mechanisms of psychosocial adjustment in patients seeking "face-lift" operation. *Psychosom Med* 1965;27:183–192.
30. Goin MK, Burgoyne RW, Goin JM, Staples FR. A prospective psychological study of 50 female face-lift patients. *Plast Reconstr Surg* 1980;65:436–442.
31. Sarwer DB, Wadden TA, Pertschuk MJ, Whitaker LA. Body image dissatisfaction and body dysmorphic disorder in 100 cosmetic surgery patients. *Plast Reconstr Surg* 1998;101(6):1644–1649.
32. Sarwer DB, Wadden TA, Whitaker LA. An investigation of changes in body image following cosmetic surgery. *Plast Reconstr Surg* 2002;109:363–369.
33. Dunofsky M. Psychological characteristics of women who undergo single and multiple cosmetic surgeries. *Ann Plast Surg* 1997;39(3):223–228.
34. Binder WJ, Bloom DC. The use of custom-designed midfacial and submalar implants in the treatment of facial wasting syndrome. *Arch Facial Plast Surg* 2004;6:394–397.
35. Sommer B, Zschocke I, Bergfeld D, et al. Satisfaction of patients after treatment with botulinum toxin for dynamic facial lines. *Dermatol Surg* 2003;29:456–460.
36. Harth W, Linse R. Botulinophilia: contraindication for therapy with botulinum toxin. *Int J Clin Pharmacol Ther* 2001;39(10):460–463.
37. Koch RJ, Newman JP, Safer DL. Psychological predictors of patient satisfaction with laser skin resurfacing. *Arch Facial Plast Surg* 2003;5:445–446.
38. Fried RG, Cash TF. Cutaneous and psychosocial benefits of alpha hydroxyl acid use. *Percept Mot Skills* 1998; 86:137–138.
39. Edgerton MT, Langmann MW, Pruzinsky T. Patients seeking symmetrical recontouring for "perceived" deformities in the width of the face and skull. *Aesthetic Plast Surg* 1990;14:59–73.
40. Krowchuk DP. Managing acne in adolescents. *Pediatr Clin North Am* 2000;47:841–857.
41. White GM. Recent findings in the epidemiologic evidence, classification, and subtypes of acne vulgaris. *J Am Acad Dermatol* 1998;39:S34–37.
42. Koo J. The psychosocial impact of acne: patients' perceptions. *J Am Acad Dermatol* 1995;32:S26–30.
43. Baldwin HE. The interaction between acne vulgaris and the psyche. *Cutis* 2002;70:133–139.
44. Kellett SC, Gawkrodger DJ. The psychological and emotional impact of acne and the effect of treatment with isotretinoin. *Br J Dermatol* 1999;140:273–282.
45. Gupta MA, Gupta AK. Depression and suicidal ideation in dermatology patients with acne, alopecia areata, atopic dermatitis, and psoriasis. *Br J Dermatol* 1998;139:846–850.
46. Papadopoulos L, Walker C, Aitken D, Bor R. The relationship between body location and psychological morbidity in individuals with acne vulgaris. *Psychology, Health, and Medicine* 2000;5(4):431–438.
47. Cotterill JA, Cunliffe WJ. Suicide in dermatological patients. *Br J Dermatol* 1997;137:246–250.
48. Krowchuk DP, Stancin T, Keskinen R, et al. The psychosocial effects of acne in adolescents. *Pediatr Dermatol* 1991;8:332–338.
49. Mallon E, Newton JN, Klassen A, et al. The quality of life in acne: a comparison with general medical conditions using generic questionnaires. *Br J Dermatol* 1999; 140:672–676.
50. Mulder MMS, Sigurdsson V, van Zuuren EJ, et al. Psychosocial impact of acne vulgaris. *Dermatology* 2001;203:124–130.

51. Rubinow DR, Peck GL, Squillace KM, et al. Anxiety and depression in cystic acne patients after successful treatment with isotretinoin. *J Am Acad Dermatol* 1987;17:25–32.
52. MacDonald Hull S, Cunliffe WJ, Hughes BR. Treatment of the depressed and dysmorphic acne patient. *Clin Exp Dermatol* 1991;16:210–211.
53. Layton AM. Optimal management of acne to prevent scarring and psychological sequelae. *Am J Clin Dermatol* 2001;2:135–141.
54. Cash TF, Santos M. *Remembrance of things past: The vestigial psychological effects of adolescent acne in early adulthood.* Unpublished manuscript. Norfolk, VA: Old Dominion University, 2004.
55. Papadopoulos L, Bor R, Legg C. Coping with the disfiguring effects of vitiligo: a preliminary investigation into the effects of cognitive-behavioural therapy. *Br J Med Psychol* 1999;72:385–396.
56. Kovacs SO. Vitiligo. *J Am Acad Dermatol* 1998;38:647–666.
57. Hartmann A, Brocker EB, Becker JC. Hypopigmentary skin disorders: current treatment options and future directions. *Drugs* 2004;64:89–107.
58. Kent G, Al'Abadie M. Psychologic effects of vitiligo: a critical incident analysis. *J Am Acad Dermatol* 1996;35: 895–898.
59. Rapp SR, Feldman SR, Exum ML, et al. Psoriasis causes as much disability as other major medical diseases. *J Am Acad Derma* 1999;41:401–407.
60. Novartis. Eczema patients face a lifetime of isolation, bullying, discrimination, and under-performance at school and work (2004). www.novartis.com. International Study of Life with Atopic Eczema. Paper presented at the European Academy of Dermatology and Venereology; Florence, Italy.
61. Koo J, Lebwohl A. Psychodermatology: the mind and skin connection. *Am Fam Physician* 2001; 64:1873–1878.
62. Gupta MA, Gupta AK. Psychiatric and psychological comorbidity in patients with dermatological disorders: epidemiology and management. *Am J Clin Dermatol* 2003;4:833–842.
63. Grossbart TA, Sherman C. Skin deep: A mind/body program for healthy skin. Santa Fe, NM: Health Press, 1992.
64. Chiang JK, Barsky S, Bronson DM. Tretinoin in the removal of eyeliner tattoo. *J Am Acad Dermatol* 1999;40(1):999–1001.
65. Zwerling CS, Christensen FH, Goldstein NF. *Micropigmentation*. Thorofare, NJ: Slack, 1986.
66. Kligman AM, Freeman B. History of baldness: from magic to medicine. *Clin Dermatol* 1988;6(4):83–88.
67. Morris D. *Bodywatching: A Field Guide to the Human Species*. New York: Crown, 1985.
68. Cash TF. The psychosocial consequences of androgenetic alopecia: a review of the research literature. *Br J Dermatol* 1999;141:398–405.
69. Cash TF. The psychology of hair loss and its implications for patient care. *Clin Dermatol* 2001; 19(2):161–166.
70. Cash TF. Psychological effects of androgenetic alopecia among men. *J Am Acad Dermatol* 1992;26:926–931.
71. Cash TF, Price V, Savin R. The psychosocial effects of androgenetic alopecia on women: comparisons with balding men and female control subjects. *J Am Acad Dermatol* 1993;29:568–575.
72. Kaufman KD, Olsen EA, Whiting D, et al. Finasteride in the treatment of men with androgenetic alopecia. *J Am Acad Dermatol* 1998;39:578–589.
73. Pharmacia & Upjohn Co. Rogaine® Extra Strength for Men (5% Minoxidil Topical Solution) for non-prescription use. Data presented at FDA Non-prescription Drug Advisory Committee Meeting. July 16, 1997. Pharmacia & Upjohn, Kalamazoo, Mich.
74. McNulty P, Buesching DP, Patrick DL, Gagnon DD. Change in quality of life in a study of male minoxidil users. *Drug Inf J* 1993;27(3):871.
75. American Society for Aesthetic Plastic Surgery. *ASAPS 2004 Statistics on Cosmetic Surgery*. New York: ASAPS, 2005.
76. American Psychiatric Association. *Diagnostic and Statistical Manual of Mental Disorders*. 4th ed. Washington, DC: American Psychiatric Association Press, 2000.
77. Morselli E. Sulla dismorfofobia e sulla tafefobia. *Bolletinno della R Accademia di Genova* 1886;6:110–119.
78. American Psychiatric Association. *Diagnostic and Statistical Manual of Mental Disorders*. 3rd ed. Washington, DC: American Psychiatric Association Press, 1987.
79. Cotterill JA. Dermatological non-disease: A common and potentially fatal disturbance of cutaneous body image. *Br J Dermatol* 1981;104:611–619.
80. Edgerton MT, Jacobson WE, Meyer E. Surgical-psychiatric study of patients seeking plastic (cosmetic) surgery: ninety-eight consecutive patients with minimal deformity. *Br J Plast Surg* 1960;13: 136–145.
81. Knorr NJ, Edgerton MT, Hoopes JE. The "insatiable" cosmetic surgery patient. *Plast Reconstr Surg* 1967; 40(3):285–289.
82. Sarwer DB, Crerand CE, Gibbons LM. Body dysmorphic disorder and aesthetic surgery. In: Nahai F, ed. *The Art of Aesthetic Surgery: Principles and Techniques*. St. Louis: Quality Medical Publishing. In press.
83. Otto MW, Wilhelm S, Cohen LS, Harlow BL. Prevalence of body dysmorphic disorder in a community sample of women. *Am J Psychiatry* 2001;158:2061–2063.
84. Faravelli C, Salvatori S, Galassi F, Aiazzi L, Drei C, Cabras P. Epidemiology of somatoform disorders: a community survey in Florence. *Soc Psychiatry Psychiatr Epidemiol* 1997;32(1):24–29.
85. Bohne A, Keuthen NJ, Wilhelm S, et al. Prevalence of symptoms of body dysmorphic disorder and its correlates: a cross-cultural comparison. *Psychosomatics* 2002;43(6):486–490.
86. Bohne A, Wilhelm S, Keuthen NJ, Florin I, Baer L, Jenike MA. Prevalence of body dysmorphic disorder in a German college student sample. *Psychiatry Res* 2002;109(1):101–104.
87. Cansever A, Uzun O, Donmez E, Ozsahin A. The prevalence and clinical features of body dysmorphic disorder in college students: a study in a Turkish sample. *Compr Psychiatry* 2003;44(1):60–64.
88. Sarwer DB, Cash TF, Magee L, et al. Female college students and cosmetic surgery: an investigation of experiences, attitudes, and body image. *Plast Reconstr Surg* 2005; 115(3):931–938.

89. Crerand CE, Sarwer DB, Magee L, et al. Rate of body dysmorphic disorder among patients seeking facial plastic surgery. *Psychiatric Annals* 2004;34(12):958–965.
90. Aouizerate B, Pujol H, Grabot D, et al. Body dysmorphic disorder in a sample of cosmetic surgery applicants. *Eur Psychiatry* 2003;18(7):365–368.
91. Vindigni V, Pavan C, Semenzin M, et al. The importance of recognizing body dysmorphic disorder in cosmetic surgery patients: do our patients need a preoperative psychiatric evaluation? *Eur J Plast Surg* 2002;25:305–308.
92. Ishigooka J, Iwao M, Suzuki M, et al. Demographic features of patients seeking cosmetic surgery. *Psychiatry Clin Neurosci* 1998;52:283–287.
93. Vargel S, Ulusahin A. Psychopathology and body image in cosmetic surgery patients. *Aesthetic Plast Surg* 2001;25(6):474–478.
94. Phillips KA, Dufresne RG, Wilkel C, Vittorio CC. Rate of body dysmorphic disorder in dermatology patients. *J Am Acad Dermatol* 2000;42:436–441.
95. Dufresne RG, Phillips KA, Vittorio CC, Wilkel CS. A screening questionnaire for body dysmorphic disorder in a cosmetic dermatologic surgery practice. *Dermatol Surg* 2001;27:457–462.
96. Uzun O, Basoglu C, Akar A, et al. Body dysmorphic disorder in patients with acne. *Compr Psychiatry* 2003; 44(5):415–419.
97. Sarwer DB, Whitaker LA, Pertschuk MJ, Wadden TA. Body image concerns of reconstructive surgery patients: an under-recognized problem. *Ann Plast Surg* 1998; 40:404–407.
98. Phillips KA, Grant JE, Siniscalchi J, Albertini RS. Surgical and nonpsychiatric medical treatment of patients with body dysmorphic disorder. *Psychosomatics* 2001;42(6):504–510.
99. Cunningham SJ, Feinmann C. Psychological assessment of patients requesting orthognathic surgery and the relevance of body dysmorphic disorder. *Br J Orthod* 1998;25:293–298.
100. Cunningham SJ, Bryant CJ, Manisali M, Hunt NP, Feinmann C. Dysmorphophobia: recent developments of interest to the maxillofacial surgeon. *Br J Oral Maxillofac Surg* 1996;34:368–374.
101. Phillips KA, Diaz S. Gender differences in body dysmorphic disorder. *J Nerv Ment Dis* 1997;185(9):570–577.
102. Perugi G, Akiskal HS, Giannotti D, et al. Gender-related differences in body dysmorphic disorder (dysmorphophobia). *J Nerv Ment Dis* 1997;185(9):578–582.
103. Phillips KA, McElroy SL, Keck PE, et al. Body dysmorphic disorder: 30 cases of imagined ugliness. *Am J Psychiatry* 1993;150(2):302–308.
104. Phillips KA, McElroy SL. Insight, overvalued ideation, and delusional thinking in body dysmorphic disorder: theoretical and treatment implications. *J Nerv Ment Dis* 1993;181(11):699–702.
105. Phillips KA, McElroy SL, Keck PE, Hudson JI, Pope HG Jr. A comparison of delusional and non-delusional body dysmorphic disorder in 100 cases. *Psychopharmacol Bull* 1994;30(2):179–186.
106. Phillips KA, Castle DJ. Body dysmorphic disorder. In: Castle DJ, Phillips KA, eds. *Disorders of Body Image.* Hampshire, England: Wrighton Biomedical Publishing, 2002:101–120.
107. Phillips KA, Taub SL. Skin picking as a symptom of body dysmorphic disorder. *Psychopharmacol Bull* 1995;31:279–288.
108. Koblenzer CS. Psychodermatology of women. *Clin Dermatol* 1997;15:127–141.
109. Rosen JC, Reiter J, Orosan P. Cognitive-behavioral body image therapy for body dysmorphic disorder. *J Consult Clin Psychol* 1995;63(2):263–269.
110. Phillips KA. *The Broken Mirror.* New York: Oxford University Press, 1996.
111. Phillips KA. Quality of life for patients with body dysmorphic disorder. *J Nerv Ment Dis* 2000; 188(9):170–175.
112. Veale D. Outcome of cosmetic surgery and "DIY" surgery in patients with body dysmorphic disorder. *Psychiatr Bull R Coll Psychiatr* 2000;24:218.
113. Veale D, Boocock A, Gournay K, et al. Body dysmorphic disorder: a survey of fifty cases. *Br J Psychiatry* 1996;169:196–201.
114. Gunstad J, Phillips KA. Axis I comorbidity in body dysmorphic disorder. *Compr Psychiatry* 2003; 44(4):270–276.
115. Hollander E, Cohen L, Simeon D. Body dysmorphic disorder. *Psychiatr Ann* 1993;23(7):359–364.
116. Neziroglu FA, McKay D, Todaro J, Yaryura-Tobias JA. Effect of cognitive behavior therapy on persons with body dysmorphic disorder and comorbid Axis II diagnoses. *Behav Ther* 1996;27:67–77.
117. Phillips KA, McElroy SL. Personality disorders and traits in patients with body dysmorphic disorder. *Compr Psychiatry* 2000;41(4):229–236.
118. Sarwer DB. Awareness and identification of body dysmorphic disorder by aesthetic surgeons: results of a survey of American Society for Aesthetic Plastic Surgery members. *Aesthetic Surgery Journal* 2002; 22:531–535.
119. Leonardo J. New York's highest court dismisses BDD case. *Plastic Surgery News* 2001 July:1–9.
120. Yazel L. The serial-surgery murder. *Glamour* May 1999:108–114.
121. Sarwer DB, Didie ER. Body image in cosmetic surgical and dermatological practice. In: Castle DJ, Phillips KA, eds. *Disorders of Body Image.* Hampshire, England: Wrighton Biomedical Publishing, 2002:37–53.
122. Sarwer DB, Pertschuk MJ. Cosmetic Surgery. In: Kornstein SG, Clayton AH, eds. *Textbook of Women's Mental Health.* New York: Guilford, 2002:481–496.
123. Sarwer DB. Psychological considerations in cosmetic surgery. In: Goldwyn RM, Cohen MN, eds. *The Unfavorable Result in Plastic Surgery.* Philadelphia: Lippincott Williams & Wilkins, 2001:14–23.
124. Hollander E, Allen A, Kwon J, et al. Clomipramine vs. Desipramine crossover trial in body dysmorphic disorder. *Arch Gen Psychiatry* 1999;56:1033–1039.
125. Hollander E, Liebowitz M, Winchel R, et al. Treatment of body-dysmorphic disorder with serotonin reuptake blockers. *Am J Psychiatry* 1989;146(6):768–770.
126. Perugi G, Giannotti D, Di Vaio S, Frare F, Di Vaio S, Cassano GB. Fluvoxamine in the treatment of the body dysmorphic disorder (dysmorphophobia). *Int Clin Psychopharmacol* 1996;11:247–254.
127. Phillips KA. Body dysmorphic disorder: clinical aspects and treatment strategies. *Bull Menninger Clin* 1998;62(4 Suppl 1):A33–A48.

128. Phillips KA, Dwight MM, McElroy SL. Efficacy and safety of fluvoxamine in body dysmorphic disorder. *J Clin Psychiatry* 1998;59(4):165–171.
129. Phillips KA, Albertini RS, Siniscalchi JM, etal. Effectiveness of pharmacotherapy for body dysmorphic disorder: a chart review study. *J Clin Psychiatry* 2001;62:721–727.
130. Phillips KA, Albertini RS, Rasmussen SA. A randomized placebo-controlled trial of fluoxetine in body dysmorphic disorder. *Arch Gen Psychiatry* 2002;59:381–388.
131. Phillips KA, Najjar F. An open-label study of citalopram in body dysmorphic disorder. *J Clin Psychiatry* 2003;64(6):715–720.
132. Looper KJ, Kirmayer LJ. Behavioral medicine approaches to somatoform disorders. *J Consult Clin Psychol* 2002;70(3):810–827.
133. Neziroglu FA, Yaryura-Tobias JA. Exposure, response prevention, and cognitive therapy in the treatment of body dysmorphic disorder. *Behav Ther* 1993;24:431–438.
134. Veale D, Gournay K, Dryden W, et al. Body dysmorphic disorder: a cognitive behavioural model and pilot randomised controlled trial. *Behav Res Ther* 1996;34(9):717–729.
135. Wilhelm S, Otto MW, Lohr B, Deckersbach T. Cognitive behavior group therapy for body dysmorphic disorder: a case series. *Behav Res Ther* 1999;37:71–75.
136. Sarwer DB, Gibbons LM, Crerand CE. Cognitive behavioral treatment of body dysmorphic disorder. *Psychiatric Annals* 2004;34(12):934–941.
137. Neziroglu FA, Khemlani-Patel S. A review of cognitive and behavioral treatment for body dysmorphic disorder. *CNS Spectr* 2002;7:464–471.
138. Sarwer DB, Crerand CE, Didie ER. Body dysmorphic disorder in cosmetic surgery patients. *Facial Plast Surg* 2003;19(1):113–122.
139. Napoleon A. The presentation of personalities in plastic surgery. *Ann Plast Surg* 1993;31(3):193–208.
140. Cash TF, Fleming EC. The impact of body image experiences: development of the Body Image Quality of Life Inventory. *Int J Eat Disord* 2002;31(4):455–460.
141. Wilhelm S, Otto MW, Zucker BG, Pollack MH. Prevalence of body dysmorphic disorder in patients with anxiety disorders. *J Anxiety Disord* 1997;11(5):499–502.

Chapter 15

Cosmetic Surgery of the Body

David B. Sarwer, PhD, Elizabeth R. Didie, PhD, and Lauren M. Gibbons, BA

This chapter reviews the research that has examined the psychological characteristics of patients before, and after, undergoing cosmetic procedures of the body. The greater part of this work has focused on the preoperative and postoperative characteristics of women who have undergone cosmetic breast augmentation. As a result, the majority of the chapter will address these issues. Given the relatively high rates of complications associated with breast augmentation, it is surprising that few studies have investigated the relationship between postoperative complications and psychological outcomes. We also will discuss the thought-provoking results from several epidemiological studies that have found a relationship between cosmetic breast implants and suicide.

Body contouring procedures such as lipoplasty and abdominoplasty have long been popular; however, the psychological aspects of these procedures have received little attention. Less common procedures, such as body contouring implants, as well as cosmetic genital procedures, also have received little empirical study. Intuitively, individuals who seek these procedures may display psychological characteristics that are different from those of individuals who seek the more common procedures. The chapter will conclude with a discussion of eating disorders and muscle dysmorphia (thought to be a subtype of body dysmorphic disorder). These syndromes may be both the most common and relevant psychiatric disorders among individuals who pursue cosmetic procedures for the body.

COSMETIC BREAST AUGMENTATION

The American Society of Plastic Surgeons reported that 264,041 women underwent cosmetic breast augmentation surgery in 2004 (1). This represents an increase of almost 600% in the past decade. These numbers do not capture procedures being performed by the increasing number of non-plastic surgeon physicians who offer breast augmentation. Thus, while the numbers are substantial, they likely underestimate the number of augmentation procedures performed annually.

The dramatic increase in the popularity of cosmetic breast augmentation is somewhat remarkable considering that in 1992 the Food and Drug Administration issued a moratorium on the use of silicone–gel filled implants. Then FDA Commissioner David Kessler called for further study of the physical safety and psychological benefits of breast implants. Several studies and literature reviews since have suggested that silicone breast implants are not associated with specific diseases, including cancer and connective tissue disease (2–6). Yet, in 2003, following an application from a breast implant manufacturer to return silicone–gel filled implants to the American

This chapter was supported, in part, by funding from National Institute of Diabetes and Digestive and Kidney Diseases (Grant #K23 DK60023-03) to Dr. Sarwer.

marketplace, the FDA upheld its previous decision, arguing that sufficient data on potential long-term complications were still lacking. Silicone–gel filled implants remain widely available in almost every other country throughout the world. Their fate in the United States, however, remains uncertain at the present time.

Over the last several decades, numerous studies have investigated the psychological characteristics of women who undergo cosmetic breast augmentation. Some studies have provided important descriptive information on the psychological characteristics of women interested in the procedure. Others have investigated the psychological changes typically experienced postoperatively.

Demographic and Descriptive Characteristics

The stereotypical breast augmentation patient is widely thought to be a single, European–American woman in her early 20s to mid-20s who is interested in breast augmentation surgery as a way to facilitate the development of a romantic relationship. Several studies, however, have suggested that the typical patient is quite different from this stereotype. She is most often European–American, but is frequently in her late 20s or early 30s and is married with children (7–17). While these characteristics may describe the "typical" patient, women from their late teens to mid-40s of varying ethnic backgrounds and relationship status present for breast augmentation surgery. Furthermore, the characteristics of these women likely vary based upon region of the country, characteristics of a surgeon's practice, as well as other variables.

Women who receive breast implants differ from other women on a variety of unique characteristics. Women with breast implants are more likely to have had more sexual partners, report a greater use of oral contraceptives, be young at their first pregnancy, and have a history of terminated pregnancies as compared to other women (18–21). They have been found to be more frequent users of alcohol and tobacco (19–21). They also have a higher divorce rate (16–17). Finally, they have been found to have a below average body weight (18–23), leading to concern that some of these women may be experiencing eating disorders (discussed in more detail below).

Motivations for Breast Augmentation

Several factors likely motivate women to undergo cosmetic breast augmentation (24). Intrapsychic factors describe the internal motivations for surgery and the resulting effects of surgery on psychological status. Interpersonal factors concern the importance of the appearance of the breasts in marital, sexual, and social relationships. With regard to these factors, women who seek breast augmentation report anticipating improved quality of life, body image, and self-esteem, as well as increased marital and sexual satisfaction postoperatively (11,16–17,22,25–29). Informational and medical factors also are thought to play a role in the decision to seek augmentation. Women who undergo breast augmentation obtain a great deal of information about breast implants from the mass media (22,30–31) and appear to be aware of many of the risks associated with implants (22,26,32).

Studies of Preoperative and Postoperative Psychological Status

Numerous studies have investigated the preoperative psychological status of women interested in breast augmentation. They were undertaken, in large part, to further understand the psychological characteristics of the typical patient, but also to potentially identify women who were psychologically inappropriate for surgery. As has been reviewed in greater detail elsewhere (24), the early generations of research in this area primarily relied on clinical interviews to assess preoperative and postoperative psychological functioning. Later studies have been more likely to use valid and reliable psychometric measures to assess relevant characteristics. The methodology employed has, more often than not, predicted the outcome of the investigation.

Clinical Interview Studies

Initial investigations of the psychological characteristics of breast augmentation patients relied heavily on unstructured clinical interviews of women prior to surgery. Appearance-related concerns were frequently interpreted as symbolic displacements of intrapsychic conflicts by psychiatrists who were trained in the psychoanalytic model of personality and psychopathology, the dominant theoretical orientation at that time. Not surprisingly, breast augmentation patients, as well as most cosmetic surgery candidates, were seen as highly psychopathological (15–17,33). Clinical interview investigations have described breast augmentation patients as experiencing increased symptoms of depression, anxiety, guilt, and low self-esteem (15–17,33). In one such investigation, 55% were described as being "in need of therapy" (17) and 70% in another study as "deviating from the normal picture" (15). The majority were reported to have personality disorders (34).

Interview-based reports tended to focus on the character structure of prospective breast augmentation patients. Relatively few examined the effects of breast augmentation on psychological functioning. The majority of these studies have reported improvements in self-esteem and depressive symptoms postoperatively (8,33) or at least no change from the preoperative status (15).

Psychometric Investigations

Studies that used standardized psychometric tests typically have found significantly less psychopathology than the interview-based investigations. Two studies of breast augmentation patients that used psychometric measures, including the Minnesota Multiphasic Personality Inventory, found little evidence of psychopathology (10,13). In contrast, only one investigation found greater symptoms of depression in breast augmentation patients as compared to controls (11). Investigations that used other standardized measures also found few differences in personality characteristics as compared to controls (13).

Studies that have used psychometric measures to assess changes in psychological status following cosmetic surgery have typically reported improvements in a variety of domains. Few, however, have examined postoperative changes among breast augmentation patients. The two reports of breast augmentation patients that used psychometric measures found mixed results. One found a decrease in symptoms of depression from preoperative status (35); the other reported increased symptoms of depression in 30% of patients in the immediate postoperative period (36).

Summary

The results of the clinical interview and psychometric investigations are contradictory. Unfortunately, both sets of investigations have suffered from a variety of methodological limitations that makes drawing definitive conclusions from this research difficult, if not impossible. The clinical interviews were typically not standardized and did not include inter-rater reliability of the symptoms or diagnoses. Furthermore, the theoretical biases of the psychiatrist–interviewers may have influenced the degree of psychopathology reported. The psychometric investigations suggest far less psychopathology among breast augmentation patients; however, this research also suffers from methodological problems. Several failed to include preoperative assessments and reported only postoperative results, including those immediately after surgery, when women may not have yet achieved their final aesthetic result. Most psychometric investigations did not include appropriate control or comparison groups. Therefore, it is unclear if the frequency of psychological conditions found among surgical candidates represents increased psychopathology above and beyond that found in the general population.

Despite the methodological problems and contradictory findings, two tentative conclusions can be drawn (37–39). First, breast augmentation candidates likely present for surgery with a variety of psychological symptoms and conditions. Whether some of these conditions serve as contraindications for surgery has yet to be established. Second, although an increasing number of studies have demonstrated improvements in psychological functioning following cosmetic procedures, relatively few have specifically investigated this issue in breast augmentation patients. Therefore, it is likely premature to definitively conclude that cosmetic breast augmentation confers psychological benefits.

Studies of Body Image Dissatisfaction

Within the past decade, an increasing amount of attention has been paid to the relationship between body image and cosmetic surgery (38–41). Body image dissatisfaction has long been thought to motivate many appearance-enhancing behaviors, from weight loss and exercise to clothing and cosmetic purchases (42). A theoretical model has been proposed which suggests that body image dissatisfaction may be the primary motivational factor in the pursuit of cosmetic surgery (41). Several empirical studies have suggested that cosmetic surgery patients report increased body image dissatisfaction prior to surgery (22,40,43–46). Others have found improvements in body image postoperatively (26,47–51).

Several clinical reports over the past several decades have described the body image concerns of breast augmentation patients (10–11,13,28). Breast augmentation candidates typically report less dissatisfaction with their breasts compared to breast reduction patients (52). However, greater than 50% of breast augmentation patients reported significant behavioral avoidance, such as camouflaging their breasts or avoidance of being seen undressed, in response to negative feelings about their breasts.

Two more recent studies have compared breast augmentation candidates to small-breasted women not seeking breast augmentation. Women who sought breast augmentation, as compared to controls recruited from a university community, reported greater dissatisfaction with their breasts, as well as greater investment in their overall appearance and greater concern with their appearance in social situations (45). Augmentation candidates also rated their ideal breast size, as well as the breast size preferred by women, as significantly larger than did controls. Finally, prospective patients reported more frequent teasing about their physical appearance and more frequent use of psychotherapy than did controls. These later results suggest that some women interested in breast augmentation may be experiencing negative emotional consequences as a result of their breast dissatisfaction.

In the second study, breast augmentation candidates were compared to healthy women similar in age, body mass, and breast size recruited from a gynecology outpatient clinic (22). Women interested in breast augmentation again reported greater dissatisfaction with their breasts. As compared to controls, however, they did not report greater investment or dissatisfaction with their overall appearance. Women pursuing breast augmentation reported being motivated for surgery by their own feelings about their breasts, as also found in other studies (26). Romantic partners and sociocultural ideas of beauty played less of an influential role in the decision to seek surgery.

Women who undergo breast augmentation experience improvements in their body image postoperatively, as suggested by clinical reports (10,12,15) and empirical studies (26,48,50). In one of the largest studies of psychosocial outcomes following breast augmentation, greater than 90% of patients reported an improved body image 2 years postoperatively (26). The beneficial role of breast implants on body image may be best illustrated by women who have had their implants removed. These women report less subsequent satisfaction with their appearance, fewer positive appearance-related thoughts, and greater discrepancy between their ideal and current body size (53). Removal of breast implants without replacement, much like a loss of a breast to cancer without subsequent reconstruction, appears to a have a dramatic, adverse impact on women's body image.

Psychological Functioning and Postoperative Complications

Clinical reports suggest that the majority of women are satisfied with the outcome of breast augmentation surgery (12,35,54–55). For example, one prospective investigation (26) found surgery satisfaction rates to be 94%, 92%, and 91% at 6 months, 12 months, and 24 months, respectively, after surgery. As detailed above, an increasing number of studies suggest that women experience psychological improvements postoperatively (26,48,50). These benefits, however, may be tempered by the experience of a postoperative complication. Between 10% and 25% of women are reported to experience a surgical or implant-related complication (56–58). The most common complications are implant leakage or rupture/deflation, capsular contracture, discomfort or pain, breast asymmetry, scarring, loss of nipple sensation, and breast-feeding difficulties (2–6,56–60).

In two studies, approximately 10% of women who receive breast implants for cosmetic purposes experience a significant complication within 5 years of implantation (56–57). (For women who received implants for reconstructive purposes, the rate of complications was 34%.) In a study of 749 women who received breast implants in the United States before 1991 (before the FDA ban on silicone–gel filled implants), 23.8% of women experienced complications severe enough to require additional surgery (57). The most common complication was capsular contracture (73.6% of complications, 17.5% of women), followed by implant rupture (24.2% of complications, 5.7% of women), hematoma (24.2% of complications, 5.7% of women), and wound infection (10.7% of complications, 2.5% of women). Other large-scale studies in Europe have corroborated these findings (3–4,58–60).

The relationship between postoperative complications and patient satisfaction is unclear. At least three studies have suggested that the experience of a complication is negatively related to postoperative satisfaction (26,32,61). In contrast, while approximately 10–20% of women experienced complications serious enough to require additional surgery (e.g., deflation, rupture, capsular contracture, or asymmetry), less than 3% expressed dissatisfaction with their implants (62). Intuitively, women who experience a postoperative complication may be more likely to have a less positive psychological outcome. However, this issue has received little empirical attention. In a large prospective study, Cash et al. (26) found that while women typically report improvements in self-image and body image after breast augmentation, those who experienced postoperative complications reported less favorable changes in body image. At 6 months after surgery, women who experienced a "socially detectable" complication, such as significant capsular contracture, expressed less surgical and body image satisfaction compared to women with non-socially detectable or no complications. By 24 months after surgery, the groups did not differ in satisfaction, however, "socially detectable" complications viewed the risk–benefit ratio of surgery less favorably compared to those with less visible or no complications. Women who had their breast implants removed as a result of complications have reported a decrease in musculoskeletal symptoms and body pain, as well as an increase in general mental health and vitality (63). However, as noted above, these women frequently report a more negative body image (53). Additional research is needed to determine if the experience of postoperative complications tempers the psychological benefits of the procedure.

Breast Implants and Suicide

In the past few years, a new concern about breast implants has developed. At least four large epidemiological studies in the United States and Europe designed to investigate the relationship between breast implants and mortality found an unexpected relationship between breast implants and suicide (64–67). Across the four studies, the suicide rate (as obtained from patients' death records) was two to three times greater among patients with breast implants as compared to either patients who underwent other cosmetic surgical procedures or population estimates.

None of the studies identified a causal relationship between breast implants and suicide. However, the findings left the nature of the relationship open for speculation by both the scientific and lay communities. As there is no evidence that silicone alters neurotransmitter activity or other brain chemistry, it is unlikely that the implants specifically "caused" these women to commit suicide. The relationship is most likely explained by some unidentified psychological variable(s).

Some women may enter into the surgery with unrealistic expectations about the effect that breast augmentation will have on their lives. When these expectations are not met, they may become despondent, depressed, and potentially suicidal. Alternatively, women who experience postoperative complications, particularly those that are not found to be statistically associated with breast implants (such as autoimmune and connective tissue diseases), may become depressed as a result of a lack of perceived attention from the medical community. Although speculative, both of these hypotheses have some intuitive appeal.

Some women may have had preoperative personality characteristics that predisposed them to commit suicide. Many of these characteristics, such as increased alcohol consumption and higher divorce rates are, in and of themselves, associated with an increased risk of suicide. Joiner (68) has argued that these and other personality and demographic characteristics could actually account for an even higher suicide rate than found in the epidemiological investigations. He further suggests that postoperative improvements in body image may produce a protective effect from the otherwise increased risk. Jacobsen et al. found an increased prevalence of preoperative psychiatric hospitalizations in women who received breast implants as compared to women who underwent other forms of cosmetic surgery or breast reduction (65). These results suggest that the increased suicide rate among women who have breast implants likely reflects some underlying psychopathology rather than a direct relationship with the implants (69–70). Obviously, additional prospective epidemiological and psychological studies involving valid and reliable methodologies are needed to confirm the finding and further investigate this issue.

LIPOPLASTY AND ABDOMINOPLASTY

The United States is currently experiencing an obesity epidemic. Approximately two-thirds of American adults are now considered to be overweight or obese, as defined by a body mass index (BMI) of 25 kg/m^2 or greater (71). Obesity is associated with increased body image dissatisfaction (72) as well as several significant comorbidities, including coronary heart disease, hypertension, type II diabetes, osteoarthritis, and sleep apnea. Americans spend billions of dollars annually on diet and exercise programs in an effort to lose weight. Unfortunately, successful long-term weight control efforts are elusive for most individuals. Although designed for body contouring purposes, many individuals erroneously believe that lipoplasty (liposuction) and adominoplasty are weight control strategies that may serve as a permanent solution to weight problems.

Lipoplasty

Lipoplasty is traditionally one of the most common cosmetic surgical procedures. In 2004, 324,891 people elected to undergo lipoplasty in order to alter their appearance, making it the second most popular procedure for men and women in the United States (1). The areas of the body treated with lipoplasty frequently vary by gender.

Not surprisingly, women often request lipoplasty for the lateral thighs ("saddle bags") and hips, whereas men request the procedure for their "love handles."

As with most cosmetic procedures, patient selection is essential for optimal outcomes. The physically best patient has a normal or slightly elevated BMI with localized areas of fat that have been resistant to diet and exercise. While these features paint the picture of a patient's physicality, far less is known about the psychological characteristics of the typical liposuction patient. Unlike the sizable literature on the psychological characteristics of breast augmentation patients, few, if any, studies have specifically investigated the preoperative and postoperative psychological status of liposuction patients.

As with all forms of cosmetic surgery, patients' expectations of the postoperative result are critical to a successful outcome. A patient that expects to have dramatic changes in his or her body shape following liposuction may be immensely disappointed. Despite the popularity of the procedure, numerous misconceptions remain among the general public. Many patients erroneously believe that liposuction is only used to remove excess fat from the torso, when the procedure is frequently used throughout the body. More relevant to the issue of patient expectations, many patients mistakenly believe that liposuction leads to significant weight loss and, therefore, is a treatment for excess body weight. Surprisingly, the typical weight loss experienced following liposuction has not been well documented. One pilot study of 14 moderately overweight women (BMI = 27 kg/m^2) reported a mean weight loss of 5.1 kg by 6 weeks postoperatively, with an additional 1.3 kg weight loss by 4 months (73). Studies investigating changes in lipids and insulin sensitivity following liposuction have been equivocal (74–76). A recent study of 15 obese women who lost approximately 10 kg of fat mass following large volume liposuction found no significant improvements in obesity-related metabolic abnormalities, including insulin sensitivity as well as plasma glucose, insulin, and lipid concentrations (75).

Furthermore, many patients erroneously believe that fat deposits will *never* return to the treated areas. Fat can indeed return to some degree if the patient gains weight. While liposuction reduces the number of fat cells in a local area of the body, the remaining fat cells may still expand if body weight increases. Similarly, many patients likely believe that successful liposuction will result in "washboard abs" and smooth thighs. Unfortunately, if fat cells are not removed in a consistent fashion, some residual pockets of fat may remain. Most patients, however, maintain an improved and more proportional shape, even if they do gain some weight postoperatively. Given the common misconceptions regarding liposuction, an assessment of patients' knowledge of the procedure, their postoperative expectations, and informing patients of the need for appropriate weight control efforts following surgery is recommended. (See Chapters 16 and 19.)

Approximately three quarters of all liposuction patients report satisfaction with the postoperative result (77–78). Almost one-third of patients, however, complained that too little fat was removed (77). Between 40% to 50% reported weight gain after surgery and up to 29% claimed that their fat returned to the site of the surgery (77–78). Unfortunately, these studies provided no information on patients' preoperative and postoperative expectations or body weight. Given the popularity of the procedure, coupled with the increased empirical attention to psychosocial factors in other forms of cosmetic surgery, studies of these variables in lipoplasty patients are clearly warranted.

"Abdominal etching" is a subtype of lipoplasty specifically designed to enhance muscular definition. First designed in the early 1990s in order to enhance the abdominal appearance of body builders or athletes (79), the procedure can create the illusion of a "six-pack" of abdominal muscles by removing fat in certain areas and differing depths in the abdomen. The ideal candidate for this procedure is sufficiently muscular, with a low percentage of body fat. The number of individuals who undergo this procedure each year is unknown.

Individuals with excessive weight or shape concerns, or those with formal eating disorders, require particular attention prior to lipoplasty. Women and men with anorexia nervosa or bulimia nervosa, as discussed in detail below, may mistakenly seek lipoplasty as an inappropriate compensatory behavior to control their shape and weight. In a case report of two women with bulimia nervosa who underwent lipoplasty, the request for surgery was accompanied with an unrealistic expectation that surgery would result in an improvement of eating disorder symptoms (80). The women had 19% and 21% body fat preoperatively, which is considered normal for women of their age. Postoperatively, both women reported a worsening of their bulimic and depressive symptoms, and one woman reported a weight gain of 25 lbs in 3 months (80). Unfortunately, little else is known about the relationship between eating disorders and lipoplasty. As discussed in Chapter 16, prospective patients should routinely be asked about their history of weight fluctuations, dieting and purging behaviors, and amenorrhea (for women).

In summary, a sizable number of men and women undergo lipoplasty annually. However, little is known about the preoperative and postoperative psychosocial status of these individuals. Given the close relationship of body image dissatisfaction to body weight, many of these patients may experience significant body image dissatisfaction prior to surgery. Perhaps of greater concern is the occurrence of formal eating disorders within this population. The popularity of the procedure underscores the importance of additional empirical and clinical attention to these issues.

Abdominoplasty

The number of men and women who seek abdominoplasty, or a "tummy tuck," has increased steadily over the past decade. The American Society of Plastic Surgeons (ASPS) reported that its surgeon members performed 107,019 cosmetic abdominoplasties in 2004 (1). This represents a 71% increase in the past 4 years, making it one of the most rapidly growing surgical procedures.

One factor that may be contributing to the popularity is that increasing numbers of individuals with extreme obesity that are now undergoing bariatric surgery ("stomach stapling") for weight loss. Bariatric procedures typically result in a weight loss of approximately one-third of an individual's initial body weight. In addition, the procedure often results in significant improvements in obesity-related comorbidities and psychosocial status (81). Unfortunately, many patients are left with folds of skin and fat on the abdomen, arms, and thighs following the massive weight loss. This additional tissue may contribute to increased body image dissatisfaction (72) and, as a result, may lead patients to seek abdominoplasty and other related procedures. The ASPS reported that approximately 56,000 individuals underwent abdominoplasty and other body contouring procedures following the massive weight loss associated with bariatric surgery (1). Case reports suggest that these individuals experience improvements in body image, self-esteem and some of the physical discomfort associated with the excess skin (82). Formal studies, however, have yet to be undertaken.

To our knowledge, only one study has documented the psychosocial changes associated with abdominplasty. Bolton et al. (47) asked 30 women to complete measures of body image and quality of life preoperatively and postoperatively. Eight weeks after the surgery, women reported significant improvements in overall body image dissatisfaction, abdominal dissatisfaction, and self-conscious avoidance of body exposure during sexual activity. Patients did not report significant improvements in self-concept or general life satisfaction. These results are consistent with the other postoperative studies of cosmetic surgery patients, which found that the impact of cosmetic surgery procedures resulted in improvement in body image discontent, but not necessarily more general psychosocial functioning (50).

OTHER BODY ENHANCEMENT PROCEDURES

There are an almost limitless number of procedures that can be done to enhance the body. Many of these are relatively uncommon, but often receive a great deal of mass media attention. We will focus our discussion here on body contouring implants and genital enhancement procedures. In addition, we will briefly discuss tattoos and body piercing as a means of appearance enhancement.

Body Contouring Implants

In the past decade or so, cosmetic surgery has been somewhat redefined. Originally designed for reconstructive purposes, pectoral, calf, or gluteal implants are now used for cosmetic enhancement. Individuals can now augment their legs, arms, buttocks, and chests with silicone–gel filled implants personally tailored for size and shape. The number of individuals undergoing these procedures remains small. The American Society for Aesthetic Plastic Surgery (ASAPS) reported, for example, that only 2,141 buttock augmentations were performed in 2004 (83).

Although these procedures appear to be gaining in popularity, little is known about the psychological motivations and characteristics of those who seek them or the psychological changes that may occur postoperatively. Many of the features shaped by these implants are typically covered by clothing. As a result, the changes in appearance are not readily visible to most people seen by the patient each day. Thus, it is quite possible that some individuals who undergo these procedures may be suffering from body dysmorphic disorder (see Chapter 14) or its associated disorder, muscle dysmorphia (discussed below).

Genital Enhancement

An unknown number of men and women are dissatisfied with the appearance of their genitalia and some now pursue what has been called "genital enhancement" or "genital beautification" procedures. (From a surgical prospective, these procedures are similar to those undertaken for individuals undergoing sexual reassignment surgery discussed in Chapter 13. Little is known, however, about the psychological characteristics of people who undergo these procedures for purely cosmetic reasons.) Men may undergo a variety of procedures to lengthen or widen their genitals. Women may seek surgery to reduce the size of the labia minora. Although these "defects" are sometimes thought of as functional (impeding urination or adversely affecting sexual functioning), there is also a significant aesthetic component. Patients typically report that they are motivated for surgery out of embarrassment, either when undressed, such as in health club locker rooms or sexual situations, or when wearing tight clothing (84–85).

The number of these procedures performed each year is unknown. However, there are many Web sites and Internet advertisements, typically sponsored by surgeons, devoted to these procedures. Considering the nature of these procedures, it is possible that a significant percentage of these patients are suffering from body dysmorphic disorder or other psychiatric disorders with a delusional or psychotic component. For some, the concern about the appearance of the genitals becomes quite excessive. The plastic surgery literature includes several case reports of individuals who have performed "do-it-yourself" surgeries, such as injecting their genitals with various oils and substances (86–88).

Tattoos and Body Piercing

Once limited to soldiers and prison populations, tattoos are now routinely seen in mainstream culture. It is estimated that up to 20 million Americans have tattoos (89). A recent report found that 10% to 13% of adolescents (12 yrs to 18 yrs) and 3%

to 8% of the general population had tattoos (90). More than half of tattoos are found on women (91). Despite the increasing popularity of tattoos, requests for tattoo removal appear to be on the rise as well, perhaps because of the development of more effective laser removal tools (91). Similar to other cosmetic procedures, tattoo removal seems to be a consequence of a desire to improve one's self-image, and not a consequence of external motivations. In a study of 105 individuals seeking tattoo removal, 61% reported embarrassment as a consequence of their tattoo(s) and 26% reported a lower body image (91).

Accurate estimates of the number of Americans who have undergone body piercing are lacking. Body piercing is likely even more prevalent than tattoos, as piercings are less expensive and less difficult to obtain. Furthermore, body piercings are typically considered less permanent than tattoos, as holes in the skin can close after jewelry is removed. However, piercings can result in lifelong complications such as scarring and blood-borne infectious diseases (92), as well as more temporary complications such as abscesses (93). Mayers et al. found that 51% of 454 college students had at least one body piercing (including ear), and 17% of these individuals had experienced a medical complication (e.g., bleeding, local trauma, and bacterial infections) as a consequence of their piercing(s) (94). Tongue piercings may be particularly prone to infection and can result in swelling, chipped or fractured teeth, speech impediment, and/or nerve damage (95).

Carroll et al. (90) has argued that the presence of tattoos and/or body piercings in adolescents should be considered a marker for other risk-taking behaviors. In a sample of 484 adolescents, those with tattoos and/or body piercings were more likely to have engaged in risky behaviors such as drug use and sexual activity and be at increased risk for disordered eating and suicide (90). Furthermore, among college women and men, Crawford and Cash found that pierced and/or tattooed students scored higher on a measure of excitement seeking, were more likely to smoke cigarettes, and engage in binge drinking, relative to their "unmarked" peers (96). The pierced/tattooed students also reported more body image dissatisfaction, despite being pleased with their "body art." Perhaps body dissatisfaction is an impetus to obtain body art to "improve" one's appearance.

PSYCHIATRIC DISORDERS AND COSMETIC SURGERY OF THE BODY

As with the cosmetic procedures of the face, it is likely that all of the major psychiatric diagnoses can be found within the population of individuals who seek cosmetic procedures of the body. Eating disorders and muscle dysmorphia, which is thought to be a subtype of body dysmorphic disorder (BDD), may be the most common conditions among these patients.

Eating Disorders

Overvalued ideas of shape and weight are hallmark features of anorexia nervosa and bulimia nervosa. The overemphasis on body image leads men and women with these disorders to engage in the restriction of food intake and/or to use inappropriate compensatory methods (e.g., purging, excessive exercise) to control weight gain or to alter the shape of their bodies. The formal diagnostic criteria for anorexia nervosa and bulimia nervosa are found in Tables 15-1 and 15-2, respectively.

The distinguishing feature of anorexia nervosa is a fanatical pursuit of thinness related to an overwhelming fear of becoming fat (97). Patients with bulimia nervosa are generally distinguished from those with anorexia on the basis of relatively normal weight and the presence of binge eating and purging (97). The normal weight of

▶ **TABLE 15-1   Anorexia Nervosa: DSM IV-TR Diagnostic Criteria**

(1) The refusal to maintain a body weight over a minimally normal weight for age and height (e.g., weight loss leading to maintenance of body weight less than 85% of that expected, or failure to make expected weight gain during period of growth, leading to body weight less than 85% of that expected)

(2) Intense fear of gaining weight or becoming fat, even though underweight

(3) Disturbance in the way that one's body weight or shape is experienced, undue influence of body weight or shape on self-evaluation, or denial of the seriousness of the current low body weight

(4) In postmenarchal females, amenorrhea (e.g., the absence of 3 consecutive menstrual cycles) is present

Specifying Type

Restricting type: During the current episode of anorexia nervosa, the person has not regularly engaged in binge-eating or purging behavior (i.e., self-induced vomiting or the misuse of laxatives, diuretics, or enemas)

Binge-Eating/Purging Type: During the current episode of anorexia nervosa, the person has regularly engaged in binge-eating or purging behavior (i.e., self-induced vomiting or the misuse of laxatives, diuretics, or enemas)

Reprinted with permission from the *Diagnostic and Statistical Manual of Mental Disorders-IV-TR.* Copyright 2000. American Psychiatric Association.

bulimic patients frequently makes them more difficult to identify than anorexic patients.

Given the disproportionate amount of concern that eating disorder patients place on their appearance, these disorders may be more frequent among those who seek cosmetic surgery. Eating disordered patients may erroneously believe that surgery will improve their immense dissatisfaction with their bodies and fragmented self-esteem.

Eating disorders may be a particular concern for women who are seeking breast augmentation surgery. As noted above, breast augmentation patients are frequently

▶ **TABLE 15-2 Bulimia Nervosa: DSM IV-TR Diagnostic Criteria**

(1) The presence of recurrent episodes of binge eating

Binge eating is characterized by the following:
   a. eating, in a discrete period of time (e.g., within any 2-hour period), an amount of food that is definitely larger than most people would eat during a similar period of time and under similar circumstances.
   b. a sense of lack of control over eating during the episode (e.g., a feeling that one cannot stop eating or control what or how much one is eating)

(2) The recurrent inappropriate compensatory behavior in order to prevent weight gain, such as self-induced vomiting; misuse of laxatives, diuretics, enemas, or other medications; fasting or excessive exercise

(3) The binge eating and inappropriate compensatory behaviors both occur, on average, at least twice a week for 3 months

(4) Self-evaluation is unduly influenced by body shape and weight

(5) The disturbance does not occur exclusively during episodes of anorexia nervosa

Specifying Type:

Purging Type: During the current episode of bulimia nervosa, the person has regularly engaged in self-induced vomiting or the misuse of laxatives, diuretics, or enemas

Nonpurging Type: During the current episode of bulimia nervosa, the person has used other inappropriate compensatory behaviors, such as fasting or excessive exercise, but has not regularly engaged in self-induced vomiting or the misuse of laxatives, diuretics, or enemas

Reprinted with permission from the *Diagnostic and Statistical Manual of Mental Disorders-IV-TR.* Copyright 2000. American Psychiatric Association.

below average weight (18–23) and report greater exercise compared to physically similar women not seeking breast augmentation (22). At present, however, there is limited information on the rate of eating disorders among breast augmentation patients.

The study of the relationship between eating disorders and other cosmetic procedures has been restricted to case reports. Women with both anorexia and bulimia have experienced an exacerbation of their eating disorder symptoms following breast augmentation, lipoplasty, rhinoplasty, and chin augmentation (80,98–99). Interestingly, a case report of five breast reduction patients (also see Chapter 12) with bulimia suggested that four of the five women experienced an improvement in their eating disorder symptoms and psychological distress postoperatively (100). Prior to surgery, several of these women reported weight gain in an effort to camouflage the size of their breasts by gaining excess weight. Others reported restrictive eating with the hopes that weight loss would reduce fat tissue in the breasts. Breast reduction appeared to address these concerns and, based on patient reports, the women did not feel compelled to engage in these maladaptive eating behaviors. Impressively, the improvement in eating disorders symptoms was maintained 10 years postoperatively (101).

Muscle Dysmorphia

As noted above, the rising popularity of body contouring implants and abdominal etching procedures to increase the appearance of muscularity may be suggestive of the psychiatric condition, muscle dysmorphia. Considered a form of BDD (see Chapter 14 for a detailed discussion of BDD among cosmetic surgery patients), muscle dysmorphia refers to a preoccupation with being insufficiently large and muscular (102). Patients with muscle dysmorphia tend to weight lift and diet in compulsive manner as well as engage in other checking and camouflaging behaviors (i.e., layering clothing to appear larger). Additionally, patients with this disorder may abuse anabolic steroids in order to compensate for their perceived lack of muscularity. Like those with BDD, individuals with muscle dysmorphia also typically experience significant social and occupational impairment, often because their exercise and eating regimens are so time consuming.

The prevalence of muscle dysmorphia in the general population is unknown. Estimates suggest that 5% of nonprofessional weight-lifters (recruited from community gyms) to 9% of individuals with BDD have muscle dymorphia (103). Although stereotypically considered a disorder of men, 85% of female body builders reported severe preoccupation with being muscular and lean to the point of impaired social or occupational functioning (102). On the other hand, Pickett, Lewis, and Cash found that competitive male bodybuilders had a better body image evaluation than did noncompetitive weightlifters and physically active controls (104). The bodybuilders also had better social self-esteem than controls, but also had higher levels of eating pathology.

Not surprisingly, muscle dysmorphia and eating disorders often occur together (102). Although a preoccupation with exercise and weight training is usually the primary concern, individuals with muscle dysmorphia often report secondary preoccupations with diet and eating habits (102). Thirteen percent of men and 47% of women with muscle dysmorphia described past histories of eating disorders (102). Other common comorbid conditions include substance abuse (e.g., anabolic steroids, amphetamines, ephedrine), and obsessive–compulsive disorder (102).

Studies have yet to investigate the relationship between muscle dysmorphia and cosmetic surgery. Preoccupation with appearance and a history of disordered eating should be investigated in all patients with extreme muscularity and among those who seek body contouring procedures (see Chapter 16).

CONCLUSIONS

This chapter reviewed the psychological factors associated with cosmetic procedures of the body. A great deal of attention has been directed toward understanding the psychological characteristics of patients who undergo these procedures. Given the methodological limitations of the early studies, firm conclusions are difficult to draw. In recent years, body image has taken more of a central focus in the study of these patients. Patients who seek these procedures typically report increased body image dissatisfaction prior to surgery and improvements in body image at least 2 years postoperatively. While encouraging, four epidemiological studies have recently identified a relationship between breast implants and suicide. Although the exact nature of that relationship is yet unclear, it reminds us of the powerfully strong interaction between the outward appearance and internal perceptions of the body experienced by many cosmetic surgery patients.

In the last several years, other cosmetic procedures of the body, such as body contouring implants and genital beautification, have increased in popularity. Unfortunately, there is scant information on the psychological aspects of these procedures. Given the body image concerns among patients who seek any of the wide range of body contouring procedures, there is some concern about the occurrence of eating disorders, such as anorexia and bulimia, as well as muscle dysmorphia. The increasing popularity of all of these procedures likely will lead to additional research on the psychological characteristics of the patients who seek them, as well as the psychological changes thought to occur postoperatively.

REFERENCES

1. *2005 Report of the 2004 National Clearinghouse of Plastic Surgery Statistics*. Arlington Heights, IL: American Society of Plastic Surgeons, 2005.
2. Bondurant S, Ernester VR, Herdman R. Committee for the Safety of Silicone Breast Implants, Division of Health Promotion and Disease Prevention. *Safety of Silicone Breast Implants*. Washington, DC: National Academy Press, 2000.
3. Holmich LR, Kjoller K, Fryzek JP, et al. Self-reported diseases and symptoms by rupture status among unselected Danish women with cosmetic silicone breast implants. *Plast Reconstr Surg* 2003;111:723–732.
4. Jensen B, Wittrup IH, Friss S, et al. Self-reported symptoms among Danish women following cosmetic breast implant surgery. *Clin Rheumatol* 2002;21:35–42.
5. Sanchez-Guerrero J, Colditz GA, Karlson EW, et al. Silicone breast implants and the risk of connective-tissue diseases and symptoms. *N Engl J Med* 1995;332:1666–1670.
6. Silverman BG, Brown SL, Bright RA, et al. Reported complications of silicone gel breast implants: an epidemiologic review. *Ann Intern Med* 1996;124(8):744–756.
7. Edgerton MT, McClary AR. Augmentation mammaplasty: psychiatric implications and surgical indications. *Plast Reconstr Surg* 1958;21:279.
8. Edgerton MT, Meyer E, Jacobson WE. Augmentation mammaplasty II: further surgical and psychiatric evaluation. *Plast Reconstr Surg* 1961;27:279.
9. Druss RG. Changes in body image following augmentation breast surgery. *Int J Psychoanal Psychother* 1973; 2:248.
10. Baker JL, Kolin IS, Bartlett ES. Psychosexual dynamics of patients undergoing mammary augmentation. *Plast Reconstr Surg* 1974;53:652.
11. Schlebusch L. Negative bodily experience and prevalence of depression in patients who request augmentation mammaplasty. *S Afr Med J* 1989;75:323.
12. Young VL, Nemecek JR, Nemecek DA. The efficacy of breast augmentation: breast size increase, patient satisfaction, and psychological effects. *Plast Reconstr Surg* 1994;94:958–969.
13. Shipley RH, O'Donnell JM, Bader KF. Personality characteristics of women seeking breast augmentation. *Plast Reconstr Surg* 1977;60:369.
14. Goin JM, Goin MK. *Changing the Body: Psychological Effects of Plastic Surgery*. Baltimore: Williams & Wilkins, 1981.
15. Sihm F, Jagd M, Pers M. Psychological assessment before and after augmentation mammaplasty. *Scand J Plast Surg* 1978;12:295.
16. Beale S, Lisper H, Palm B. A psychological study of patients seeking augmentation mammaplasty. *Br J Psychiatry* 1980;136:133–138.
17. Schlebusch L, Levin A. A psychological profile of women selected for augmentation mammaplasty. *S Afr Med J* 1983;64:481.
18. Brinton LA, Brown SL, Colton T, et al. Characteristics of a population of women with breast implants compared with women seeking other types of plastic surgery. *Plast Reconstr Surg* 2000;105:919–927.

19. Cook LS, Daling JR, Voigt LF, et al. Characteristics of women with and without breast augmentation. *JAMA* 1997;277:1612–1617.
20. Fryzek JP, Weiderpass E, Signorello LB, et al. Characteristics of women with cosmetic breast augmentation surgery compared with breast reduction surgery patients and women in the general population of Sweden. *Ann Plast Surg* 2000;45(4):349–356.
21. Kjoller K, Holmich LR, Fryzek JP, et al. Characteristics of women with cosmetic breast implants compared with women with other types of cosmetic surgery and population-based controls in Denmark. *Ann Plast Surg* 2003;50(1):6–12.
22. Didie ER, Sarwer DB. Factors that influence the decision to undergo cosmetic breast augmentation surgery. *J Womens Health* 2003;12:241–253.
23. Sarwer DB, LaRossa D, Bartlett S, et al. Body image concerns of breast augmentation patients. *Plast Reconstr Surg* 2003;112:83–90.
24. Sarwer DB, Nordmann JE, Herbert JD. Cosmetic breast augmentation surgery: a critical overview. *J Womens Health* 2000;9:843–856.
25. Birtchnell S, Whitfield P, Lacey JH. Motivational factors in women requesting augmentation and reduction mammaplasty. *J Psychosomatic Res* 1990;34:509–514.
26. Cash TF, Duel LA, Perkins LL. Women's psychosocial outcomes of breast augmentation with silicone gel-filled implants: a 2-year prospective study. *Plast Reconstr Surg* 2002;109(6):2112–2121.
27. Kaslow F, Becker H. Breast augmentation: psychological and plastic surgery considerations. *Psychotherapy* 1992;29:467–473.
28. Kilmann PR, Sattler JI, Taylor J. The impact of augmentation mammaplasty: a follow-up study. *Plast Reconstr Surg* 1987;80:374–378.
29. Meyer L, Ringberg A. Augmentation mammaplasty-psychiatric and psychosocial characteristics and outcome in a group Swedish women. *Scand J Plast Reconstr Surg* 1987;21:199–208.
30. Larson DL, Anderson RC, Maksud D, et al. What influences public perceptions of silicone breast implants? *Plast Reconstr Surg* 1994;94:318–325.
31. Palcheff-Wiemer M, Concannon MJ, Cohn VS, et al. The impact of the media on women with breast implants. *Plast Reconstr Surg* 1993;92:779–785.
32. Handel N, Wellisch D, Silverstein MJ, et al. Knowledge, concern and satisfaction among augmentation mammaplasty patients. *Ann Plast Surg* 1993;30:13–22.
33. Ohlsen L, Ponten B, Hambert G. Augmentation mammaplasty: a surgical and psychiatric evaluation of the results. *Ann Plast Surg* 1978;2:42–52.
34. Napoleleon A. The presentation of personalities in plastic surgery. *Ann Plast Surg* 1993;31:193–208.
35. Schlebusch L, Marht I. Long-term psychological sequelae of augmentation mammaplasty. *S Afr Med J* 1993;83:267–271.
36. Meyer L, Ringberg A. Augmentation mammaplasty—psychiatric and psychosocial characteristics and outcome in a group of Swedish women. *Scand J Plast Reconstr Surg* 1987;21:199.
37. Honigman R, Phillips KA, Castle DJ. A review of psychosocial outcomes for patients seeking cosmetic surgery. *Plast Reconstr Surg* 2004;113:1229–1237.
38. Sarwer DB, Crerand CE. Body image and cosmetic medical treatments. *Body Image: An International Journal of Research* 2004;1:99–111.
39. Sarwer DB, Gibbons LM, Crerand CE. Body disorder and aesthetic surgery. In: Nahai F, ed. *The Art of Aesthetic Surgery: Principles and Techniques.* St. Louis, MO: Quality Medical Publishing. In press.
40. Sarwer DB, Pertschuk MJ, Wadden TA, et al. Psychological investigations in cosmetic surgery: a look back and a look ahead. *Plast Reconstr Surg* 1998;101:1136–1142.
41. Sarwer DB, Wadden TA, Pertschuk MJ, et al. The psychology of cosmetic surgery: a review and reconceptualization. *Clin Psychol Rev* 1998;18:1–22.
42. Sarwer DB, Didie ER. Body image in cosmetic surgical and dermatological practice. In: Castle DJ, Phillips KA, eds. *Disorders of Body Image.* Petersfield, UK: Wrighton Biomedical Publishing Ltd., 2002:37–53.
43. Pertschuk MJ, Sarwer DB, Wadden TA, et al. Body image dissatisfaction in male cosmetic surgery patients. *Aesthetic Plast Surg* 1998;22:20–24.
44. Sarwer DB, Whitaker LA, Wadden TA, et al. Body image dissatisfaction in women seeking rhytidectomy or blepharoplasty. *Aesth Surg J* 1997;17:230–234.
45. Sarwer DB, LaRossa D, Bartlett SP, et al. Body image concerns of breast augmentation patients. *Plast Reconstr Surg* 2003;112:83–90.
46. Simis KJ, Verhulst FC, Koot HM. Body image, psychosocial functioning, and personality: how different are adolescents and young adults applying for plastic surgery? *J Child Psychol Psychiatry* 2001;42(5):669–678.
47. Bolton MA, Pruzinsky T, Cash TF, et al. Measuring outcomes in plastic surgery: body image and quality of life in abdominoplasty patients. *Plast Reconstr Surg* 2003;112:619–625.
48. Banbury J, Yetman R, Lucas A, et al. Prospective analysis of the outcome of subpectoral breast augmentation: sensory changes, muscle function, and body image. *Plast Reconstr Surg* 2004;113(2):701–707.
49. Dunofsky M. Psychological characteristics of women who undergo single and multiple cosmetic surgeries. *Ann Plast Surg* 1997;39(3):223–228.
50. Sarwer DB, Wadden TA, Whitaker LA. An investigation of changes in body image following cosmetic surgery. *Plast Reconstr Surg* 2002;109:363–369.
51. Simis KJ, Hovius SE, de Beaufort ID, et al. After plastic surgery: adolescent-reported appearance ratings and appearance-related burdens in patient and general population groups. *Plast Reconstr Surg* 2002;109(1):9–17.
52. Sarwer DB, Bartlett SP, Bucky LP, et al. Bigger is not always better: body image dissatisfaction in breast reduction and breast augmentation patients. *Plast Reconstr Surg* 1998;101(7):1956–1963.
53. Walden KJ, Thompson JK, Wells KE. Body image and psychological sequelae of silicone breast explantation: preliminary findings. *Plast Reconstr Surg* 1997;100(5):1299–1306.

54. Park AJ, Chetty U, Watson ACH. Patient satisfaction following insertion of silicone breast implants. *Br J Plast Surg* 1996;49:515–518.
55. Wells KE, Cruse CW, Baker JL, et al. The health status of women following cosmetic surgery. *Plast Reconstr Surg.* 1994;93:907–912.
56. Cunningham BL, Lokeh A, Gutowski KA. Saline-filled breast implant safety and efficacy: a multicenter retrospective review. *Plast Reconstr Surg* 2000;105(6):2143–2149.
57. Gabriel SE, Woods JE, O'Fallon WM, et al. Complications leading to surgery after breast implantation. *N Engl J Med* 1997;336(10):677–682.
58. Kjoller K, Holmich LR, Jacobsen PH, et al. Epidemiological investigation of local complications after cosmetic breast implant surgery in Denmark. *Ann Plast Surg* 2002;48(3):229–237.
59. Fryzek JP, Signorello LB, Hakelius L, et al. Self-reported symptoms among cosmetic breast implant and breast reduction surgery. *Plast Reconstr Surg* 2001;107:206–213.
60. Fryzek JP, Signorello LB, Hakelius L, et al. Local complications and subsequent symptom reporting among women with cosmetic breast implants. *Plast Reconstr Surg* 2001;107:214–221.
61. Fiala TG, Lee WPA, May JW. Augmentation mammoplasty: results of a patient survey. *Ann Plast Surg* 1993;30:503–509.
62. Strom SS, Baldwin BJ, Sigurdson AJ, et al. Cosmetic saline breast implants: a survey of satisfaction, breast-feeding experience, cancer screening and health. *Plast Reconstr Surg* 1997;100(6):1553–1557.
63. Rohrich RJ, Kenkel JM, Adams WP, et al. A prospective analysis of patients undergoing silicone breast implant explantation. *Plast Reconstr Surg* 2000;105(7):2529–2537.
64. Brinton LA, Lubin JH, Burich MC, et al. Mortality among augmentation mammoplasty patients. *Epidemiology* 2001;12(3):321–326.
65. Jacobsen PH, Holmich LR, McLaughlin JK, et al. Mortality and suicide among Danish women with cosmetic breast implants. *Arch Intern Med* 2004;164:2450–2455.
66. Koot VC, Peeters PH, Granath F, et al. Total and cause specific mortality among Swedish women with cosmetic breast implants: a prospective study. *BMJ* 2003;326(7388):527–528.
67. Pukkala E, Kulmala I, Hovi SL, et al. Causes of death among Finnish women with cosmetic breast implants, 1971–2001. *Ann Plast Surg* 2003;51(4):339–342.
68. Joiner TE. Does breast augmentation confer risk of or protection from suicide? *Aesthetic Surgery Journal* 2003;23:370–375.
69. McLaughlin JK, Lipworth L, Tarone RE. Suicide among women with cosmetic breast implants: a review of the epidemiologic evidence. *J Long Term Eff Med Implants* 2003;13(6):445–450.
70. Sarwer DB. Discussion of Causes of Death among Finnish Women with Cosmetic Breast Implants, 1971–2001. By E Pukkala et al. *Ann Plast Surg* 2003;51:343–344.
71. Hedley AA, Ogden CL, Johnson CL, et al. Prevalence of overweight and obesity among US children, adolescents and adults, 1999–2002. *JAMA.* 2004; 291:2847–2850.
72. Sarwer DB, Thompson JK, Cash TF. Obesity and body image in adulthood. *Psych Clin NA.* 2005;28:69–87.
73. Giese SY, Bulan EJ, Commons GW, et al. Improvements in cardiovascular risk profile with large-volume liposuction: a pilot study. *Plast Reconstr Surg* 2001;108(2):510–519
74. Baxter RA. Serum lipid changes following large-volume suction lipetomy. *Aesthetic Surg J* 1997;17:213–215.
75. Klein S, Fontana L, Young VL, et al. Absence of an effect of liposuction on insulin action and risk factors for coronary heart disease. *N Engl J Med* 2004;350:2549–2557.
76. Samdal F, Birkeland KI, Ose L, et al. Effect of large-volume liposuction on sex hormones and glucose- and lipid metabolism in females. *Aesthetic Plast Surg* 1995;19(2):131–135.
77. Dillerud E, Haheim LL. Long-term results of blunt suction lipectomy assessed by a patient questionnaire survey. *Plast Reconstr Surg* 1993;92:35.
78. Rohrich RJ, Broughton G, Horton B, et al. The key to long-term success in liposuction: a guide for plastic surgeons and patients. *Plast Reconst Surg* 2004;114:1945–1952.
79. Mentz HA, Gilliland MD, Patronella CK. Abdominal etching: differential liposuction to detail abdominal musculature. *Aesthetic Plast Surg* 1993;17:287–290.
80. Willard SG, McDermott BE, Woodhouse L, et al. Lipoplasty in the bulimic patient. *Plast Reconstr Surg* 1996;98:276–278.
81. Sarwer DB, Wadden TA, Fabricatore AN. Psychosocial and behavioral aspects of bariatric surgery. *Obes Res* 2005;13:639–648.
82. Rhomberg M, Pulzi P, Piza-Katzer H. Single-stage abdominoplasty and mastopexy after weight loss following gastric banding. *Obes Surg* 2003;13:418–423.
83. American Society for Aesthetic Plastic Surgeons. *The 2004 ASAPS Statistics.* New York: ASAPS, 2005.
84. Choi HY, Kim KT. A new method for aesthetic reduction of labia minora (the Deepithelialized Reduction Labioplasty). *Plast Reconstr Surg* 2000;105:419–422.
85. Perovic SV, Radojicic ZI, Djordjevic ML, et al. Enlargement and sculpturing of a small and deformed glands. *J Urol* 2003;170:1686–1690.
86. Behar TA, Anderson EE, Barwick WJ, et al. Sclerosing lipogranulomatosis: a case report of scrotal injection of automobile transmission fluid and literature review of subcutatneous injection of oils. *Plast Reconstr Surg* 1991;91:352–361.
87. Bhagat R, Holmes IH, Andrzjej K, et al. Self-injection with olive oil: a cause of lipoid pneumonia. *Chest* 1995;107:875–876.
88. Cohen JL, Kreoleian CM, Krull EA. Penile paraffinoma: self-injection with mineral oil. *J Am Acad Dermatol* 2001;45:S222–224.
89. Greif J, Hewitt W, Armstrong ML. Tattooing and body piercing: body art practices among college students. *Clin Nurs Res* 1999;8(4):368–385.
90. Carroll ST, Riffenburgh RH, Roberts TA, et al. Tattoos and body piercings as indicators of adolescent risk-taking behaviors. *Pediatrics* 2002;109:1021–1027.

91. Armstrong ML, Stuppy DJ, Gabriel DC, et al. Motivation for tattoo removal. *Arch Dermatol* 1996; 132(4):412–416.
92. Wright J. Modifying the body: piercing and tattoos. *Nurs Stand* 1995;10(11):27–30.
93. Tweeten SS, Rickman LS. Infectious complications of body piercing. *Clin Infect Dis* 1998; 26:735.
94. Mayers LB, Judelson DA, Moriarty BW, et al. Prevalence of body art (body piercing and tattooing) in university undergraduates and incidence of medical complications. *Mayo Clin Proc* 2002;77:29–34.
95. Farah CS, Harmon DM. Tongue piercing: case report and review of current practice. *Aust Dent J* 1998; 43(6):387–389.
96. Crawford Y, Cash TF. Tattooing and body piercing among college students: relationships with personality and body image. Unpublished manuscript. Norfolk, VA: Old Dominion University.
97. American Psychiatric Association. *Diagnostic and Statistical Manual of Mental Disorders.* 4th ed. Text Revision. Washington DC: American Psychiatric Association, 2000.
98. McIntosh VV, Britt E, Bulik CM. Cosmetic breast augmentation and eating disorders. *N Z Med* 1994; 107:151–152.
99. Yates A, Shisslak CM, Allender JR, et al. Plastic surgery and the bulimic patient. *Int J Eat Disord* 1988; 7:557–560.
100. Losee JE, Serletti JM, Kreipe RE, et al. Reduction mammaplasty in patients with bulimia nervosa. *Ann Plast Surg* 1997;39:443–446.
101. Losee JE, Jiang S, Long DE, et al. Macromastia as an etiologic factor in bulimia nervosa: 10-year follow-up after treatment with reduction mammoplasty. *Ann Plast Sur.* 2004;52:452–457.
102. Pope HG, Gruber AJ, Choi P, et al. Muscle dysmorphia: an underrecognized form of body dysmorphic disorder. *Psychosomatics* 1997;38:548–557.
103. Olivardia R. Mirror, mirror on the wall, who's the largest of them all? The features and phenomenology of muscle dysmorphia. *Harv Rev Psychiatry* 2001;9:254–259.
104. Pickett T, Lewis RA, Cash TF. Men, muscles, and body image: comparisons of competitive bodybuilders, weight trainers, and athletically active controls. *Br J Sport Med.* 2005;39:217–222.

Chapter 16

Psychological Assessment of Cosmetic Surgery Patients

David B. Sarwer, PhD

As discussed throughout this book, the psychological evaluation of patients who present for plastic surgery is a central part of the management and treatment of these individuals. This is particularly true for patients interested in elective cosmetic procedures. As these patients do not have an illness or injury, the goal of treatment is not simply a return to a previously "normal" appearance. Rather, the goal typically is an improvement in a physical appearance that is already within the range of "normal." As a result, the impact of these procedures falls in both the psychological and physical realms.

This chapter considers the psychological assessment of cosmetic surgery patients from two different perspectives. It begins by discussing the psychological evaluation of these individuals as conducted by the plastic surgeon or other medical specialist who performs cosmetic surgical and nonsurgical treatments. The goal of this assessment is not to have the medical professional play the role of the mental health professional. Rather, it is to provide information to assist the professional in evaluating the psychological functioning of patients and to provide guidance in determining when a referral to a qualified psychologist or psychiatrist may be appropriate or necessary. The second half of the chapter discusses the psychological evaluation of these patients as conducted by the mental health professional. This information is presented to provide mental health professionals with a template to appropriately assess these patients, as well as to illustrate to the referring medical professional the nature of these evaluations.

PSYCHOLOGICAL ASSESSMENT OF COSMETIC SURGERY PATIENTS BY THE PLASTIC SURGEON

The psychological assessment and screening of patients interested in cosmetic surgery is critical for at least two reasons (1–4). First, such screening can help determine if patients' preoperative motivations and postoperative expectations are realistic. Second, the screening is vital in identifying patients who have psychiatric conditions that may contraindicate treatment. A comprehensive assessment of prospective patients can help identify those, who at a minimum, may become a clinical management problem. In the worst case scenario, these may be the patients who threaten or follow through with threats of legal action or violence following surgery. Goldwyn and Gorney presented an interesting discussion of

This chapter was supported, in part, by funding from National Institute of Diabetes and Digestive and Kidney Diseases (Grant #K23 DK60023-03).

specific "patient types" and the implications of treating these individuals in Chapters 2 and 19, respectively.

All of the major psychiatric diagnoses can likely be found within the growing numbers of individuals who now seek cosmetic surgical and nonsurgical (or minimally invasive) treatments (3–6). Conditions such as untreated major depression, uncontrolled schizophrenia, and active substance abuse are relatively easy to identify and contraindicate treatment, just as they contraindicate many medical treatments. The relationship between less severe psychopathology, such as mild depression or anxiety, and postoperative outcomes is less clear. In the absence of definitive prospective studies of this relationship, patients who have these conditions should be evaluated on a case-by-case basis. As discussed in previous chapters, conditions such as post traumatic stress disorder and social phobia in reconstructive surgery patients, and body dysmorphic disorder and eating disorders in cosmetic patients, may be overrepresented among these patient populations. As a result, they warrant additional attention both pre- and postoperatively.

The preoperative psychological assessment of patients by the treating medical professional should be a central part of the initial consultation. The assessment should focus on several areas: motivations and expectations, appearance and body image concerns, and psychiatric status and history (1–4). Questionnaire 16-1 at the end of this chapter may be useful in assessing these areas. Patients' behavior in the office, as well as interactions with the professional staff, should be carefully monitored and used to help evaluate appropriateness for treatment. Providing referrals to mental health professionals when needed is an important, yet often overlooked, part of patient selection that is discussed below. In addition, the unique issues of male and adolescent patients are briefly discussed.

Motivations and Expectations

The patient's motivations for surgery should be evaluated during the initial consultation. Motivations have been categorized as internal (undergoing the surgery to improve one's self-esteem) or external (undergoing the surgery for some secondary gain, such as obtaining a promotion or starting a new romantic relationship) (7–9). To assess the nature of patients' motivations, it may be useful to start the initial consultation by asking why patients are interested in surgery at this time. This question may help determine if patients are interested in treatment for themselves and their own sense of self-esteem or if they are seeking treatment to please others. While a clear distinction between internal and external motivations is difficult, internally motivated patients are thought to be more likely to meet their goals for surgery (10). At least three studies have suggested that being motivated for surgery in order to please a romantic partner is associated with a poor postoperative outcome (11–13).

Postoperative expectations have been categorized as surgical, psychological, and social (14). Surgical expectations address the specific concerns about physical appearance, both pre- and postoperative, and are discussed in detail below. Psychological expectations include potential improvements in psychological functioning that may occur after surgery. Social expectations address the potential social benefits of cosmetic surgery.

Many people interested in cosmetic treatments believe that the procedures will make them more attractive to current or potential romantic partners. At least two studies have suggested that following cosmetic facial procedures, patients are considered to be more physically attractive by others (15–16). There is presently no empirical evidence, however, to suggest that patients' social relationships improve after surgery. Thus, prospective patients should be aware that an improvement in appearance likely will not result in a change in the social responses of others. In fact, negative postoperative reactions from romantic partners, parents, or close friends may undermine psychosocial outcomes. In their review of studies investigating psychological outcomes following cosmetic surgery, Honigman et al. (17) found three studies that suggested that unrealistic expectations are associated with poor postoperative outcomes (11–12,18). In contrast, patients who are internally motivated and who have realistic expectations may be the most likely to be satisfied with their postoperative result. Questionnaire 16-1 provides several suggestions to assess the motivations and postoperative expectations of prospective patients.

Physical Appearance and Body Image

Given the relationship between body image and cosmetic surgery (5,19–20), the assessment of patients' body image concerns is a critical part of the evaluation. While the surgeon may know that patients are interested in specific procedures based on information in patients' histories, it is useful to have patients articulate, in their own words, what they dislike about their appearance. Patients should be able to describe with little effort specific concerns that are visible. Previous studies have found no relationship between degree of physical deformity and degree of emotional distress in cosmetic surgery patients (10,21–22). Patients who are markedly distressed about slight defects that are not readily visible may be suffering from body dysmorphic disorder (BDD).

As discussed in Chapter 14, between 7% and 15% of patients who seek cosmetic surgery or related medical treatments are thought to suffer from BDD (23–29). The vast majority of persons with BDD reported experiencing no improvements in their symptoms following these treatments (30–31). Therefore, BDD is often considered a contraindication for cosmetic procedures (2–4,32). Psychopharmacologic and psychotherapeutic treatments are thought to be more effective interventions for these patients (33).

The degree of dissatisfaction also should be thoroughly assessed. While some body image dissatisfaction is typical among most patients, those who report extreme dissatisfaction may be suffering from BDD. Asking more specific questions about the extent of the dissatisfaction, as found in Questionnaire16-1, can indicate the degree of distress and impairment a person may be experiencing. Patients who state that they think about their appearance problem for long periods of time throughout the day, often at the expense of being able to think about other things, may be suffering from BDD. Some patients may unintentionally reveal the extent of their preoccupation by presenting the surgeon with numerous photographs of models or celebrities who have the feature(s) they desire. Others may take photographs of themselves and, either through crude pencil drawings or elaborate computer enhancements, attempt to depict the desired changes. Although these pictures may be instructive to the surgeon in specific circumstances, such behaviors only hint at the hours which patients likely have spent thinking about their appearance.

Patients also should be asked how their feelings about their appearance impact their daily functioning. These questions can indicate the degree of impairment patients may be experiencing. Those who report that their appearance concerns prevent them from maintaining employment or relationships, or concerns that prevent them from engaging in daily activities most people would do without a second thought, may have BDD. It is important to remember, however, that BDD symptoms fall on a continuum. Severe cases where individuals are unable to maintain employment or rarely leave their homes are relatively easy to recognize. In less severe forms of the disorder, individuals are able to work and maintain relationships, but their quality of life suffers dramatically. For example, they avoid various social situations or endure them with considerable self-consciousness, or they spend substantial time checking and re-checking their appearance in mirrors.

In addition, patients should be asked what types of things they have done previously to improve their appearance. Forty-five percent of cosmetic surgery patients report that they have undergone a previous cosmetic procedure (34). These numbers, however, likely do not account for other less invasive treatments and homemade remedies patients may have tried. Among persons with BDD, 76% of 250 adults sought and 66% obtained nonpsychiatric medical treatments including cosmetic surgery and dermatological treatments (30).

To assist further in the assessment of BDD, practitioners may wish to familiarize themselves with the Body Dysmorphic Disorder Questionnaire (35), provided in Questionnaire 16-2 at the end of this chapter. This brief self-report measure derived from DSM-IV diagnostic criteria, assesses appearance concerns and their impact on daily functioning. The measure is intended as a screening tool and not as a diagnostic instrument. A modified version of the BDDQ, the BDDQ-Dermatology Version also is available (25). In Chapter 4 in this volume, Cash presents another, more recent and detailed version of this questionnaire, the Body Image Disturbance Questionnaire (36). All of these measures may be useful in both clinical and research settings.

Cosmetic surgeons are clearly aware of the presence of individuals with BDD in their patient population. A survey of cosmetic surgeons suggested that they believed that 2% of patients seen for an initial cosmetic consultation suffered from BDD (37). Greater than 80% of surgeons indicated that they had observed some of the characteristic symptoms of the disorder in patients—excessive concern with a minor appearance flaw, excessive requests for surgery, and dissatisfaction with a previous surgery. The vast majority of surveyed surgeons (84%) reported that they had refused to operate on a patient suspect of having BDD; 64% had scheduled a second consultation; and 50% had referred patients for a mental health consultation. In addition, 84% of surgeons indicated that they had operated on a patient whom they believed was appropriate for surgery, only to realize after the operation that the patient may have had BDD. Of surgeons who had this experience, 82% reported that the patient had a poor outcome with regard to BDD symptoms. Forty-three percent indicated that the patient was more preoccupied with the defect than before surgery, and 39% reported that the patient was now preoccupied with a different physical feature. Despite surgeons' apparent awareness of the problems associated with treating patients with BDD, only 30% believed that it was always a contraindication to a cosmetic treatment.

Psychiatric History and Status

Another important step in determining the psychological appropriateness of patients is obtaining a psychiatric history. This information should be routinely collected as part of the medical history and physical exam, no differently than obtaining a general medical history. If this information is typically collected on a preprinted form completed by the patient before the consultation, these questions should be repeated during the initial face-to-face meeting with the patient. Some patients are reluctant to candidly report mental health histories, in part out of fear that previous or ongoing psychiatric treatment will preclude cosmetic treatment. A recent investigation found that 19% of cosmetic surgery patients reported a mental health history, which was significantly greater than 4% of noncosmetic plastic surgery patients (38). Furthermore, 18% of cosmetic surgery patients reported using a psychiatric medication (almost exclusively anti-depressant medications) at the time of their initial consultation, which also was significantly greater than 5% of noncosmetic surgery patients. Many of these patients likely received these medications from their primary care physician and not from a psychiatrist. Clinical experience, as well as investigations from other surgical populations (39), suggests that primary care professionals often prescribe sub-therapeutic dosages of these medications. In situations where patients are receiving these medications from nonpsychiatrists, and psychopathology is suspected, a consultation with a mental health professional is recommended (1–4,38). Questionnaire 16-1 provides a series of questions to help assess a patient's psychiatric treatment history.

In addition to BDD, mood and eating disorders may be overrepresented among patients who seek cosmetic surgery and related treatments (6,20). Patients' mood, affect, and overall presentation will provide important clues to the presence of a mood disorder. If one is suspected, neurovegetative symptoms, including sleep, appetite, and concentration, should be assessed. If patients endorse difficulties in any of these areas, they should be asked about the frequency of crying or irritability, social isolation, feelings of hopeless, and the presence of suicidal thoughts. As discussed in detail in the previous chapter, four epidemiological studies have found a relationship between cosmetic breast augmentation and suicide (40–43). The most recent of these studies also identified a higher rate of psychiatric hospitalizations among women who received breast implants as compared to those who underwent other plastic surgical procedures (41). Although the specific psychiatric diagnoses were not identified, McLaughlin et al. have argued that mental health consultations should be considered for women interested in breast augmentation and considered to be at high risk by the surgeon (44). Affirmative answers to several of the questions assessing the presence of depression in Questionnaire 16-1 should necessitate such consultations.

Eating disorders, as discussed in Chapter 15, may occur with greater frequency among women who seek procedures such as liposuction or breast augmentation. To help assess for the presence of an eating disorder, the height and weight of all patients should be obtained and used to calculate body mass index (the patient's weight [in kilograms] divided by their height [in meters] squared). Patients with a BMI <20 kg/m^2 should be asked about a history of recent weight fluctuations, ongoing dieting efforts, binge eating, and purging or other compensatory behaviors. Women also should be asked about amenorrhea (see Questionnaire 16-1).

Patients with a history of psychopathology and who are not currently engaged in psychiatric treatment may warrant a psychiatric consultation preoperatively to further assess their current status. Patients currently under psychiatric care should be asked if their mental health professional is aware of their interest in surgery. After securing the patients' written consent, the surgeons should contact these professionals to confirm that the proposed treatment is appropriate at this time. Patients who have not mentioned their interest in cosmetic surgery to their mental health provider, or refuse to allow the surgeon to contact that person, should be viewed with caution. While such secretiveness was once commonplace among cosmetic surgery patients, in the current environment of greater acceptance of cosmetic surgery, it may reflect a degree of paranoid thinking suggestive of psychopathology. These patients warrant a psychiatric consultation. Patients who are dissatisfied with their postoperative result have used their psychiatric history as part of their legal action against the surgeon, arguing that their psychiatric condition prevented them from fully understanding the procedure and its potential outcomes. These occurrences underscore the importance of assessing and documenting the psychiatric status of all patients undergoing cosmetic surgery. Chapter 19 provides a further discussion of this issue.

Observing Office Behavior

Patients' behavior during their office visits should be observed closely. A 30-minute to 45-minute consultation is a relatively brief period of time to learn about patients' psychiatric status. Patients typically are on their best behavior during their initial visit and will often expend a great deal of effort to present themselves to the surgeon as "appropriate" for surgery. They often will neglect to share vital information with the surgeon and his or her staff that might play an important role in evaluating their appropriateness for a procedure. Therefore, every bit of information obtained either during the consultation, or observed during interactions with the nursing or office staff, should be used in making a determination of appropriateness for surgery.

As Goldwyn noted in Chapter 2, nursing staff and office assistants often witness different aspects of patients' behavior during other interactions in the office. These individuals may gather valuable insight into patients' psychological functioning that may alert the surgeon to a potential problem. Patients who have difficulty following the office routine warrant further attention. Those who frequently cancel or change appointments, ask for appointments outside of office hours, or who do not wish to talk to anyone other than the surgeon should be reconsidered for surgery. Patients who raise concerns among the staff should, at a minimum, be seen for a second preoperative consultation. If concerns persist, these patients should be referred to a psychologist or psychiatrist for a consultation.

Mental Health Referrals

If the surgeon and/or staff have concerns about the psychological status of prospective patients, a referral to a psychologist or psychiatrist for an evaluation should be made. Given the relationship between body image dissatisfaction and cosmetic surgery (see Chapters 14 and 15), a psychologist or psychiatrist with interest or expertise in body image may be the ideal consultant. These mental health professionals often work with other forms of psychopathology with a body image component, such as eating disorders or BDD. Professionals who work in other areas of health psychology also may have some experience with body image issues. Regardless of the expertise of the consultant, it is important that the surgeon communicate to the consultant the specific nature of the referral question. A well-qualified mental health professional with a good understanding of the psychological aspects of cosmetic (as well as noncosmetic) surgery can be a valuable asset to a plastic surgeon's practice.

Patients will often react to mental health referrals with anger. Many will frequently refuse to accept the referral. Patients who refuse to see the consultant are probably not good candidates for treatment. In this current competitive environment, many patients will eventually find a physician who will treat them, thereby not receiving the mental health care they need. Hopefully, some patients will hear the concerns of the surgeon they initially consulted and realize that cosmetic treatment is not appropriate at this time. Therefore, it is important that the surgeon treat the referral to the psychologist or psychiatrist like any other referral to a medical professional. This frequently will help de-stigmatize the mental health professional to the patient and make the referral more acceptable to him or her.

It is important to communicate to the patient the reason for the consultation. It may be useful to say:

> Undergoing a cosmetic medical treatment is an important decision. You are considering making changes to your appearance that are more or less permanent. These treatments often lead to changes in how you feel about your appearance—some which may be positive and others that may be less positive. I think it is important that we both are 100% sure that this treatment is right for you at this time. Therefore, because I care about your well-being, I would like you to see a psychologist (psychiatrist) who often works with us to help us decide if this is the right time.

Such a statement underscores the importance of the consultation to the patient in a nonthreatening manner and hopefully prevents the patient from responding with anger or hostility.

Patients also may need to be referred to a mental health professional postoperatively. On occasion, patients are dissatisfied with what the surgeon considers to be a successful procedure. In other instances, patients are experiencing an exacerbation of psychopathology that was not detected preoperatively. (These same situations also may occur with patients who undergo reconstructive procedures.) Patients in both examples warrant further assessment and, often, psychotherapeutic care.

Either based on the information gathered during the initial consultation, or following a consultation with a mental health professional, physicians who offer cosmetic treatments may find themselves in the unusual position of wanting to say

"No" to patients who have requested treatment. Training in both the medical and mental health professions, both directly and indirectly, teaches the professional to help anyone and everyone who seeks treatment. Nevertheless, there will be patients who ask for the wrong kind of help. Some will ask for cosmetic surgery when a mental health treatment is more appropriate. Others may ask for a treatment outside of the professional's area of expertise. Still others may simply rub the professional the wrong way, making an appropriate professional relationship difficult. In these cases, the professional should remember that a cosmetic treatment is an *elective* treatment for both parties involved. Patients can elect to have them; professionals can elect to say no.

When the treating professional elects to say no to a proposed treatment, this should be done clearly and with sensitivity. The reasons for saying no should be clearly stated in person. The conversation should be thoroughly documented in the chart and followed by a letter to the patient. As discussed in Chapter 19, professionals who do not deal with these issues directly and avoid these patients can put themselves at greater risk for legal actions.

CASE EXAMPLE

The following case illustrates a patient who raised concerns with both the surgeon and his staff and was thought to be inappropriate for surgery.

Case 1: Louise

Louise is a 45-year-old European–American woman who presented to a plastic surgeon with concerns about some wrinkling of her perioral region. She is married, works as a high school teacher, and has two college-age children. She came to her initial appointment well dressed and well groomed. She indicated that the wrinkling around her mouth made a scar from a childhood bicycle accident more visible than it had been earlier in her life. The surgeon had little difficulty observing some modest wrinkling of the perioral region, but believed that the scar had healed well and was more or less invisible from conversational distance. The surgeon indicated that laser treatment might improve some of the wrinkling, but would likely have little effect on the scar and her overall appearance.

The day after the consultation, Louise phoned the surgeon and asked him to repeat his impression of her appearance and treatment recommendations to her once again. As customary to his practice, he sent Louise a letter detailing his impression and recommended course of treatment. Upon receiving the letter, Louise called the surgeon again and, in a 30-minute phone conversation, went over the letter with the surgeon line by line. In response to her apparent preoccupation with a slight defect in her appearance, as well as her obsessive behavior regarding his impressions, the surgeon referred Louise for a psychological evaluation prior to agreeing to treat her.

Male and Adolescent Patients

Men represented 13% of all cosmetic surgery patients in 2004 (34). Plastic surgeons historically have viewed male patients with skepticism. In the first report of male patients in the literature, all 18 were diagnosed as psychotic, neurotic, or personality disordered (45). This study, however, was done over 45 years ago, when the number of male patients was significantly smaller than it is today. Subsequent studies have found few differences between male and female patients (22,46). Yet, the perception of male patients as being psychopathological has endured. As men still represent a relatively small percentage of persons who undergo cosmetic surgery, a psychopathological male patient may be more likely to remain in the mind of a surgeon as compared to a problematic female patient. These perceptions may reflect a gender stereotypic bias that males who wish to surgically alter their appearance are inherently suspect, as "normal" men are not concerned about such matters—only some psychopathology would motivate such a gender atypical request. It is important for the surgeon to be aware of this possible bias and consider the patient as an individual in evaluating the advisability of surgery.

In 2004, 326,233 individuals 18 years of age or younger underwent a cosmetic procedure (34). This represents an increase of approximately 7% since 2000. While the majority of these procedures are done to treat acne and other skin problems, procedures such as liposuction and breast augmentation are relatively popular and performing them on adolescents is somewhat controversial. As with many rapidly developing areas of Western culture, however, the hype surrounding these procedures has already outpaced thoughtful consideration of the appropriateness of cosmetic surgery on individuals whose bodies and body images are still developing. Unfortunately, there has been scarcely any research on the psychological characteristics of adolescents who seek cosmetic surgery (47).

Optimistically, one could argue that adolescent patients are just like adults—that the majority are psychologically appropriate for surgery and may experience psychological benefit postoperatively. Realistically, given the central role of body image in the pursuit of cosmetic surgery, coupled with the often turbulent nature of body image during adolescence, it is clear that more research in this area is needed before we can confidently state that cosmetic surgery is psychologically beneficial to the majority of adolescents who pursuit it.

Assessing motivations for treatment may be particularly important. Some teens may be driven by pressure from parents to improve their appearance, particularly in families in which one or both parents have had cosmetic procedures. To address this potential situation, the ASPS suggests that the teenager, and not the parent, must be the person who initiates the request for cosmetic surgery. Asking the adolescent when he or she first started thinking about surgery may help determine if the interest in surgery is internally derived or strongly influenced by external pressures. Even if the adolescent's interest in surgery is internally derived, the parents' attitudes toward surgery should be assessed. Parents are occasionally not supportive of an adolescent's interest in surgery, but have agreed to pursue it (and most often pay for it) simply to appease the teen's unrelenting requests. This family dynamic may reflect some psychopathology in the teen or the family and, therefore, warrants further assessment prior to surgery.

Adolescents' interest in cosmetic surgery, like that of adults, may be influenced by the mass media, either through the unrealistic images of beauty or through stories promoting the benefits of cosmetic surgery. Adolescents also may feel some pressure from their peers to have surgery (see Chapter 3 for a discussion of this issue). Such pressure may be both direct and indirect. A peer may suggest cosmetic surgery to a teen unhappy with his or her appearance, or an adolescent may live in a community in which cosmetic surgery is seen as a "rite of passage" or is commonly given as a "Sweet 16" birthday or high school graduation present. In any case, these issues should be discussed as part of the preoperative consultation.

PSYCHOLOGICAL ASSESSMENT OF THE COSMETIC SURGERY PATIENT BY THE MENTAL HEALTH PROFESSIONAL

Mental health professionals may encounter individuals interested in cosmetic surgery in a variety of contexts. Patients in a general psychotherapy practice, particularly those who have body image concerns, may have considered (or have undergone) cosmetic procedures. A plastic surgeon or other physician who offers cosmetic treatments also may ask a mental health professional to consult on a patient either preoperatively or postoperatively.

These patients represent an interesting and unique experience for the mental health professional. Before agreeing to accept these consultations, the professional should examine his or her own beliefs about cosmetic surgery and its ability to positively impact peoples' lives. Professionals who do not believe that changing the outward appearance can improve internal perceptions of one's self probably should not conduct these assessments. On the other hand, professionals also should understand that such treatments are not beneficial to everyone. Thus, consulting professionals should either believe in, or be open to, the idea that cosmetic treatments can produce psychological benefits. Finally, prior to the onset of the consultation, mental health professionals should remind patients that, as consultants, they will be sharing the results of their evaluation and their recommendations of the appropriateness of treatment with the referring physician.

Preoperative Consultations

The vast majority of patients interested in cosmetic surgical and nonsurgical procedures are thought to be psychologically appropriate for such treatments (3–6). Most patients typically have specific appearance concerns, internal motivations, and realistic postoperative expectations. Thus, most do not need a psychological evaluation prior to undergoing a cosmetic treatment. Few, if any, cosmetic surgeons require that all patients undergo a psychological evaluation. Nevertheless, many physicians will elect not to perform procedures on patients who are thought to have an untreated or impairing psychiatric problem.

Patients who display symptoms of psychopathology during their initial consultation with the cosmetic surgeon, as well as those with a history of psychopathology, are most likely to be referred to the mental health professional. Many of the early descriptions of cosmetic surgery patients are complete with elaborate interpretations of the role of unconscious conflicts and poor parental relationships in the decision to seek surgery. There is no evidence, however, to suggest that such interpretations are necessarily valid or useful in determining patients' appropriateness for surgery (48–49). Thus, a detailed assessment of patients' parental relationships and decades-old historical experiences is unlikely to provide useful information to either the mental health professional or to the referring surgeon in determining appropriateness for surgery. Rather, a more straightforward evaluation of patients' current functioning, as found in a general cognitive-behavioral assessment (50), is recommended.

The cognitive-behavioral assessment of the cosmetic surgery patient focuses on the patients' thoughts, behaviors, and experiences that have contributed to their dissatisfaction with their appearance as well as the decision to seek treatment. This involves the assessment of the "ABCs" of patients' interest in surgery—the antecedents (A) to the decision to seek a cosmetic treatment, the behavioral responses (B) to their concerns about their appearance, and expected consequences (C) of their decision to seek surgery. The evaluation should determine if the patients' thoughts and behaviors are maladaptive to the point that they reflect some form of psychopathology that would contraindicate cosmetic treatment.

In addition to utilizing the basic principles of cognitive-behavioral assessment, the assessment by the mental health professional, like that of the treating physician, should focus on the patients' motivations for, and expectations about, cosmetic surgery, their appearance and body image concerns, as well as their psychiatric history and status. These areas of evaluation overlap with those recommended for the treating physician, however, the expertise of the mental health professional will allow for a more detailed assessment than is typically undertaken in the initial consultation with the physician.

Motivations and Expectations

Similar to the treating surgeon, the mental health professional should inquire about patients' motivations and expectations for cosmetic surgery. In assessing patients' motivations for surgery, the mental health professional may want to begin by asking, "When did you first think about changing your appearance?" Similarly, it may be instructive to ask, "What other things have you done to improve your appearance?" In addition to providing important clinical information, these questions also may reveal the presence of some obsessive or delusional thinking, as well as compulsive or bizarre behaviors, related to physical appearance. It is not uncommon for cosmetic surgery patients to report that they have tried several "do-it-yourself" treatments, such as non-FDA approved cosmetic treatments available on the Internet, in an attempt to improve their appearance. Many of these were likely not helpful and some may have been potentially dangerous.

The role of patients' social relationships in the decision to seek surgery should be assessed. Patients should be asked how romantic partners, family members, and close friends feel about the decision to change a physical feature. While these individuals likely influence patients' decision-making process, their role may not be as great as intuitively thought. Breast augmentation patients reported that their decision to seek surgery was influenced more by their own feelings about their appearance than it was influenced by the thoughts of their romantic partners (51–52). Nevertheless, as discussed above, patients who seek treatment specifically to please a current partner, or attract a new one, are thought to be less likely to be satisfied with their postoperative outcomes.

As discussed in Chapter 3, the relatively recent explosion in the number of television shows about cosmetic surgery, as well as surgeons' "infomercials," may play a role in patients' interest in surgery. These programs, coupled with the mass media's nonstop promotion of unrealistic and unattainable ideals of physical beauty, likely influence individuals' beliefs about how cosmetic treatments can change patients' lives. Thus, the mental health professional should inquire about patients' general expectations about how the change in appearance, which may be rather subtle and potentially unnoticed by others, will influence their lives.

Physical Appearance and Body Image

Pruzinsky (14) has suggested the use of Lazarus' BASIC ID (53)—Behavior, Affect, Sensation, Imagery, Cognition, Interpersonal, and Drugs—as a template to assess the body image concerns of cosmetic surgery. In addition, Cash's (54) model of the historical and proximal influences on body image, described in Chapter 4, can provide an additional framework for this part of the assessment. Several of the paper-and-pencil measures discussed in Chapter 4 also may provide additional information on the nature and degree of body image dissatisfaction.

Prospective patients should be able to articulate specific concerns about their appearance that should be visible to the mental health professional with little effort. Patients who are markedly distressed about slight defects that are not readily visible may be suffering from BDD. The nature of the appearance defect may be difficult for mental health professionals to assess for at least two reasons. First, appropriate ethical care would prohibit mental health professionals from asking patients to remove articles of clothing to observe the defect. Second, the judgment of an appearance defect as "slight or imagined" is highly subjective. What a mental health professional judges to be a slight defect well within the range of normal may be a defect that a cosmetic surgeon judges to be easily correctable. As a result, the degree of emotional distress and impairment, rather than the specific nature of the defect, may be more accurate indicators of BDD in these patients (1–6,55).

Nevertheless, some heightened body image dissatisfaction is considered "normal" for persons interested in cosmetic surgery. As discussed above, numerous studies have found that cosmetic surgery candidates report heightened body image dissatisfaction, particularly with the feature considered for surgery (28,46,51,56–58). Some of the thoughts and behaviors that contribute to both the development and maintenance of this dissatisfaction are likely maladaptive. Many patients believe that others take notice of their appearance defects; others report increased anxiety or avoidance of specific social situations because of self-consciousness about their appearance. Thus, the degree and psychosocial consequences of their dissatisfaction should be assessed. Asking about the amount of time spent thinking about a feature or the activities missed or avoided, similar to those questions found in Questionnaire 16-1, may indicate the degree of distress and impairment a person is experiencing and may help determine the presence of BDD. As discussed above, self-report measures of BDD symptoms (in Questionnaire 16-2 of this chapter and Table 4-1) also may be helpful in this regard.

Psychiatric History and Status

The assessment of the patients' psychiatric history and current status, as would be done in any mental health consultation, is a central part of the evaluation. With the exception of BDD (see Chapter 14), there currently are no conclusive data on the prevalence of psychiatric diagnoses among persons who seek or undergo cosmetic surgery. As noted above, it is likely that all of the major psychiatric diagnoses can be found in this patient population. Particular attention should be paid to disorders with a body image component, such as eating disorders and somatoform disorders, as well as mood and anxiety disorders. The presence of these disorders, however, may not be an absolute contraindication for cosmetic surgery. In the absence of sound data on the relationship between psychopathology and surgical outcome, appropriateness for surgery should be made on a case-by-case basis and include careful collaboration between the mental health professional and referring surgeon.

As discussed above, approximately 20% of patients who seek cosmetic medical treatment report using a psychiatric medication (38). As mental health professionals frequently observe, patients who receive these medications from primary care physicians often do not experience complete relief from their symptoms. Thus, a psychopharmacologic evaluation should be considered if symptoms do not appear to be well controlled. If patients are in treatment with another mental health professional, the consultant should contact this professional and discuss patients' appropriateness for cosmetic treatment.

Concluding the Evaluation

At the conclusion of the evaluation, the mental health professional should share his or her clinical impressions with the patient, as well as the recommendation to the referring physician about the appropriateness for surgery. The results of the evaluation can be communicated to the referring physician with a phone call and/or letter summarizing the assessment and recommendations. Obviously, referring physicians will make the ultimate decision about whether to go forward with surgery. Nevertheless, it is good practice to share the results of the consultation with the patient.

The following summarizes Louise's evaluation and early treatment with the mental health professional.

Case 1 (continued): Louise

Louise accepted the surgeon's referral to the psychologist with some reluctance, believing that she was "not crazy" and telling the surgeon that she was considering a consultation with her sister's surgeon. She arrived at her psychological consultation well dressed and well groomed, but clearly anxious. She indicated that she had been self-conscious of the appearance of the scar on her lip since the time of the accident. She believed that the scar left her looking "deformed," although it was not readily visible. Louise indicated that her concern with the scar had affected both her professional and personal life. She indicated that, in the past, she was frequently late to teach her first class of the day, as she would often "get stuck" at home applying and reapplying her makeup to hide her scar. To address this problem, she asked the principal to give her an open hour to start the day. She also indicated that she would only approach her students from her left side, the side away from the scar. Louise reported that she rarely left her house on the weekends because of concerns about her scar. She recalled one recent instance when, while buying some popcorn at a movie, she was convinced that the employee behind the counter was staring at her scar.

Louise entered into psychotherapeutic treatment for BDD. Her beliefs about her appearance, however, were quite fixed. She was convinced that she would only feel better about her appearance if the scar was removed. She was reluctant to engage in any behavioral exercises designed to challenge her belief that people were noticing her scar. The depths of her preoccupation became quite clear in her third treatment session. Louise indicated that she could not imagine leaving her house without makeup. She was presented with the fictional scenario where she received a phone call in the middle of the night from the emergency room informing her that one of her children has been involved in a car accident and that she needed to come to the hospital immediately. When asked if she could go to the hospital without makeup, she said "no."

Postoperative Consultations

Mental health professionals also may be asked to consult with patients postoperatively. This typically occurs in one of two scenarios—a patient is dissatisfied with a technically successful procedure or a patient is experiencing an exacerbation of psychopathology that was not detected preoperatively. Patients in each of these examples typically warrant psychotherapeutic care. As discussed in detail in Chapter 4, cognitive-behavioral models of body image therapy (54) are often useful with these individuals, although more diagnosis-specific treatments also may be required (e.g., for depression, social or generalized anxiety, etc.).

The following case describes a patient who was dissatisfied with her postoperative result.

Case 2: Marie

Marie is a 35-year-old, European–American woman. She is single and works in the marketing department of a local shopping center. She was referred for psychological treatment by her plastic surgeon. She arrived at her assessment well dressed and well groomed. Although she did not appear to be anxious, she displayed obsessive thinking when discussing her previous cosmetic surgery. Marie reported that she had undergone liposuction of her midsection 2 years ago. Following her surgery, she reported gaining approximately 15 pounds following the death of her mother. In Marie's estimation, the surgeon removed too much fat from her midsection so that when she regained her weight, her breasts, shoulders, and arms were proportionally larger than her "thin" midsection. She shared her concerns with the surgeon, who noted Marie's heightened anxiety. He indicated that there was nothing else he could do for her surgically, recommended that she try to lose the weight she had gained, and referred her for psychological assessment and treatment to address her dissatisfaction and anxiety. Marie was not satisfied with his response and believed that she was now far less attractive than she was prior to surgery. Although the psychologist did not see Marie undressed, her body appeared proportional in clothing. (The surgeon confirmed that she was proportional when undressed.) Marie entered into psychological treatment to address her concerns with her body.

CONCLUSIONS

The psychological assessment of patients interested in cosmetic surgery is a critical part of the patient selection process. Failure to identify patients who are psychologically inappropriate for treatment can create significant problems for the treating physician and his or her staff, as well as for the patient. As part of the initial consultation, patients should be asked about their motivations and expectations for treatment. Their appearance and body image concerns should be assessed carefully and the potential presence of BDD, mood, and eating disorders should be determined. In addition, a psychiatric history should be obtained on all patients. Treatment providers are encouraged to identify an appropriate mental health professional as a consultant and refer patients to this individual as needed.

Given the increasing popularity of cosmetic surgery, it is likely that most mental health professionals will encounter patients interested in changing their bodies through cosmetic surgery. In addition to utilizing the basic principles of cognitive-behavioral assessment, preoperative assessments should focus on several additional areas. Like the evaluation by the treating physician, the mental health professional should complete a more detailed assessment of the patient's motivations and expectations for surgery, appearance concerns, and psychiatric history and status. Successful collaboration between the cosmetic surgeon and mental health professional can increase the likelihood that the greatest number of patients receives appropriate treatment for their appearance and body image concerns.

Questions for the Prospective Cosmetic Surgery Patient

Motivations and Expectations
- Why are you interested in surgery now?
- How do you anticipate your life will be different following surgery?
- How do people in your life feel about your getting cosmetic surgery?
- Is there anything about getting cosmetic surgery that worries you?
- How will you know if you are happy with the results of surgery?

Physical Appearance and Body Image
- What is it that you dislike about your appearance?
- How unhappy do you become when you think about your appearance?
- When does the feature bother you the most?
- Do you ever camouflage or hide the feature from others?
- Do you ever feel like you spend too much time thinking about your appearance?
- Do your feelings about your appearance keep you from doing certain activities?
- What other things have you done to improve your appearance?

Psychiatric History and Status
- Have you ever had any significant problems with depression or anxiety?
- Have you ever, or are you currently, under the care of a mental health professional?
- Have you ever, or are you currently, taken an antidepressant or other psychiatric medication?
- If yes, who is prescribing this medication?

For individuals who, based on their presentation, are suspected of being depressed, ask:
- How are you sleeping? Are you having any difficulties falling asleep, staying asleep, or waking up prematurely?
- Have you noticed any changes in your appetite?
- How is your concentration?

If patient endorses any of these neurovegative symptoms, ask the following:
- Are you crying more than usual?
- Are you more irritable than usual?
- Are you interacting with friends and family members?
- Do you feel hopeless or helpless?
- Do you have any thoughts about hurting yourself or ending your life?

For individuals with a BMI <20 kg/m², ask the following to assess for the presence of an eating disorder:
- Have you experienced a weight loss of greater than 10 lbs in the past 6 months?
- Are you actively trying to lose weight at this time?
- Do you ever eat large amounts of food and feel "out of control" of your eating?
- After eating, do you ever make yourself vomit, take laxatives, exercise excessively or engage in any other behavior to compensate for what you just ate?

Body Dysmorphic Disorder Questionnaire

Please read each question carefully and circle the answer that is true for you. Also write in answers where indicated.

1. Are you worried about how you look?

   Yes   No

   —If yes: Do you think about your appearance problems a lot and wish you could think about them less?

   Yes   No

   —If yes: Please list the body areas you don't like: _____

   _____

   _____

Examples of disliked body areas include: your skin (for example, acne, scars, wrinkles, paleness, redness); hair; the shape or size of your nose, mouth, jaw, lips, stomach, hips, etc.; or defects of your hands, genitals, breasts, or any other body part.

NOTE: If you answered "No" to either of the above questions, you are finished with this questionnaire. Otherwise continue.

2. Is your *main* concern with how you look that you aren't thin enough or that you might get too fat?

   Yes   No

3. How has this problem with how you look affected your life?

   • Has it often upset you a lot?

   Yes   No

   • Has it often gotten in the way of doing things with friends or dating?

   Yes   No

   —If yes: Describe how: _____

   _____

   • Has it caused you any problems with school or work?

   Yes   No

   —If yes: What are they? _____

   _____

   • Are there things you avoid because of how you look?

   Yes   No

   —If yes: What are they _____

   _____

4. On an average day, how much time do you usually spend thinking about how you look? (Add up all the time you spend in a day, then circle one.)

   a. Less than 1 hour a day

   b. 1–3 hours a day

   c. More than 3 hours a day

Reprinted with permission of the author from Phillips KA. *The Broken Mirror: Understanding and Treating Body Dysmorphic Disorder*. New York: Oxford University Press, 1996.

REFERENCES

1. Grossbart TA, Sarwer DB. Cosmetic surgery: Surgical tools—Psychosocial goals. *Semin Cutan Med Surg* 1999;18:101–111.
2. Sarwer DB. Psychological considerations in cosmetic surgery. In: Goldwyn RM, Cohen MI, eds. *The Unfavorable Result in Plastic Surgery.* 3rd ed. Philadelphia: Lippincott Williams & Wilkins, 2001.
3. Sarwer DB, Crerand CE, Didie ER. Body dysmorphic disorder in cosmetic surgery patients. *Facial Plast Surg* 2003;19:7–17.
4. Sarwer DB, Crerand CE, Gibbons LM. Body dysmorphic disorder. In: Nahai F, ed. *The Art of Aesthetic Surgery.* St. Louis: Quality Medical Publishing. In press.
5. Sarwer DB, Crerand CE. Body image and cosmetic medical treatments. *Body Image: An International Journal of Research* 2004;1:99–111.
6. Sarwer DB, Magee L, Crerand, CE. Cosmetic surgery and cosmetic medical treatments. In: Thompson JK, ed. *Handbook of Eating Disorders and Obesity.* Hoboken, NJ: John Wiley and Sons, 2004:718–737.
7. Edgerton MT, Knorr NJ. Motivational patterns of patients seeking cosmetic (aesthetic) surgery. *Plast Reconstr Surg* 1971;48:551–557.
8. Goin JM, Goin MK. *Changing the Body: Psychological Effects of Plastic Surgery.* Baltimore, MD: Williams & Wilkins, 1981.
9. Meyer E, Jacobson WE, Edgerton MT, Canter A. Motivational patterns in patients seeking elective plastic surgery. *Psychol Med* 1960;22:193–202.
10. Edgerton MT, Langman MW, Pruzinsky T. Plastic surgery and psychotherapy in the treatment of 100 psychologically disturbed patients. *Plast Reconstr Surg* 1991;88:594–608.
11. Beale S, Lisper H, Palm B. A psychological study of patients seeking augmentation mammaplasty. *Br J Psychol* 1980;136:133–138.
12. Edgerton MT, Meyer E, Jacobson WE. Augmentation mammaplasty: II. Further surgical and psychiatric evaluation. *Plast Reconstr Surg* 1961;27:279–301.
13. Wright MR, Wright WK. A psychological study of patients undergoing cosmetic surgery. *Arch Otolaryngol* 1975;101:145–151.
14. Pruzinsky T. Cosmetic plastic surgery and body image: critical factors in patient assessment. In: Thompson JK, ed. *Body Image, Eating Disorders, and Obesity.* Washington, DC: American Psychological Association, 1996:109–127.
15. Cash TF, Horton CE. Aesthetic surgery: effects of rhinoplasty on the social perceptions of patients by others. *Plast Reconstr Surg* 1983; 72:543–550.
16. Kalick SM. Aesthetic surgery: how it affects the way patients are perceived by others. *Ann Plast Surg* 1979;2:128–134.
17. Honigman R, Phillips KA, Castle DJ. A review of psychosocial outcomes for patients seeking cosmetic surgery. *Plast Reconstr Surg* 2004;113,1229–1237.
18. Napoleleon A. The presentation of personalities in plastic surgery. *Ann Plast Surg* 1993;31:193–208.
19. Pruzinsky T, Edgerton MT. Body image change in cosmetic plastic surgery. In: Cash TF, Pruzinksy T, eds. *Body Images: Development, Deviance, and Change.* New York: Guilford Press, 1990:217–236.
20. Sarwer DB. Cosmetic surgery and body image change. In: Cash TF, Pruzinsky T, eds. *Body Images: A Handbook of Theory, Research and Clinical Practice.* New York: Guilford Press, 2002:422–430.
21. Boone OB, Wexler MR, Kaplan-DeNour AK. Rhinoplasty patients' critical self-evaluation of their noses. *Plast Reconstr Surg* 1996;98:436–439.
22. Hay GG. Psychiatric aspects of cosmetic nasal operations. *Br J Psychol* 1970;116:85–97.
23. Aouizerate B, Pujol H, Grabot D, et al. Body dysmorphic disorder in a sample of cosmetic surgery applicants. *Eur Psychiatry* 2003;18:365–368.
24. Crerand CE, Sarwer DB, Magee L, et al. Rate of body dysmorphic disorder among patients seeking facial plastic surgery. *Psychiatric Ann* 2004;34:958–965.
25. Dufresne RG, Phillips KA, Vittorio CC, Wilkel CS. A screening questionnaire for body dysmorphic disorder in a cosmetic dermatologic surgery practice. *Dermatol Surg* 2001;27:457–462.
26. Ishigooka J, Iwao M, Suzuki M, et al. Demographic features of patients seeking cosmetic surgery. *Psychiatry Clin Neurosci* 1998;52:283–287.
27. Phillips KA, Dufresne RG, Wilkel C, Vittorio CC. Rate of body dysmorphic disorder in dermatology patients. *J Am Acad Dermato* 2000;42:436–441.
28. Sarwer DB, Wadden TA, Pertschuk MJ, Whitaker LA. Body image dissatisfaction and body dysmorphic disorder in 100 cosmetic surgery patients. *Plast Reconstr Surg* 1998;101:1644–1649.
29. Uzun O, Basoglu C, Akar A, et al. Body dysmorphic disorder in patients with acne. *Compr Psychiatry* 2003; 44:415–419.
30. Phillips KA, Grant JE, Siniscalchi J, Albertini RS. Surgical and nonpsychiatric medical treatment of patients with body dysmorphic disorder. *Psychosomatics* 2001;42:504–510.
31. Veale D, Boocock A, Gournay K, et al. Body dysmorphic disorder: a survey of fifty cases. *Br J Psychiatr* 1996; 169:196–201.
32. Sarwer DB, Didie ER. Body image in cosmetic surgical and dermatological practice. In: Castle D, Phillips KA, eds. *Disorders of Body Image.* Stroud, England: Wrighton Biomedical Publishing, 2002:37–53.
33. Sarwer DB, Gibbons LM, Crerand CE. Cognitive behavioral treatment of body dysmorphic disorder. *Psychiatric Ann* 2004;34:934–941.
34. *2005 Report of the 2004 National Clearinghouse of Plastic Surgery Statistics.* Arlington Heights, IL: American Society of Plastic Surgeons, 2005.
35. Phillips KA. *The Broken Mirror: Understanding and Treating Body Dysmorphic Disorder.* New York: Oxford University Press, 1996.

36. Cash TF, Phillips KA, Santos MT, Hrabosky JI. Measuring "negative body image": validation of the body image disturbance questionnaire in a non-clinical population. *Body Image: An International Journal of Research* 2004;1:363–372.
37. Sarwer DB. Awareness and identification of body dysmorphic disorder by aesthetic surgeons: results of a survey of American Society for Aesthetic Plastic Surgery members. *Aesth Surg J* 2002;22:531–535.
38. Sarwer DB, Zanville HA, LaRossa D, et al. Mental health histories and psychiatric medication usage among persons who sought cosmetic surgery. *Plast Reconstr Surg* 2004;114:1927–1933.
39. Sarwer DB, Cohn NI, Gibbons LM, et al. Psychiatric diagnoses and psychiatric treatment among bariatric surgery candidates. *Obes Surg* 2004;14:1148–1156.
40. Brinton LA, Lubin JH, Burich MC, et al. Mortality among augmentation mammoplasty patients. *Epidemiology* 2001;12:321–326.
41. Jacobsen PH, Holmich LR, McLaughlin JK, et al. Mortality and suicide among Danish women with cosmetic breast implants. *Arch Intern Med* 2004;164:2450–2455.
42. Koot VC, Peeters PH, Granath F, et al. Total and cause specific mortality among Swedish women with cosmetic breast implants: a prospective study. *BMJ* 2003;326:527–528.
43. Pukkala E, Kulmala I, Hovi SL, et al. Causes of death among Finnish women with cosmetic breast implants, 1971–2001. *Ann Plast Surg* 2003;51:339–342.
44. McLaughlin JK, Wise TN, Lipworth L. Increased risk of suicide among patients with breast implants: do the epidemiologic data support psychiatric consultation? *Psychosomatics* 2004;45:277–280.
45. Jacobson WE, Edgerton MT, Meyer E, et al. Psychiatric evaluation of male patients seeking cosmetic surgery. *Plast Reconstr Surg* 1960;26:356–372.
46. Pertschuk MJ, Sarwer DB, Wadden TA, Whitaker LA. Body image dissatisfaction in male cosmetic surgery patients. *Aesthetic Plast Surg* 1998;22:20–24.
47. Sarwer DB. Plastic Surgery in Children and Adolescents. In: Thompson JK, Smolak L, eds. *Body Image, Eating Disorders, and Obesity in Children and Adolescents: Theory, Assessment, Treatment, and Prevention*. Washington, DC: American Psychological Assocation Press, 2001:341–366.
48. Sarwer DB, Wadden TA, Pertschuk MJ, Whitaker LA. The psychology of cosmetic surgery: a review and reconceptualization. *Clin Psychol Rev* 1998;181–22.
49. Sarwer DB, Pertschuk MJ, Wadden TA, Whitaker LA. Psychological investigations of cosmetic surgery patients: a look back and a look ahead. *Plast Reconstr Surg* 1998;101:1136–1142.
50. Sarwer DB, Sayers SL. Behavioral interviewing. In: Bellack AS, Hersen M, eds. *Behavioral Assessment: A Practical Handbook*. 4th ed. New York: Pergamon, 1998:63–78.
51. Didie ER, Sarwer DB. Factors which influence the decision to undergo cosmetic breast augmentation surgery. *J Womens Health* 2003;12:241–253.
52. Cash TF, Duel LA, Perkins LL. Women's psychosocial outcomes of breast augmentation with silicone gel-filled implants: a 2-year prospective study. *Plast Reconstr Surg* 2002;109:2112–2121.
53. Lazarus AA. Multimodal behavior therapy: treating the "BASIC ID." *J Nerv Ment Dis* 1973;156:404–111.
54. Cash TF. Cognitive-behavioral perspectives on body image. In: Cash TF, Pruzinsky T, eds. *Body Image: A Handbook of Theory, Research, and Clinical Practice*. New York: Guilford Press, 2002:38–46.
55. Sarwer DB, Pertschuk MJ. Cosmetic surgery. In: Kornstein SG, Clayton AH, eds. *Textbook of Women's Mental Health*. New York: Guilford Press, 2002:481–496.
56. Sarwer DB, Bartlett SP, Bucky LP, et al. Bigger is not always better: body image dissatisfaction in breast reduction and breast augmentation patients. *Plast Reconstr Surg* 1998;101:1956–1961.
57. Sarwer DB, LaRossa D, Bartlett SP, et al. Body image concerns of breast augmentation patients. *Plast Reconstr Surg* 2003;112:83–90.
58. Sarwer DB, Whitaker LA, Wadden TA, Pertschuk MJ. Body image dissatisfaction in women seeking rhytidectomy or blepharoplasty. *Aesthetic Surg J* 1997;17,230–234.

Ethical and Professional Issues in Plastic Surgery

Chapter 17

Ethical and Professional Considerations in Craniofacial Reconstructive Surgery

Ronald P. Strauss, DMD, PhD, Margot B. Stein, PhD, and Carla Fenson, M.Ed

Bioethical cases often make mass media headlines because they highlight important controversies in contemporary life. Issues regarding new medical technology, and how they affect freedom and dignity, are worthy of consideration by society at large and are regularly discussed in the most public political and social forums. However, the ethical dilemmas faced by surgeons and physicians in daily clinical practice rarely receive such attention. Indeed, such issues may even pass as mundane, often unrecognized as ethical dilemmas because they have become such a part of clinical routine.

What do we mean when we ask "what is an ethical question?" An ethical question is one that entails judgment about what is right and what is wrong. Ethical issues may relate to how the professional can most fairly and equitably respond to the needs or concerns of a patient or client. Ethical issues raise moral or values-based questions. In the context of craniofacial surgery, little attention has been given to the ethical and moral issues that arise in the course of relatively customary and routine clinical practice. We seek to highlight those situations in craniofacial surgery that raise profound ethical and social questions that have rarely been the subject of professional or media inquiry.

The primary goal of this chapter is to present a framework for understanding the nature of ethical issues that arise in the course of providing craniofacial surgery. A large portion of the chapter focuses on presenting cases deriving from real clinical situations to promote consideration of these issues. We understand that the use of case situations to explore ethical matters has some serious limitations. Cases are vignettes that simplify facts and occur out of context. They lack the texture of the doctor–patient relationship and rarely allow for nuanced situational analysis. Yet, they also present an excellent opportunity to examine how clinicians approach decision making and help to clarify professional and personal values. Examples or cases are often useful in making ethical issues real and allowing for debate and consideration of various options (1).

GENERAL PERSPECTIVES ON BIOETHICAL ISSUES

The Structure and Function of Ethics Committees

Physicians do not make bioethical decisions in a vacuum. The patient, family, the law, and health professional cultures all importantly contribute to ethical deliberation. Once a situation is identified as an ethical dilemma, it may then be examined from a variety of perspectives. The clinician who faces an ethical dilemma often

Acknowledgments: The authors would like to thank Ms. Cassandra Aspinall for granting us permission to include Case 7, which she graciously shared with the authors.

quickly becomes aware that no choice to be made will fully satisfy all parties. Indeed, this is the inherent nature of a dilemma. There is legitimacy to several "sides" in ethical debates. Clinicians who are accustomed to coping with uncertainty in their clinical lives may find themselves frustrated at their inability to resolve an ethical dilemma to their satisfaction. Thinking about an ethical dilemma may occur most effectively in social and interpersonal interaction, rather than in isolation. Consequently, many hospitals and academic health centers have established ethics committees to help deal with these issues.

The ethics committee characteristically includes various representatives—thoughtful physicians, spiritual leaders, community representatives, and lay members. Such committees serve two primary functions. First, ethics committees adjudicate ethical complaints from patients, families, health professionals, or health insurers against members of the professional staff. In this function, the ethics committee may serve a monitoring and conflict resolution role. When conflicts persist, final settlements may occur under the guidance of hospital administrators, in complaints to licensing boards, or through the legal system. Second, ethics committees serve as consultants to physicians or other professionals who are facing difficult ethical dilemmas. They provide professionals access to a forum in which they can present a situation and hear the various responses or positions in a supportive and confidential setting.

For example, a physician might present a dilemma regarding a patient to an ethics committee to gather information about how to proceed with treatment. The ability to solicit such advice without worry about violations of confidentiality is truly critical; therefore, ethics committees are conducted under a cloak of privacy. However, in this role, the ethics committee rarely offers the physician a clear resolution of the ethical dilemma. Rather, the consultation may be used to outline possible viewpoints and to define possible courses of action in a given situation. Clinicians may feel anxiety or disappointment when they realize that the ethics committee cannot just advise "what to do" in a given situation. The ultimate decision most often resides with the health professional or with the health care team.

Bioethical Decision Making

Bioethical decisions, particularly those involving the treatment of children with craniofacial anomalies, have a critical impact on health outcomes and on individual and family quality of life. Such decisions often raise questions that call for a distinction between what is "right" and what is "wrong." In the conduct of clinical care, judgments about fairness, human duty, and personal morals are ethical decisions. These are not merely technical questions meant for experts in ethics; health professionals in clinical practice make these decisions on a regular basis (2–4).

In some respects, ethical issues in craniofacial care are particular instances of social and moral decisions that occur in the conduct of other human matters. For example, issues involving access to costly craniofacial services are merely a subset of issues that relate to how a society allocates scarce resources. Ethical debate will sometimes consider whether individual benefit should be maximized or whether the needs of the society at large should receive priority. In the conduct of ethical decision making, it may not be possible to reconcile fully the desires of individuals with the needs of the society at large.

Guiding Ethical Principles

Several ethical principles may influence the values expressed in craniofacial ethical decisions. Often ethical decisions involve the distinction between autonomy, beneficence, and non-maleficence. Issues of competence and justice are also worthy of consideration. (These issues are also discussed in the context of cosmetic procedures in Chapter 18.)

Autonomy and Beneficence

Autonomy implies the ability of an individual to determine how he or she is to be treated by others. It means that a person can freely act to define the treatment, outcomes, and processes used in his or her health care. Autonomy implies the ability to make reasonable informed decisions in one's self-interest. Beneficence is a principle by which professionals provide what they believe is best for another person. In the case of health care, a professional will judge what form of treatment is offered in a patient's best interest. Sometimes the professional's idea of the best course of treatment may differ from the patient's or from the family's. When this occurs, who decides on the final course of action? Issues of autonomy and beneficence arise frequently in communicating surgical treatment plans and in negotiating an agreed upon course of care. The professional's sharing of information and the patient's and family's desires for information shape how the patient's best interest will be defined.

Non-maleficence

Health professionals are often seen as being held to a principle of non-maleficence, or the expectation that they will do everything possible to avoid harm, as compared to creating good or well-being. In the surgical care of children with craniofacial anomalies, should the surgeon provide an operation to a patient just because the family or patient requests it? Should the surgeon only provide the patient with the treatment options the surgeon believes are optimal and withhold other possibilities? Should a surgeon who does not believe he or she can perform an operation without significant risk of harm refer the patient elsewhere? Should he or she explain her decision in doing so?

Competence

Another concept that affects clinical decision making is competence, which implies the legal ability to make health care decisions. Adults are assumed to be competent unless their legal decision-making rights have been granted to others, such as a legal guardian or one with the power of attorney. Adults who, because of limited intellectual capacity or other disabilities, are unable to engage in the informed consent process, may be considered incompetent to make their own health care decisions. Children or adolescents (below the age of 18) are not generally considered competent to make independent decisions without a guardian's involvement. Thus, adolescents are asked to provide assent for treatment while parents or guardians ultimately provide informed consent. The principle of competence highlights the difference between the law and ethics. It may be legal for a professional to perform a procedure on a patient, but it may not be ethical to do so.

Justice

In bioethical decision making, justice involves three related concepts: treating people fairly; giving people what they deserve; and giving people what they are entitled to. These concepts are tied to distributive justice or approaches towards allocating resources in a society (4). In the case of craniofacial surgery, the costly nature of care and the relatively small number of professionals who offer it contribute to its perception as a scarce resource. Various allocation rationales may be proposed to decide who receives craniofacial surgical care and who does not. Does the sickest person receive care first? Is care distributed on a first-come, first-served basis or is it given by merit?

It is also important to recall that, for most clinicians, this issue of justice is considered in the context of a given doctor–patient relationship. In contrast, on a public health or policy level, health professions are called upon to protect society and to act to maximize fairness. On occasion, the individual and societal goals may be at odds with one another.

SPECIFIC BIOETHICAL ISSUES IN CRANIOFACIAL CARE

The remainder of this chapter presents cases that are representative of ethical dilemmas that occur in the context of providing craniofacial services. The discussion that follows each case necessarily offers only a limited set of options and viewpoints. Nevertheless, they illuminate the mechanism of ethical discourse. The discussants are not formally trained ethicists; rather, they are thoughtful health professionals and social scientists with extensive clinical experience concerning the issues discussed. This resembles the reality of most ethics committees, few of which have formally educated biomedical ethicists and typically call upon members of the local community who may bring a fair and considered perspective to ethical discourse.

As noted earlier, solutions to these dilemmas are rarely, if ever, clear and definitive. However, thoughtful discussion and contemplation of these situations, which following the guidance of the ethical principles discussed above, can facilitate greater insight and sensitivity as craniofacial teams struggle to do what is in the best interests of their patients.

CASE EXAMPLES

Case 1: Robby—When Is Enough, Enough?

> Robby is a 16-year-old boy with a history of unilateral complete cleft lip and palate. He plays basketball on his high school's varsity team and plans to go to college after graduation. He has an obvious maxillary deficiency and lip and nose deformity that can be repaired with two surgical procedures that should optimally be done in the next 1 to 2 years. Robby's parents have said that they want the best possible result for Robby because for him "the sky is the limit." At this visit with the treatment team, Robby says, "enough is enough, I don't want any more surgery. I don't want to miss basketball practice and I am sick of doctors and hospitals."

Is it the treatment team's role to advocate for more surgery? What are the alternatives?

Robby has been presented the option of surgery that technically may be considered as elective, but is intended to correct an obvious lip and nose deformity often associated with social stigma, painful self-consciousness, and diminished self-esteem (the psychological effects of craniofacial conditions are reviewed in Chapter 5). The current standard of care suggests that the necessary corrective surgical procedures should be performed within 2 years or by the time he is 18. His parents understandably wish to do all they can to help their son put his best possible face to the world, literally and figuratively.

Robby presents an interesting and not unusual dilemma for those who work with adolescent candidates for craniofacial surgery. The central issues raised by this case include patient autonomy, adequately informed consent, and what Ward has termed "partnership without coercion" (2, p. 8). These issues are closely intertwined with key features of adolescent development and related family dynamics that can challenge all participants in medical treatment during this stage of life (5,6). Before proceeding to discuss these issues it is helpful to consider briefly some salient features of adolescent development.

Sixteen-year-old Robby is in middle adolescence, a developmental stage that is characterized by more sophisticated mental reasoning. These abilities include improved perspective taking that makes it easier to place a specific issue within its broader context ("the big picture") and an intensified quest for personal competence and mastery in daily life. In addition, because most adolescents have relatively little life experience to use as a reference, they tend to emphasize the present over the future. For many, adolescence also is marked by an emotional intensity that can be expressed in passionate commitment to personal beliefs and ideals that sometimes may cloud rational judgment. Thus, the teenager is often involved in a continuous dance between the personal and the public, the self and the community, self-focus and altruism (7–11).

The right of the patient to determine the nature and timing of his treatment is obviously a central issue in this case. But can the principle of patient autonomy exist in a vacuum? In other words, should the surgeon's sense of duty to the patient's long-term welfare be put aside in favor of Robby's right to choose? Because Robby is not yet an adult, do his wishes need to be weighed against research-based medical opinion and the wishes of his parents, who, it may be assumed, know their child and his needs well and wish to protect his future? How do we reconcile the well-founded concerns of all involved?

One could argue that the principle of autonomy can be meaningful only when the patient is adequately informed about procedures and treatment outcomes. For the purpose of this example, let's assume that his previous surgeries are consistent with the typical standard of care and are otherwise unremarkable. Nevertheless, we do not know how Robby has interpreted his treatment course and what meaning it has for him at this time. We may assume that he is a busy high school junior, who plays sports, is facing increasing academic demands, and is likely concerned about his social life as well. In this context, it may be realistic to conclude that time and timing with regard to his surgery are significant considerations for him.

It would be helpful to know more about Robby's understanding of the proposed surgery and what it and his recovery will involve. Perhaps he has some unexpressed or even unrecognized worries about this procedure. Teenagers may be poorly informed, harbor misconceptions, be reluctant to ask potentially embarrassing questions, and, instead, may adopt an air of bravado so as not to appear vulnerable to others (8,11–14). Therefore, it may be helpful if the surgeon first spends time talking with Robby alone, to explore, in greater depth, his concerns about surgery. This may provide an opportunity to address questions that he may have and is not comfortable addressing without explicit permission and support. Is Robby satisfied with his appearance at this point in time? If left to his own devices, how would he time his own surgery? What does he think might be the trade-offs were he to postpone surgery more than 2 years? How might he feel about his decision 5 years from how if postponement resulted in a less successful outcome? Such a discussion makes it possible for the surgeon to go beyond the potentially paternalistic definition of disclosure as to what the surgeon thinks Robby should know, enabling him to discover what Robby wants and needs to know. One might ask whether this more extended discussion is not only desirable but indispensable if, as in Great Britain, children between 16 and 18 are assumed to have the same degree of competence to consent as an adult (4, p. 7).

Of course, the surgeon may provide Robby with excellent pertinent information, listen to his concerns and respond appropriately, and yet still meet with refusal to proceed. Middle and late adolescents often use their rapidly developing conceptual and reasoning skills to challenge adult authority and to question whether "father (or mother or doctor) knows best." This challenge may be rationally or emotionally based, or a combination of the two. The primacy of emotion for a 16-year-old to 18-year-old may trump the primacy of medical reasoning (6,9–10,12,15).

In this case, should the surgeon ally with Robby's parents and together try to convince him to proceed with surgery despite his clearly stated resistance? The surgeon and parents may share the belief that "the sky is the limit" and that to postpone a medical procedure beyond its optimal timing would be irresponsible and ultimately unfair to Robby, whose judgment may seem clouded by short-term considerations. This raises the issue of parental perceptions of surgical necessity. One might wish to know more about the relationship between Robby and his parents and how they communicate with each other. What are their expectations for Robby, not only for his physical appearance but other aspects of his future functioning? In terms of Robby, what does "the sky is the limit" mean? What is their problem-solving style when faced with disagreement in their family? Are they willing to engage with their son in a lengthy conversation without a perception of what the "right" outcome should be? If Robby remains adamant in his opposition to surgery even though his parents feel that it would be in his best interest to move ahead with it, should the surgeon comply with the parents' wishes and perform the surgery? Could his actions be justified by the principle of benevolence or could they be considered as coercive?

The manner in which surgeon and parents engage Robby in this conversation, and whether or not they listen respectfully to what he has to say, can have long-term consequences apart from surgical outcomes. The terms of engagement in this case could affect his trust in health professionals, his attitude toward medical interventions, his faith in his own judgment and ability to solve problems, as well as his relationship with his parents.

Case 2: Eric—The Alienated Adolescent

Eric is a 14-year-old boy who presents to the craniofacial clinic in full "skateboarder" attire and with multiple ear piercings. Eric has come to clinic with his mother and younger sister who have remained in the waiting room at Eric's request. He is being seen to plan an alveolar bone graft to close an anterior oro-nasal fistula. In the course of his examination, Eric tells the surgeon that he often smokes marijuana in the evenings and, on occasion, has tried "designer drugs" at parties. He is interested in having surgery and is not concerned that his substance use is a problem. His mother has never mentioned his use of drugs before and the surgeon wonders if she even knows.

Should this information be shared with the craniofacial team? Should it be shared with his mother? What factors might influence this decision?

The profile of an "alienated adolescent" draws upon a set of stereotypes about adolescent culture and alternative lifestyles. It is important that the dress and accessories of Eric's appearance not guide the surgeon's judgment. Each patient deserves individual attention and all attempts to avoid prejudicial assumptions are warranted. That being said, it is clear that Eric has chosen to share a set of relevant facts regarding his substance use. Were he truly alienated, would he share such potentially powerful or damaging information? Does this indicate his level of trust and confidence in the surgeon and his assumption that his revelations will be kept confidential? Could it be that he is sharing this information as a form of help seeking? It may be that he is hoping to hear that his substance use is not a problem but is testing to see whether the surgeon shares that conclusion. Indeed, most adolescents assume that responsible, adult authority figures are likely to find illicit substance use to be dangerous and deplorable.

The quandary in this case relates to whether the surgeon can best help Eric by keeping his confidence and working with him directly or by sharing the information with his mother in the expectation that she will respond appropriately and find assistance for her son. The violation of Eric's private communication may result in his disappointment and possibly in his refusal to continue with his care. However, it would be worth exploring his expectations directly with him. What did he think would happen with this information once shared? What information does he want shared and with whom? Does he understand the surgeons need or desire to share the information with his mother? How would he respond to such sharing of the information? Does he understand the ramifications of illicit substance use? This discussion may provide the surgeon with a "teachable" moment in which Eric can be educated in the legal risks and biomedical or psychological dangers of drug use and possibly, help him engage his parents in an important discussion of these issues. Hopefully, one outcome of the interaction with Eric will be a referral for assistance and a commitment to follow him over time.

One potential approach is to have a preliminary discussion with both Eric and his mother in which the ground rules for sharing and disclosure are considered. A parent might find benefit in their child having a trusted mature adult confidant, that he or she might waive their expectation for physician–parent communication regarding private information. However, without that discussion, the surgeon might be in a quandary about what information to disclose and what to hide.

If the surgeon is convinced that Eric is in imminent danger of doing damage to himself or others (if he is dealing drugs as well), either physically or psychologically, it is important that the surgeon take steps to avoid such harm. If Eric's substance use is increasing or becoming a larger feature of his life, then parental disclosure becomes absolutely necessary. Parents may operate with the expectation that a physician is obliged to disclose all potential harms to the parent and they may not understand his or her reluctance to share concerns about something as important as substance use.

This dilemma puts the principles of autonomy, confidentiality, and competence in potential conflict. Professionals must consider the ramifications of disclosure and nondisclosure and decide which will maximize the patient's future health and well-being. If surgical outcomes can be negatively impacted by substance use, then surgical planning will absolutely require behavioral change. The team's mental health professional may prove to be a resource in evaluating the patient and guiding physician decision making.

Case 3: Jane—de Lange Syndrome—To Operate or Not?

Tommy and Jonelle Jones, low-income and uninsured parents, have contacted the Craniofacial Center with a referral from their family doctor. Shortly after her delivery at a small rural hospital, their daughter Jane, now 2 years old, was diagnosed with de Lange syndrome. Her symptoms include hand abnormalities, sporadic seizures, gastric reflux, and a cleft of the hard and soft palate. She is able to be fed without a feeding tube.

Early testing suggests that she has severe mental retardation and has no sign of intelligible speech. At her diagnostic evaluation, the speech pathologist expressed little confidence that she will ever develop verbal speech. The parents have asked the team whether it is a good idea to surgically close her cleft palate. The team's plastic surgeon has said that she is willing to do cleft palate surgery. The team's speech pathologist says she can find no rationale for such surgery.

What are the major bioethical issues facing the team? How do they agree on an appropriate treatment plan for Jane?

This case raises several of the most poignant and complex issues that are frequently presented to craniofacial teams. These include the dependence of parents of a child with special needs on health care providers and the faith they place in their craniofacial team, and, obviously, Jane's (and the parents') quality of life. In addition, the team must struggle with issues related to effective communication and consensus building.

The Jones family is scarcely atypical; they are a young family of limited means and no health insurance. They may not have the knowledge and self-assurance to firmly and successfully advocate for what they perceive as Jane's basic needs. Although most parents tend to defer rapidly to the recommendations of their health providers, this deference tends to be even more pronounced among those who find themselves in the Jones' situation.

Do the team members defer to the speech pathologist's professional opinion that Jane probably never will develop speech? Though it is always possible that the speech pathologist is correct in her prediction, other professionals who work with persons with handicapping conditions often believe that a little skepticism regarding this belief is healthy and in the best interest of the child and family. While the speech pathologist may be well within the bounds of professionalism in maintaining that she finds no rationale for surgery, other team members might find this an inadequate basis for withholding corrective surgery.

In Jane's case, her cleft of the hard and soft palate affects more than speech; there are quality of life issues that involve the mechanics of daily functioning and appearance concerns. If her cleft is not surgically repaired, she will likely have greater needs for assistance with food preparation and feeding throughout childhood. This will place additional stress on her parents.

Does the fact that Jane has a severely handicapping condition raise additional ethical issues? Sometimes the issue of impaired cognitive abilities, like financial issues, is an "elephant in the room" during team discussions. As such, cognitive limitation often influences individual decisions without ever being explicitly raised. In some societies, the dearth of adequate health care is so severe that triage, in a case like this, is unavoidable. In the United States, some surgeons may privately consider how to best allocate resources in the craniofacial setting, but few, if any, teams have arrived at a policy on which to base such decisions. Under current law and values, would denying Jane optimal care on the basis of her "severe mental retardation" constitute a violation of her civil rights?

Last but not least, is it critical for the team to reach a group consensus regarding its recommendations or should the team leader present the contradictory views of the clinicians to the parents? How team members resolve their differing opinions will be shaped by the team's operating premises. For example, is this an interdisciplinary team that follows a true collaborative model where individual members tend to learn from each other, gaining information and insights from other professions, and working together to arrive at a more complete understanding of the nature and needs of the patient and family? In contrast, is the group comprised of professionals from various disciplines who meet as a unit, but generally think and behave in a manner consistent with their specific discipline? This latter, more individualistic approach to team functioning risks fragmenting care and is less likely to foster the collaborative process necessary to arrive at a group consensus.

If the team cannot achieve consensus regarding its treatment recommendations, and is honest with the parents about the disagreement between the team plastic surgeon and the team speech pathologist, the Jones are left in a quandary. Do they break away from the team approach and try to find a surgeon who is willing to proceed with treatment? Do they feel disappointed, disheartened, angry, or betrayed by the team? Will they feel that because they have been powerlessness to obtain corrective surgery for their daughter, they themselves have betrayed her?

Case 4: Maria—Allocation of Treatment Resources

Maria is a 15-year-old girl with a bilateral cleft lip and palate. She arrives at her appointment with her mother. Maria lives with her parents and four siblings in the country. Her father works as a sharecropper. Previous exposure to the family has suggested that they are quite poor. They have no health or dental insurance.

Maria's mother enters the clinic examination room and says: "Doctor, I'm just so excited to see Maria getting ready to have her jaw fixed. She could look so pretty with a good profile and bite." Maria's treatment options include a maxillary advancement operation to bring her upper jaw into alignment and three dental implants to replace missing upper teeth. The cost of this treatment plan is quite substantial, but it is the optimal care. The alternative would be to have the team dentist make a low-cost plastic removable partial denture that would replace the missing teeth and permit her to function at this time.

What treatment should be recommended? In making a recommendation, should the issue of cost be considered?

Maria's treatment highlights one of the central ethical and financial dilemmas of health services provision in most Westernized countries today, namely access to optimal care. In contrast to many developed countries, the United States traditionally has not viewed affordable health care as an individual right that should be provided at minimal expense by society to all. As health providers, we find ourselves assessing treatment for many patients with no or limited health insurance and no other means of otherwise paying for treatment they need. Often the most sophisticated and effective treatments are also the most costly, and, consequently, often subject to formal and informal rationing. If these costly and technically advanced treatments cannot be offered to everyone regardless of ability to pay, those believing in distributive justice would insist that the process for obtaining these treatments be made as fair as possible.

If Maria is offered the low-cost plastic removable partial denture, instead of the more extensive surgical intervention, the primary ethical dilemma presented in this case appears to be avoided. Such an approach might be justifiable from a utilitarian point of view, as it would meet the basic treatment needs of the largest number of patients at a lesser cost. However, if the first priority is to offer optimal care to all patients, regardless of their ability to pay, the dilemma remains. Current standards of care would support the choice of the optimal, more expensive, and longer lasting treatment. Among other benefits, it could not be misplaced or lost, a not inconsequential factor when treating a 15-year-old. Surgical treatment would likely serve her for many years to come.

Is it the surgeon's or team's responsibility to make a decision on care based on the perceptions of the family's financial resources? Though Maria might significantly benefit from maxillary advancement surgery, could her medical bills drain the family resources to the point where other family members might need to forego basic necessities? Does this line of thinking become inappropriately paternalistic? Instead, should this decision be left solely to the family? Should the team consider waving some or all of the surgical costs and, even if so, will the hospital be responsive to the family's financial situation and adjust their fees accordingly? How does this affect the treatment of similar children in the future?

Another issue is that of distributive justice: how will the individual decision involving Maria affect other children and adult patients who will come to the team in similar situations with similar needs? Does the craniofacial team have an established policy or are such decisions made individually on an ad hoc basis? What is the rationale to subsidize some treatments and not others?

Maria's mother is a caring parent who wants the best for her children and is invested in their care. By telling her about the option of maxillary advancement surgery, she is placed in an awkward and painful position. On the one hand, the team would like to spare her the anguish of having to weigh the advantages of an optimal, but prohibitively costly treatment for a beloved child against the financial and possibly social and emotional costs to other family members. On the other hand, others might argue that from the vantage point of maximizing autonomy and related informed consent, the team's ethical obligation is clear. They might point out that based on the principle of self-determination, the mother's ability to select a treatment for her daughter is predicated on her right to be informed about the existing surgical techniques proven to be medically effective for Maria's problem. Does a surgeon have the right to act in a kind of loco parentis, deciding what Maria's mother can and cannot tolerate and what is best for her psychologically in the long term? Although the surgeon might honestly feel that he or she was operating from the principle of benevolence, his or her actions also might convey an attitude of condescension, especially for a mother who later discovers that her child was denied optimal treatment because of a failure to fully inform her of her options.

Case 5: Jonah—Down Syndrome Surgery—For Whom?

Marge has arranged for a plastic surgeon to evaluate her 10-year-old son, Jonah, for facial reconstruction. Jonah was born with Down syndrome. Marge has read about Down syndrome facial surgery in which children have tongue reductions, as well as lip, nose and eyelid procedures to help make them look more attractive and also appear "less like they have Down syndrome." Jonah has been diagnosed with mild mental retardation but is well socialized and interacts with ease. His school has suggested his placement in special education classes, but Marge wants him mainstreamed into regular classes as much as possible. She feels that if he looks better, the school might see him as more capable and place him "better." The surgeon's reading of the literature suggests that tongue reduction surgery has a short-term impact and that few surgeons are still doing facial surgery for Down syndrome. Marge pleads with the surgeon to operate on her son.

Does the surgeon agree to operate? What are the alternatives? What is the most appropriate response to Jonah's mother? What ethical or social issues are raised in this case?

In this situation, it would be worthwhile to relate to Marge the findings and controversies in the literature about surgery on individuals with Down syndrome (16–18). Given its questionable long-term medical gains, one must look closely at what the benefits of the surgery would be for Jonah. Marge feels that if Jonah's appearance is "normalized" as much as possible, he will be more readily accepted by his peers and have a better chance at being successfully mainstreamed in school. Certainly, the facial features associated with Down syndrome do convey publicly that the individual is different. The question raised here is "does one try to change Jonah's face in the hope that he will be less 'stigmatized,' or does one try to make the social and cultural environment more accommodating and accepting of Jonah?" Should the child's adjustment be facilitated by improving the interactions of other children and adults with people who do not look as they do, or by making those who look different appear as "normal" as possible, physically and behaviorally?

Certainly it would be important to consult with Jonah's school counselors and special educators to learn more about Jonah's functioning at school. Although children with Down syndrome often are successfully mainstreamed in the early years (when socialization is emphasized and academic content is concrete) cognitive limitations may limit their mainstreaming opportunities in the upper grade levels where academic demands increase. If this is the case, would changing Jonah's facial appearance necessarily help him in the long term? Surgery might help to minimize the distinctive facial characteristics; however, Jonah will still be limited cognitively. At first glance, others may see Jonah as less "affected" but he will still be affected in other ways that may invite negative attention.

Another question raised is how Jonah feels about the surgery. While his parents are the decision makers by proxy (since Jonah is under 18 and has cognitive limitations) shouldn't he still be consulted? We know that Jonah is well socialized and interacts well with others but does he *feel* different in ways that adversely affect his quality of life? Perhaps he does not want to go through with the surgery and perceives it as an ordeal. To what extent should Jonah's feelings and opinions shape the treatment decision?

Clearly there are a number of social and ethical issues raised here: This is a case that has questionable medical gain and potential medical risk to the patient. It seems that a deeper discussion with Marge about her expectations for Jonah, about Jonah's expectations for himself, and about the long-term gains from surgery, would be a good place to begin sifting through these challenging issues.

Case 6: Jennifer—Child Neglect and Parental Dominance

> The Williams family brought their 3-year-old daughter, Jennifer, to the craniofacial team for evaluation and treatment. Jennifer was born with a cleft lip and palate that has yet to be treated. The parents have recently separated after a number of years of family turmoil. Neighbors have reported to the Department of Social Services (DSS) that Mr. Williams has struck both his wife and daughter when angry or intoxicated. Jennifer has not been seen for team care on a regular basis. When the family arrives at the appointment, the tension between the parents is apparent and they are both verbally short with Jennifer. Mr. Williams tells the plastic surgeon that "he and Mrs. Williams will not go through with the evaluation unless they can be present during the team conference and for all discussions that apply to the family." The team psychologist, social worker, and pediatrician wonder if this is in the best interest of the child and the team.

What is the first issue that the team must address in Jennifer's treatment? Do the Williamses have the right to attend the team's discussion?

This case raises a set of daunting issues for any team of medical professionals. Without question, the team must maximize the child's ability to access and receive appropriate and timely care. The law, in most settings, clearly mandates that the team and its professionals must report the possibility or suspicion of abuse or neglect to the DSS. However, it appears that the family has brought the child to the team for an evaluation now with the presumption that they are willing and interested in arranging for the child's treatment. A 3-year-old child with an unrepaired cleft palate is quite unusual in most team contexts, where such a surgical procedure is generally done between 12 and 18 months of age. In this case, the team must be concerned that the surgery has not as yet occurred and that customary and appropriate care has not been obtained on a regular basis. The absence of surgical intervention to this point is suggestive of parental neglect and leads to speculation about other medical problems Jennifer may have.

It seems quite clear in this case that the team must report the parents to the DSS for past medical neglect and the suspicion of abuse. However, in doing so, they likely risk driving the family away from care at a time when they have finally arrived to seek treatment. Many families perceive these reports as a betrayal of trust that they have placed in the treatment team. The team's worst fear would be that the DSS report would drive the family away and deprive the child of essential care. Given the requirement of the team to report their concerns to the DSS, how could they best prepare the family for such a report?

A particular worry for the team might be that even though the neighbors have previously reported the father to the DSS, it is apparent that this still did not result in the child's receiving needed surgical services. This fact raises a concern about the ability of the DSS to work with the family and the child's medical needs and to intervene appropriately. The team cannot evaluate the ability of the DSS to respond effectively, yet the possibility that DSS intervention will not result in a positive outcome for the child may trouble the team decision makers. A negative assessment of the DSS is certainly premature since it is quite possible that they were unaware of the daughter's cleft palate care needs.

A second set of concerns relates to the family's determination to attend the team meeting and participate in its discussions. While families have a direct interest in the team's deliberations, their presence in the actual discussion may impede the free flow of team information sharing. Professionals might feel that they need to avoid their typical "jargon" for the benefit of the parents. More importantly, the team members might censor their comments and questions about the family's social and psychological environment in order to avoid a direct confrontation with the parents. Indeed, one might consider whether the parents' motive for being present is actually to stifle discussion of possible family/marital violence and child neglect. When team members feel under direct family scrutiny during their discussions, they may avoid the discussion of these difficult and uncomfortable issues, fearing legal or personal repercussions. In such a pressured situation, team members often substitute semi-private shadow, hallway, or sidebar conversations for frank and open team discussions. On the other hand, is it paternalistic to carry on team discussions without the presence of the parents? Is there a way to assure free professional exchange and still empower the parents?

Some teams offer parents an opportunity to meet with the team leader for an interpretive session after the team conference. During this session, parents are fully informed of the team's deliberations and given an opportunity to ask any questions. This session also allows the team leader to explain the child's needs and options for care in terms that the parents can understand. On some other teams, parents have been welcomed in the team deliberations and are active participants in the discussion. However, this practice is likely uncommon. The more typical approach is for a designated representative of the team to engage the parents before and after the team meeting and allow them every opportunity to inform team discussions. The parents' demand to attend the team meeting in this case suggests a desire to frame the team discussion under their terms and thus control and direct the team's recommendations. While the parents have a right to information and autonomy, team members have a right to be protected from coercion in the best interests of the child/patient. The final decision about treatment options certainly remains with the parents unless the DSS assumes legal authority through the courts.

Every aspect of this case suggests that this family would benefit from counseling and support. The parents have separated; they are perceived as tense with one another and short with the child. The child has not received needed medical care and therefore requires a DSS family assessment. Consultation with the team's mental health professional is also clearly needed.

Case 7: James—Language Differences and Team Communication

Mr. and Ms. Santos have a 10-year-old son, James, who was born with Crouzon's Syndrome. The family is originally from the Philippines, their primary language is Tagalog and they speak little English. In addition, they live several hours away from the clinic. James needs an advancement of his mid-face. This could be done with either distraction osteogenesis or traditional (mid-facial advancement) surgery. Because of the language barrier, the team worries about the family's ability to follow through with care during distraction. Is it appropriate to simply recommend mid-face advancement surgery without telling them about distraction?

What is the appropriate treatment recommendation? What are the family's rights? What ethical or social issues are raised in this case?

This case presents significant concerns regarding communication between the treatment team and James's parents, including questions regarding linguistic competence. Simply put, do the members of the treatment team and Mr. and Mrs. Santos have a common language in which all are fluent enough to exchange critical medical and psychosocial information? Are the parents sufficiently familiar with pertinent technical dental terminology to be able to arrive at an adequate understanding of the proposed treatment options and outcomes? Health providers sometimes erroneously assume that if the patient displays a good grasp of idiomatic language, he or she will understand technical dental/medical terminology. They then proceed to present a treatment plan without further explanation or verification of what the patient (or in this case, the parents) actually has understood. Informed consent is impossible if the patient, or the parents or guardians, lack an adequate command of both idiomatic and technical language. This dilemma can arise not only among nonnative speakers but also among native speakers with language impairments. In these cases, either a trained medical interpreter or a de facto interpreter should be present. All U.S. clinics that receive federal monies from Medicaid/Medicare are legally required to provide an interpreter. Unfortunately, cost and availability make meeting this requirement unlikely in many settings.

A second level of communication issu es in this case involves the nature of the information being provided regarding treatment options and their outcomes. Is informed consent even theoretically possible if the patient is unfamiliar with other available and possibly superior, treatment modalities? It is assumed that the physician/dentist has the duty to disclose both the risks of treatment and of nontreatment, as well as the alternative options of care. If James's surgeon decides to rely on his own professional standard of disclosure, is he being paternalistic?

Examining the key assumptions that will shape what is told to the patient may be helpful in this regard. Based on the current standards of care, it is sometimes assumed that distraction osteogenesis treatment is superior to mid-facial advancement surgery. The latter typically obtains more rapid results and is easier to explain to the patient. So, the rationale for withholding information about alternative treatment options needs to be considered. Should ease of explanation of a procedure be a critical factor in determining its selection? Or should current standards of care (e.g., the superior treatment in terms of outcome) take precedence over ease of explanation and assumed capacity to understand what is involved in a more complicated treatment? This raises the question, what are the criteria for determining whether a patient or a family is linguistically and conceptually sophisticated enough to ensure appropriate follow through? Here again, the role of a trained interpreter is crucial to an optimal treatment outcome with the caveat that he or she is rarely trained to assess linguistic competence.

How should the team proceed? The first step would be to establish reliable communication among the team, the patient, and the parents. An interpreter who is fluent in Tagalog and conversant with dental/medical terminology in both languages should be included in all consultations. This person should be able to interpret for the Santos family the treatment options and risks. An interpreter will ensure the doctor about what the family has and has not understood, what they think about it, and how they wish to proceed. Then, if the team still has concerns about the parents' ability to follow through on treatment, they might wish to explore alternative arrangements for making treatment possible. For example, are there any family members or people in the parents' community who could provide support and guidance throughout this process? In this, as in most treatment cases, communication is of the essence in obtaining the best outcomes for all concerned.

CONCLUSIONS

Ethical dilemmas that arise in the routine daily practice of craniofacial surgical and team-based care may cause clinicians frustration. The lack of easily identified solutions to ethical dilemmas is inherently stressful, as is the sense of having no clear absolute principle on which to determine appropriate action. There is great value in engaging professional peers in discussion of ethical dilemmas and cases. The cleft and craniofacial team is perfectly suited to consider ethical issues that arise in the team context. The team provides a confidential setting where honed interpersonal communications permit open interprofessional dialogue. The team or the ethics committee can provide advice or consultation to the clinician with an ethical dilemma. Once an ethical dilemma is identified as such, the team and ethics committee's guidance can help clarify the issues and make decision making more balanced and judicious.

REFERENCES

1. Strauss RP, Sharp HM, Saal HM, et al. Experiencing ethical dilemmas: cases of ethical decision-making in the care of children with major craniofacial deformities. *Cleft Palate Craniofac J* 1995;32(6):494–499.
2. Ward C. *Essays on Ethics Relating to the Practice of Plastic Surgery.* Harlow, Essex, UK: The British Association of Plastic Surgeons, Churchill Livingstone, 1995.
3. Jonsen AR, Siegler M, Winslade W. *Clinical Ethics: A Practical Approach to Ethical Decisions in Clinical Medicine.* 3rd ed. New York: McGraw-Hill, 1992.
4. Beauchamp T, Childress J. *Principles of Biomedical Ethics.* 4th ed. New York: Oxford University Press, 1994.
5. English A. Treating adolescents: legal and ethic considerations. *Med Clin North Am* 1990;74:1097–1112.
6. Moshman D. Adolescent reasoning and adolescent rights. *Hum Dev* 1993;36:27–40.
7. Anderson VA, Anderson P, Northem E, et al. Development of executive functioning through late childhood and adolescence in an Australian sample. *Dev Neuropsycho* 2001;20(1):385–406.
8. Danesi M. Adolescent language as affectively coded behavior. *Adolescence* 1989;24(94):311–320.
9. Elkind D. Egocentrism in adolescence. *Child Dev* 1967;38:1025–1034.
10. Flavel J. *Cognitive Development.* Englewood, NJ: Prentice-Hall, 1977.
11. Lapsley D, Murphy M. Another look at the theoretical assumptions of adolescent egocentrism. *Dev Rev* 1985;5:201–217.
12. Halpern-Felsher BL, Millstein SG, Ellen N, et al. The role of behavioral experience in judging risks. *Health Psychol* 2001;20:120–126.
13. Millstein SG, Halpern-Felsher BL. Judgments about risk and perceived invulnerability in adolescents and young adults. *J Res Adolesc* 2002;12(4):399–422.
14. Quadrel MJ, Fischhoff BL, David W. Adolescent (in)vulnerability. *Am Psychol* 1993;48:102–116.
15. Goldberg, E. *The Executive Brain: The Frontal Lobes and the Civilized Mind.* New York: Oxford University Press, 2001.
16. Strauss RP, Mintzker Y, Feuerstein R, et al. Social perceptions of the effects of Down's Syndrome facial surgery: a school-based study of ratings by normal adolescents. *Plast Reconstr Surg* 1988;81(6):841–846.
17. Strauss RP, Feuerstein R, Mintzker Y, et al. Ordinary faces? Down Syndrome, facial surgery, active modification and social perceptions. *Am J Ment Retard* 1989;94:115–118.
18. Strauss RP, Wexler MR, Mintzker Y. Commentary on Klaiman and Arndt—facial reconstruction in Down Syndrome: perceptions of the results by parents and normal adolescents. *Cleft Palate J* 1989;26(3):190–192.

Chapter 18

Ethical Considerations in Cosmetic Surgery

Alice M. Laneader, MBe, and Paul Root Wolpe, PhD

Altering human physical appearance is as old as recorded history. Tribal people pierce, scarify, stretch, distort, deform, tattoo, file, and remove body parts in pursuit of the beauty standards of their cultures. Similar, if not identical, behaviors are found in Westernized cultures. As detailed in Chapter 3, evolutionary psychologists have linked our desire for altering the body to innate biological drives of partner selection and reproduction. In one sense, cosmetic surgery is the application of our best technology to the aesthetic standards of modern American folk culture, no different in principle from lip plates and neck rings found in other cultures throughout the world.

We currently stand at a unique point in the history of such practices. Our unprecedented ability to manipulate human physiognomy raises new questions about the nature and limits of altering the body for purposes other than curing disease. Advances such as human reproductive cloning, genetic engineering, prosthetic organs, and brain-computer interfaces are fundamentally changing what we mean by human enhancement. These advances force us to consider the extent to which we are willing to reshape ourselves, and what changes, under which conditions, will be considered acceptable (1). Cosmetic surgery, thus, serves a harbinger of our attitudes toward a host of other technologies.

Bioethical analysis of cosmetic surgery considers a number of other problematic elements as well. Critics question the ethics of undergoing surgical risk to alter appearance rather than to cure infirmity. Many modern procedures, particularly those developed in the last decade, lack a sufficient body of evidence from clinical trials to support their efficacy and safety (2–3). Risk to patients is further increased as procedures become more ambitious and patients are placed under anesthesia for longer periods of time during the course of multiple procedures. Furthermore, there is little consideration, let alone consensus, in the field as to the differences between surgical experimentation, surgical innovation, and accepted standards of practice (2–3).

In addition to medical objections, many critics are concerned with the social and cultural aspects of cosmetic surgery. By pursuing some cultural ideal of beauty, they argue, cosmetic surgery is complicit with social messages of inadequacy, of need to conform, and of the blurring of the individual in relationship to the larger social group (4–6). Pursuing media-generated ideals of beauty, cosmetic surgery, critics argue, contributes to the oppression of women and minority groups (4,7–8). The issue brings up questions of medicine's role in perpetuating, or at least cooperating with, oppressive stereotypes, as well as the degree to which cosmetic surgery, as a medical enterprise, should resist or cater to consumer desires (8).

The field of bioethics tries to identify, edify, and make prescriptive judgments about ethical issues in medicine. In so doing, it draws upon a history of philosophical analysis of ethical principles, case studies, empirical research, and historical precedent. Bioethical dilemmas are often conceptualized upon foundational principles such as respect for autonomy, beneficence, non-maleficence, and justice. For example, the Hippocratic Oath states: "I will apply dietetic measures for the benefit of the sick according to my ability and judgment; I will keep them from harm and injustice," which emphasize the duties of beneficence and non-maleficence (9). The modern American Medical Association Council on Ethical and Judicial Affairs's "Fundamental Elements of the Patient–Physician Relationship," as well as the American Nurses Association's "Code for Nurses," both discuss the respect for human dignity drawing on principles of autonomy and justice (9). The role of bioethics is to examine medical practice, the social and cultural medical environments, and emerging medical technologies to illuminate and critique the kinds of ethical principles on which they are based and the practices they pursue.

In this chapter, we will consider the ethical challenges of cosmetic surgery. In the first section, we will examine a number of basic bioethical constructs and apply them to cosmetic surgery; we will examine the enhancement versus therapy debate, risk, patient autonomy, beneficence, and informed consent. In the second section, we will examine the social and cultural challenges that cosmetic surgery poses.

BIOETHICAL CONSTRUCTS AND COSMETIC SURGERY

Enhancement Versus Therapy

Historically, the bioethical arguments surrounding cosmetic surgery have focused on the nature of altering the human form for benefits that lie on the hazy boundary between enhancement and therapy (1,10–11). Bioethicists and clinicians often have pondered the morality of medicine's role in enhancing what is normal versus restoring health to what is diseased or disfigured. Medicine, as an enterprise, is invested with a sense of mission and duty, through which it commands rights and privileges, such as the control of dangerous substances and the right to cut into human flesh. That moral authority is based on treating the sick, and, therefore, diminishes when treating an otherwise healthy and disease-free individual (11).

The fundamental nature of the ethical debate around cosmetic surgery has not changed much since the specialty began. On one side are those who see the pursuit of aesthetic improvement as either personal vanity or a lamentable submission to the superficial priority placed on appearance in a corrupted society (12). On the other side stand those who see cosmetic treatments as a legitimate means to beautify the body and who see emotional and psychological suffering attendant to real or perceived physical unattractiveness (12). The tension that lies at the heart of the ethical debates around cosmetic surgery permeates medicine today; the rise of "lifestyle drugs," for example, demonstrate the transition of pharmaceuticals from medical treatment to consumer-based products, as accessible on the Internet as in the doctor's offices (1,8).

The majority of ethical questions attendant to cosmetic surgery arise from this tension: Should cosmetic surgery be completely a matter of consumer desire, without any need for medical justification? Does that then remove it from the realm of traditional medicine? If it is to be widely used, what are correct and incorrect applications? Should cosmetic surgery, for example, be used to help people conform to evolving media messages of what is worthy or beautiful? And if the dominant culture is what is portrayed as beautiful, should cosmetic surgery be used to alter ethnic traits? Does cosmetic surgery violate some standard of justice when it is primarily available to the wealthy? What should be the standards for pediatric usage and what is the appropriate age for informed consent?

These questions do not have definitive ethical answers. Society makes these ethical decisions through its actions, and it is clear that, at present, there is general social acceptance of cosmetic surgery as an enhancement technology. The scope of these questions is currently being expanded far beyond previous limits when issues such as the appropriateness of cosmetic surgery for ethnic alteration, the advent of face transplants, and the role of surgery for children with Down syndrome (5,7–8,13–14) are now within the purview of everyday debate. As enhancement becomes more of an accepted use for medical technologies, and as those technologies improve (thereby expanding the scope of what can be enhanced) society needs to continuously assess and redefine the line between legitimate and illegitimate application of cosmetic surgery.

Beneficence and Non-maleficence

Two important complementary principles of ethical medical care are beneficence and non-maleficence (15). Beneficence, which states an ethical duty to maximize benefit and minimize risk, is similar to but can be distinct from the principle of non-maleficence, derived from the Hippocratic dictum "do no harm." Physicians have not only the charge to not cause harm to patients, but also the responsibility to weigh patient need and risk and proceed with a plan that will assure maximum benefit to the patient. If benefit to the patient is not the ultimate outcome, the principle of beneficence is violated. The basic argument over cosmetic surgery is the argument of whether the procedures ultimately harm the patient, and whether catering to the patient's desire for cosmetic change is acting in the patient's best interest. Applying beneficence in an aesthetic surgery population can be challenging. As discussed in Chapters 14 and 15, and elsewhere (16), measuring benefit, such as quality of life, is not easy and few studies on long-term positive effects of cosmetic surgery exist. In cases of significant psychopathology, the decision to forgo the procedure should be an easy one and the principle easily applied. The deeper question is whether the act of using surgical intervention on an otherwise healthy person is a violation of the principle of non-maleficence.

Autonomy

To respect autonomy is to uphold the dignity of all human life and the understanding that we all have the right to determine what will happen to our own bodies. This principle is based upon the idea that we all have the capacity to make such a choice. Patient autonomy is defined in terms of negative and positive freedoms (17). Negative freedoms include freedom from coercion by others, while positive freedoms are those that allow for self-determination, expression, and choice. As Cohen wrote, "An autonomous patient is not only someone who can say no but also a person who is sovereign in her entire decision making capacity" (17, p. 392).

However, it is sometimes difficult to balance individual autonomy against social and cultural pressures that shape desire. Informed consent includes freedom from undue influences on one's decisions. Here begins the moral hazard of advocating cosmetic surgery based solely on patient autonomy. Every culture has its ideal standard of beauty. When the pressure to conform to that ideal is reinforced by the weight of Western advertising and popular culture, it is not unreasonable to think about certain decisions to undergo cosmetic surgery as, in some general way, coerced (18). On the other hand, all decisions we make are influenced by our culture, and if physicians become the guardians of cultural appropriateness, are they simply replacing the patient's values with their own?

Our system of medicine is predicated on the assumption that, in the absence of overt evidence of coercion and with the presentation of all relevant information, each competent, mature individual should have the right to make his or her own health care decisions. The greater fundamental question may be whether cosmetic surgery constitutes health care. This is the foundational argument for those who view the practice as outside traditional medicine.

Informed Consent

Informed consent must be obtained prior to any medical intervention. There is an important distinction to be made between ethically obtained informed consent and legally effective consent (9,19). Ethical consent denotes a decision-making process based on mutual respect and full disclosure, and usually describes a process of communication between practitioner and patient over time, rather than an informed consent "moment" where a form is signed (9,19). The legal definition of informed consent focuses on the form and its discussion, and mandates disclosure of what is "reasonably prudent" (9,19).

The process of informed consent, also discussed in the following chapter, must meet a number of requirements and include a number of elements. Patients should be informed in a clear, understandable manner, usually by the surgeon performing the procedure (19). They must have sufficient time to consider the information and to ask questions, and should not be pressured for a decision before they are ready. Included in the informed consent process should be information about the nature of the procedure; the risks of the surgery and their likelihood of occurring; alternatives to the procedure that is planned, and the risks of the alternatives. The American College of Surgeons lists the following questions as necessary to answer in an informed consent interaction (20):

- What are the indications that have led your doctor to the opinion that an operation is necessary?
- What, if any, alternative treatments are available for your condition?
- What will be the likely result if you don't have the operation?
- What are the basic procedures involved in the operation?
- What are the risks?
- How is the operation expected to improve your health or quality of life?
- Is hospitalization necessary and, if so, how long can you expect to be hospitalized?
- What can you expect during your recovery period?
- When can you expect to resume normal activities?
- Are there likely to be residual effects from the operation?

Well-informed cosmetic surgery patients report experiencing less anxiety, are more compliant with instructions, cope better with complications, and express greater satisfaction with results of the surgery (21). However, the success of the informed consent process is based largely on effective communication (both written and oral) between the surgeon and the patient as well as the patient's ability to recall and understand the information provided. As discussed by Gorney in Chapter 19 and elsewhere, informed consent often fails because of poor communication skills by surgeons and because of patients' preconceived notions and expectations (22). Perhaps as a result, the number of malpractice suits filed against cosmetic surgeons which stipulate failure to adequately confer informed consent is high in comparison to other specialties.

One final difficulty with determining a patient's ability to make an autonomous decision in the context of cosmetic surgery is the existence of underlying psychological disorders that might compel a person to seek cosmetic surgery. To ask what degree a person with body dysmorphic disorder (BDD), for example, is autonomous in consenting to an aesthetic procedure is analogous to asking to what degree someone diagnosed with anorexia nervosa is able to make an autonomous choice regarding whether or not to eat. The difference is that anorexia nervosa manifests itself through distinguishable physical features such as below average body weight, while BDD may not. If the justification for performing cosmetic surgery is to improve a patient's psychosocial functioning and overall quality of life, then one cannot ignore data (reviewed in Chapter 14 and elsewhere [16]) suggesting patients with BDD show no improvement or fare worse after surgery. As discussed in Chapter 16, surgeons have some responsibility to assess for the presence of major psychiatric disorders in a prospective patient, or at least refer the patient to a trained mental health professional if one is suspected. From a bioethical perspective, one must consider that such patients may suffer diminished autonomy due to lack of decision-making capacity, and cosmetic surgeons have an ethical responsibility to make that determination before agreeing to perform surgical procedures on those patients.

Managing Risk

Risk refers to the probability of negative consequences to a desired action. Any surgical procedure contains risk, which is usually (though not always) fairly well defined before the surgery is undertaken. While the risks of cosmetic surgery, in general, are modest compared to many other types of surgery, significant risks remain. Between 1986 and 1998, for example, 40% of medical malpractice claims filed against cosmetic surgeons in Florida involved serious, permanent damage (18). During that time, there were 39 reported deaths associated with cosmetic surgery, 18 of which occurred between 1996 and 1998 (18).

While cosmetic surgical procedures do bear less risk than many other operations, it is the responsibility of any medical field to do what is needed to minimize risk. In most medical specialties, risk is self-regulated. Professional groups typically work to assure, to the extent possible, that only qualified practitioners are allowed to practice, that clinics are held to the highest medical standards, that all adverse events are reported and catalogued, that continuing education standards are maintained, and that the public is fully informed of the risks. A study conducted by the School of Public Health at the University of Texas found that cosmetic procedures performed in doctors' offices could be safer if state governments simply required doctors to report adverse incidents involving serious injury or death (23). According to the American Society of Plastic Surgeons (ASPS), 56% of cosmetic procedures in 2003 were performed in doctors' offices (24). The lack of regulation of qualifications and comprehensive reporting requirements of medical offices and ambulatory clinics has increased the risk to cosmetic surgery patients (25). If the ethical dictum is to "do no harm," and the cosmetic surgery community recognizes this risk, then it is likely time for the discipline to require professional standards and regulate practices where cosmetic surgery is performed.

Corporatizing Medicine

The influx of managed care and the pharmaceutical industry has brought a business mentality to several medical specialties. Cosmetic surgery is "bought and sold" more often in small surgical centers doing a high number of procedures. Internal competition among surgeons, false and misleading advertising, consumerism, and a marketplace delivery system make it difficult for the field to focus on the idea of "patient first" (26–28). The commercial enterprise of cosmetic surgery, with its potential for untested and fashionable gimmicry, calls into question the nature of voluntariness and the idea of full disclosure (18).

Cosmetic surgery is a medical intervention not typically covered by insurance with patients paying out of pocket for the service. In this way, the field acts like any other marketed or fee-for-service private venture. Medicine, in general, has transformed largely into a for-profit enterprise in the United States and tends to see the people it serves as consumers as much as patients. Advertising has become more common in medicine generally. However, advertisements for cosmetic surgery in the popular media and the Internet are more likely to include false and misleading statements (26–29). Miller et al., for example, argue that cosmetic surgery lies at one end of a continuum, reflecting consumer need or sovereignty rather than the compelling nature of pathology (11). The internal duties of medicine include healing the sick and curing disease. When conducting surgery on an otherwise healthy body these duties are violated. Although one can view cosmetic surgery as the "promotion and maintenance of health" (with health defined in the broadest of terms), the practice violates the internal duties required to make the discipline a legitimate medical practice (11).

Self-regulation

Plastic surgery became a recognized specialty under the American Board of Medical Specialties in 1941. Board certification in plastic surgery is not required to perform cosmetic procedures, although it is often used as a marketing tool by those who are board-certified (12). Thus, providers of cosmetic procedures may have had little or no supervised experience in performing the surgery, no formal training in specific techniques, and may even have no formal training in surgery (18). Combined with deregulated medical marketing and minimal state regulation, cosmetic surgery today requires no clinical diagnosis and no certification of the surgeon. While this is not surprising to plastic surgeons, it is often quite surprising to consumers who are often unaware of the relative absence of requirements to perform cosmetic procedures.

This relative lack of regulation occurs in a competitive environment to acquire patients not seen in any other medical specialty, and primarily in settings that are for profit. What distinguishes cosmetic surgery from other similar medical disciplines is the product: surgery that is bought and sold to alter the appearance of a healthy individual. Without considering the merits of the activity itself, surely a competitive, consumer-driven medical environment involving risk demands a set of medical standards. While recognizing the political difficulties of achieving consensus in a group accustomed to running their services as they desire, professional ethics clearly demands that the cosmetic surgery industry should be taking aggressive measures to self-regulate.

Research in Cosmetic Surgery

Like any medical or surgical procedure, cosmetic surgery should be subjected to rigorous research protocols before it is applied to patients. Any effort to create a clinical research initiative in cosmetic surgery must adhere to the highest standards of research subject protections. Human subject research ethics and regulations have been historically written on the heels of tragic events, from the Nazi doctors's trials at Nuremberg to the United States Public Health Service study of untreated syphilis on African-American men conducted in Macon County, Alabama. More recent events, including the deaths of two young adults enrolled in clinical trials at two of America's most prestigious research universities, have generated headlines and spurred the government to increased regulatory oversight to protect human subjects enrolled in clinical research.

Research in cosmetic surgery has generated similar concern. In the early 1990s, a group of cosmetic surgeons conducted a study of 21 patients to compare two different rhytidectomy procedures (30). The surgeons used two different surgical techniques, one on either side of the face, without informing patients that they were involved in the study or that they would undergo different procedures. Patients were also not informed of the increased risk of facial paralysis associated with one of the procedures. The surgeons violated human research regulations by not submitting the study to the institution's ethical review board and for not explaining to potential patients that part of the procedure was considered experimental and results could not be guaranteed. According to ethical guidelines and regulations governing human subject research, clinical research begins when an innovative and not scientifically validated practice is applied systematically to gather generalizable knowledge about its efficacy, toxicity, or side effects (31). In this case, surgeons designed a study to compare two different procedures in order to investigate which procedure provided better aesthetic results, an activity that clearly meets the ethical and regulatory definition of clinical research (15,31).

The line between surgical innovation and human experimentation is sometimes a murky one. Nevertheless, the emphasis should always be on safeguarding the health and welfare of patients or subjects. If the call to gather more defensible scientific evidence on cosmetic surgery is heeded, so must the call to perform that research while upholding the highest standards of review and human subject protections.

Similarly, there is very little regulation of the use of specific products for cosmetic purposes. For example, many cosmetic surgeons were using botulinum toxin injections for cosmetic purposes prior to its formal approval by the Food and Drug Administration in 2002. As compared to the development of other pharmaceutical interventions, there is relatively little monitoring of the efficacy and safety of cosmetic procedures and treatments, and only limited mechanisms to prevent the use of demonstrably harmful procedures (2).

The ongoing case of silicone gel-filled breast implants also illustrates this point. The implants were initially made available prior to formal Food and Drug Administration (FDA) regulatory requirements of premarketing safety and efficacy. However, a significant risk of rupture and claims of increased autoimmune disorders by women with silicone–gel implants caused the FDA to ban their use for cosmetic purposes in 1992. An FDA Advisory Panel hearing on silicone–gel implants was held in 2003. Although the initial panel recommendation was to return silicone implants back to the market, the FDA determined that silicone–gel-filled implants would remain off the market until further data on safety of the implants was provided (32–33). While cosmetic surgeons continue to praise the aesthetic result of silicone gel-filled breast implants over saline-filled implants, additional long-term, prospective clinical trials are needed to assess both physical and psychological outcomes of both types of implants.

A current debate looms over the potential to conduct the first face transplant. Doctors in England and the United States have been preparing to remove the face from a cadaver and transplant it onto a human with facial disfigurement. According to the *American Journal of Bioethics*, surgeons from the University of Louisville believe the time has come to undertake this challenge. They argue that, years ago, internal organ transplantation was considered too risky, yet it is relatively common today. However, the ethical considerations of conducting such a face transplant can not be understated. Such a procedure would require institutional review board approval and is considered human experimentation. Risks of this procedure include chronic anti-rejection medications that may cause life threatening infections and even cancer. There also is the prospect of rejection. The Louisville team believes they are ready to proceed and argues that delay is impeding scientific advancement. The question must be asked, are we rushing forward for the purposes of science or for the patients?

SOCIAL ISSUES IN COSMETIC SURGERY

Cosmetic Surgery Consumerism and the Media

As discussed in the first chapter of this book, cosmetic surgery has exploded in popularity over the past decade. Not only have the numbers of procedures increased dramatically, but the mass media's coverage of cosmetic surgery has increased as well. As noted in several chapters, in the past few years, cosmetic surgery has become the focus of a handful of "reality" television entertainment shows that depict the cosmetic surgery experience.

This bombardment of mass media coverage likely contributes to a greater acceptance of cosmetic surgery as a means by which individuals can improve their appearance (16,34). It also raises more general questions about the role of medicine in catering to human desires. Haiken has argued that consumer pressure is responsible for the rapid growth of cosmetic surgery (8). Our culture has grown increasingly receptive to the use of medicine for nontraditional goals. When medical justifications are invoked, they tend to heavily depend on psychosocial benefits that have become a justification for a host of therapies, from the use of psychopharmaceuticals for regulating moods or medicines for treating common androgenetic alopecia to prescribing human growth hormone for "normally short" boys (1). Cosmetic surgery is perhaps the most prominent example of a new focus on lifestyle medicine, where tools that had previously been viewed by the culture as appropriate only for therapeutic goals now are finding broader application as consumer products.

This point leads us to consider the implications of our appetite for perfection both on the individual and societal level. In addition, it provides an avenue to consider the limits of proper capitulation to consumer desires. For example, it is not uncommon for parents to request cosmetic alteration the appearance of children with Down syndrome (5). Yet the physical changes cannot mask the cognitive disabilities of this condition, and the struggle to live up to some idea of "normalcy" for these patients often leads to frustration (5). If the purpose of cosmetic surgery is to enhance one's well-being and self-image, we must be sure that it meets that goal intended, and that the risks to the patient are not too great.

Cosmetic Surgery as a Gendered Activity

Feminist scholars have written extensively about the use of cosmetic surgery. Most argue that women seek surgery to attain some socially constructed image of the ideal female body (4–5,35). They have asked: As women endure a barrage of overt and subliminal media messages, how much control or autonomy do they truly have over the desire to undergo cosmetic surgery? Sullivan has argued that cosmetic surgery is not pursued by a truly autonomous individual, but by people embedded in a society's narrowing definition of beauty driven by constant influx of media images (18). The vast majority of the patients who underwent cosmetic surgery in 2004 were women (24). Few achieved the ideal images that television, magazines, and advertisements portray. Other feminists have suggested that these cultural images continue to stir a "pedagogy of defect" through which women learn that some of their body parts are faulty or imperfect (4,35). Under the pressures of media images of the female form, they argue, to say that a woman is free to choose a cosmetic procedure is a fallacy.

In contrast, other scholars wonder whether cosmetic surgery can be used (at times) as a mode of empowerment for women (4–5). The notion of "female agency" can be used to acknowledge the societal influences on the decision to seek surgery, but embrace individual choice and personal power (4). While accepting the argument about the cultural interplay around ideals of beauty, they believe that women are still powerful autonomous agents not so easily fooled. Thus, although agreeing that the desire for cosmetic surgery is a result of cultural complicity with certain female norms, they argue that women are still strong and independent, and can be empowered to make their own decisions regarding their appearance. Supporting this idea, several studies have indicated that women who seek breast augmentation surgery are more strongly motivated by their own sense of self-esteem than a desire to please romantic partners or friends (36–37). But, of course, why must their self-esteem derive from the size of their completely healthy breasts?

The experience of some Moroccan women more clearly illustrates how cosmetic surgery can be a tool of women's empowerment. Many Moroccan women are given tattoos as a sign of their ownership by others, in a manner not dissimilar to numbers tattooed on the arms of Nazi concentration camp victims (35). Some women, upon immigrating to the Netherlands, requested removal of these tattoos. The Netherlands is the only society where cosmetic surgery has been allowed under a national health plan. However, surgeries are only reimbursed if they are deemed necessary to return an individual to "normal function." The difficulty in defining normalcy has plagued the system since its inception. As cosmetic surgery became more prevalent and more requests for surgery were made, justification for providing and denying coverage became difficult. In the case of the Moroccan women, the Dutch government granted their request, based upon psychological suffering. In an act of empowerment, these Moroccan women wanted the legacy of their former enslavement removed via a cosmetic procedure.

Cosmetic Surgery and Definitions of "Normalcy"

Historically, the goal of cosmetic surgery is to improve the appearance of an individual with a "normal" appearance. "Normalcy" can be defined in either in anthropomorphic terms or in reference to psychosocial functioning and quality of life and, therefore, can be distinguished from disease or illness (10,38–39). Such definitions have significant problems. Some have argued that "normalcy" cannot be operationally defined and is based on the subjective perception of the individual (1,38). For example, a child may have protruding ears that are "normal" in terms of function, but could be considered aesthetically "abnormal" by the child, his parents, or a plastic surgeon. These judgments of normalcy lie on a continuum and may be viewed differently not only by the individual, but also society. Society may deem a cleft lip as abnormal in appearance and allow, in fact encourage, the use of cosmetic surgery to correct it, while a prominent nose may be considered within the realm of "normal" and, therefore, be seen as a less acceptable reason to undergo surgical intervention.

Daniels has tried to articulate an argument for determining normal function (38). He suggests that the goal of medicine is to bring people back to "species-typical" functioning, the basic level of functioning he believes the species is "designed for." Species-typical functioning is not a statistical average of function or form, but is defined by the way the species is designed to negotiate its environment. This moral dilemma is illustrated with the example of two boys, Billy and Johnny.

CASE EXAMPLE

Case 1: Billy and Johnny

> Billy's parents are both short and it appears that Billy will not grow to be taller than 5′3″. Johnny suffers from a tumor on his pituitary gland that leads to a deficit in growth hormone that will cause him to grow no taller than 5′3″. Both boys will have the same outcome—short stature. Is it fair or just to offer treatment with growth hormone only to Johnny and not Billy, because Johnny is "sick" while Billy is "normally" 5′3″? What if we discover the gene for Billy's short stature? Then, is short stature a "disease" amenable (eventually) to gene therapy? What it if is discovered that shorter people have cells less sensitive to growth hormone? Is Billy's short stature now considered a medical syndrome?

Daniels argues that looking at species typicality would have us judge the outcome, rather than the cause, and render these questions moot. Medicine has the obligation to restore that functioning to the degree it can, whether or not the lack of function is due to "disease."

How well does Daniels' argument extend to cosmetic surgery? For example, if a young man breaks his nose playing soccer, causing it to be misaligned from its original position, reconstructive surgery, with the goal of returning the nose to its previous appearance, is indicated. Is it fair or just to deny a second young man born with a similarly crooked nose surgical correction because it would be for mere enhancement? From this perspective, denying treatment to the second young man would be unjust. On the other hand, Daniels also argues that natural differences are acceptable, even if some are more desirable from society's standpoint (38). Thus, society does not have an obligation to help people improve beyond what is typical appearance. This defines species-typical function.

Recent pharmaceutical and biotechnological products are making the species-typical argument even more challenging. Many advances in modern medicine do not align with the ideals of mitigating and curing disease. Products for erectile dysfunction, psychopharmaceuticals to manage mood states, and the widespread use of psychiatric drugs for conditions such as attention deficit hyperactivity disorder are tolerated, and even subsidized, by society, often without convincing evidence of pathological processes at work (1). Kass, Chairman of the President's Council on Bioethics, contends that gains in health and longevity have not produced contentment but an appetite for greater perfection, and that the quest for improvement rather than treatment of disease can never ultimately be satisfied (40).

Cosmetic Surgery and Ethnicity

Cosmetic procedures also have the potential to modify the outward manifestations of ethnicity. In his book, *Making the Body Beautiful*, Gilman credits race as the impetus for the field of aesthetic surgery (7). Some have argued that cosmetic surgeons, as influential elements of society, have a responsibility to stop perpetuating potentially oppressive social ideals of beauty and ethnicity by catering to those who want to alter their appearance to emulate those ideals (41). This falls under the umbrella of what has been described as the "ethics of complicity" (42). If a particular aesthetic procedure is one that perpetuates stigmatization or discrimination, even through the promotion of the physical features of another ethnic group, then it is morally suspect to perform the surgery. For example, bleaching the skin of African-Americans to make them appear whiter, supports the cultural dominance of one ethinicity over others in a particular society.

Davis suggests that cosmetic surgery to erase ethnic features "evokes ambivalence" toward racism (5). Throughout history, minority groups have emulated the dress and appearance of majority groups as a potential pathway to assimilation (7). For example, the popularity of rhinoplasty among first and second generation Jews in the mid-20th century reflected an internalization of the Christian claim that the nose was the symbol of Jewish physiognomy and, thus, the locus both of Jews' character traits and their inability to assimilate (43). The issue is not unique to American culture; cosmetic alteration of the nose and eyes are extremely popular in Asian countries as people desire a more Western look. While it is unfair to ask the cosmetic surgeon to be the arbiter of what are deeper cultural undercurrents in society, he or she should be aware that the surgical enhancement of appearance contributes to those forces.

Cosmetic Surgery in Pediatric Populations

In 2004, 4% of all cosmetic procedures were performed on people 18 years of age or younger (24). The increase in the number of adolescent cosmetic procedures over the past several years raises some interesting questions. As discussed in Chapter 16, one issue for the cosmetic surgeon is deciding whether or not to operate on an adolescent during a period of rapid physical and psychological development. A second issue is related to the relative absence of empirical data supporting the long-term psychosocial benefits of cosmetic procedures.

In 2004, the ASPS issued a policy regarding teenage breast augmentation stating that, in accordance with the FDA approval of saline-filled implants, potential patients should be at least 18 years old (44). Hilhorst has argued that because of the psychosocial development and emotional turmoil particular to adolescents, adolescents should not undergo cosmetic surgery if they do not meet standards of stable decision making and balanced judgment (45). On the other hand, some adolescents undergo real suffering as a result of appearance-related teasing. While some argue that the more valuable lesson is to learn to stand up for oneself or to persevere in the face of adversity, the suffering is real, and surgery is sometimes a solution. The clear ethical mandate is that cosmetic surgery should never be done on adolescents casually, that it should generally be discouraged and only undertaken after thoughtful consideration and in cases of compelling need.

Cosmetic Surgery and Social Justice

It is relatively easy to criticize the American preoccupation with enhancements, such as cosmetic surgery, while living in a world riddled with disease and famine (40). Even if we, as a society, deem something as appropriate for surgical correction, what is our responsibility to assure just allocation of resources? Open debate over just allocation of medical treatment is a process that most Western, industrialized countries have had to face head-on through the establishment of universal medical coverage, but which America has avoided through its system of private insurance. Nevertheless, enhancement technology challenges our notions of distributive justice (38). Should only those with the ability to pay out of pocket have access to cosmetic surgery? And if not, where do we draw the line as to what kinds of cosmetic conditions or perceived abnormalities should our society feel an obligation to help ameliorate? The ambiguity inherent in our definitions of normalcy contributes to the difficulties in determining what health is, and, therefore, how treatment should be allocated to each member of society.

Where cosmetic surgery for enhancement alone can be clearly defined—for example, in a woman wanting to increase her otherwise normal breasts—society has clearly decided that it has no obligation to compensate the person desiring the change. However, there is a larger gray area. What kinds of appearance—buck teeth, protruding ears, mild cleft lip, port-wine stains—reach the threshold that would demand a just society help pay for amelioration? The question will only become more difficult as new enhancement pharmaceuticals and procedures are developed.

CONCLUSIONS

In this chapter we have examined the underlying ethical dilemmas facing cosmetic surgery. The role of bioethics is to pose theoretical discussion regarding the way medical care and clinical research is conducted. The increase in the demand for aesthetic procedures and the advocacy of the practice in the popular media have raised provocative questions of the circumstances under which cosmetic surgery is ethical, merely permissible, or should be resisted. Cosmetic surgery calls into question the use of medicine for reasons other than prevention of illness and treatment of disease. It also raises the question of appropriate risk—risk to the patient with procedures not scientifically validated through well designed research, risk through an increase in the number of procedures one person goes through in a given surgery, the risk to minorities including stereotyping of women and loss of ethnicity, and the risk of applying cosmetic procedures to conditions such as Down syndrome and what that says to those with such cognitive and physical conditions.

The steps needed to improve the moral standing of cosmetic surgery are clear. Scientific evidence of the safety and efficacy of cosmetic procedures and devices is needed to assure that patients are only exposed to those interventions that have been deemed safe through critical evaluation. Clear distinctions should be made between "innovation" and human experimentation. Certification requirements for all cosmetic surgeons and closer regulation of medical offices and ambulatory facilities can only increase quality and protect patients. We also need to look ahead to future dilemmas surrounding social justice and moral allocation of resources. We need to consider now, before the first face transplant, the potential for abuse and misuse of the practice.

Cosmetic surgery is a testing ground for our attempt to balance beneficence and autonomy. A person's desire for cosmetic surgery and consent to a procedure does not automatically make one an appropriate surgical candidate. A physician can respect the patient's autonomous decision, but deny surgery if the physician feels the patient will not benefit from the surgery, or that the patient is not mature or competent enough to consider all the ramifications of the procedure. Surgeons also need to be cognizant of their actions when conducting a cosmetic procedure that may enforce a cultural norm. Finally, we all need to respect advances in technology and be wary of their overuse. Cosmetic surgery has made tremendous advances over the last 40 years. Yet, it raises the eternal question of what we are really trying to achieve by altering ourselves, and whether cosmetic surgery can contribute to making us content with who we are.

REFERENCES

1. Wolpe PR. Treatment, enhancement, and the ethics of neurotherapeutics. *Brain and Cogn* 2002;50:387–395.
2. Ward CM. Surgical research, experimentation and innovation. *Br J Plast Surg* 1994;47:9–94.
3. Yarborough M. Collagen injections, a case study in the erosion of the medical profession. *Arch Otolaryngol Head Neck Surg* 1991;117:270–272.
4. Bordo S. Braveheart, Babe, and the contemporary body. In: Parens E, ed. *Enhancing Human Traits*. Washington, DC: Georgetown University Press, 1998:189–220.
5. Davis K. *Dubious Equalities & Embodied Differences: Cultural Studies on Cosmetic Surgery*. Lanham, MD: Rowman and Littlefield, 2003.
6. Angell M. *Science on Trial*. New York: W.W. Norton and Company, 1996.
7. Gilman S. *Making the Body Beautiful: A Cultural History of Aesthetic Surgery*. Princeton, NJ: Princeton University Press, 1999.
8. Haiken E. *Venus Envy*. Baltimore, MD: Johns Hopkins University Press, 1997.
9. Beauchamp TL, Walters L. *Contemporary Issues in Bioethics*. Belmont, CA: Wadsworth Publishing Company, 1994.
10. McGee G. Ethical issues in enhancement: an introduction. *Camb Q Healthc Ethics* 2000;9:299–303.
11. Miller FG, Brody H, Chung KC. Cosmetic surgery and the internal morality of medicine. *Camb Q Healthc Ethics* 2000;9:354–364.
12. Haiken E. The history of cosmetic surgery. In: Kanimer MS, Dover JS, Arndt KA, eds. *Atlas of Cosmetic Surgery*. Philadelphia: WB Saunders, 2002:3–15.
13. Wiggins OP, Barker JH, Cunningham M, et al. On the ethics of facial transplantation research. *Am J Bioeth* 2004;4:1–12.
14. The American Society of Plastic Surgery. *Science Fiction of Face Transplants May Be Closer Than You Think* [American Society of Plastic Surgery Web site]. May 6, 2004. Available at: http://www.plasticsurgery.org/news_room/press_releases/Science-Fiction-of-FaceTransplants.cfm. Accessed on January 2, 2005.
15. The National Commission for the Protection of Human Subjects of Biomedical and Behavioral Research. The Belmont Report, Ethical Principles and Guidelines for the Protection of Human Subjects of Research. April 18, 1979.
16. Sarwer DB, Crerand CE. Body image and cosmetic medical treatments. *Body Image: An International Journal of Research* 2004;1:99–111.
17. Cohen J. Patient autonomy and social fairness. *Camb Q Healthc Ethics* 2000;9:391–399.
18. Sullivan DA. *Cosmetic Surgery: The Cutting Edge of Commercial Medicine in America*. New Brunswick, NJ: Rutgers University Press, 2001.
19. Ward CM. Consenting and consulting for cosmetic surgery. *Br J Plast Surg* 1998;51:547–550.
20. Public Information from the American College of Surgeons. http://www.facs.org/public_info/operation/consent.html#princi Last accessed January 2, 2005.
21. Redden EM, Baker DM, Meisel A. The patient, the plastic surgeon and informed consent: new insights into old problems. *Plast Reconstr Surg* 1985;75:270–275.
22. Gorney M. Medical malpractice and plastic surgery: the carrier's point of view. In: Goldwyn RM, Cohen MN, eds. *The Unfavorable Result in Plastic Surgery*. Philadelphia: Lippincott Williams & Wilkins, 2001:38–43.
23. Balkrishnan R, Gill IK, Vallee JA, Feldman SR. No smoking gun: findings from a national survey of office-based cosmetic surgery adverse event reporting. *Dermatol Surg* 2003;29:1093–1099.
24. *2005 Report of the 2004 National Clearinghouse of Plastic Surgery Statistics*. Arlington Heights, IL: American Society of Plastic Surgeons, 2005.

25. The American Society of Plastic Surgery. Some Cosmetic Plastic Surgery Patients Continue to Place Themselves at Risk. [American Society of Plastic Surgery Web site]. April 27, 2004. Available at: http://www.plasticsurgery.org/news_room/press_releases/Cosmetic-Plastic-Surgery-Patients-At-Risk.cfm Accessed January 2, 2005.
26. Spilson SV, Chung KC, Greenfield ML, Walters M. Are plastic surgery advertisements conforming to the ethical codes of the American Society of Plastic Surgeons? *Plast Reconstr Surg* 2002;109:1181–1186.
27. Sullivan P. Plastic surgeons take advantage of relaxed rules, launch ad campaigns. *Can Med Assoc J* 1992;146:55–57.
28. Rohrich RJ. The market of plastic surgery: cosmetic surgery for sale—at what price? *Plast Reconstr Surg* 2001;107:1845–1847.
29. Jejurikar SS, Rovak JM, Kuzon WM, et al. Evaluation of plastic surgery information on the Internet. *Ann Plast Surg* 2002;49:460–465.
30. Ivy EJ, Lorenc PZ, Aston SJ. Is there a difference? A prospective study comparing lateral and standard SMAS face lifts with extended SMAS and composite rhytidectomies. *Plast Reconstr Surg* 1996;98:1135–1143.
31. Protection of Human Subjects. Code of Federal Regulations Title 45 Public Welfare, Department of Health and Human Services, National Institutes of Health and Office of Protection from Research Risks (currently Office of Human Research Protections) Part 46. Revised November 13, 2001. Effective December 13, 2001.
32. FDA Advisory Committee Meeting, General and Plastic Surgery Device Panels [transcript]. October 14–15, 2003.
33. FDA Decision on Silicone Gel-Filled Breast Implants [transcript]. FDA Patient Safety News: Show #25, March 2004.
34. Sarwer DB, Grossbart TA, Didie ER. Beauty and society. *Semin Cutan Med Surg* 2003;22:79–92.
35. Davis K. *Reshaping the Female Body: The Dilemma of Cosmetic Surgery.* New York: Routledge, 1995.
36. Cash TF, Duel LA, and Perkins LL. Women's psychosocial outcomes of breast augmentation with silicone gel-filled implants: a 2-year prospective study. *Plast Reconstr Surg* 2002;109:2112–2123.
37. Didie ER, Sarwer DB. Factors that influence the decision to undergo cosmetic breast augmentation surgery. *J Womens Health* 2003;12:241–253.
38. Daniels N. Normal function and the treatment-enhancement distinction. *Camb Q Healthc Ethics* 2000;9:309–322.
39. de Chalain T. Ethical resource allocation and the quest for normalcy: is pediatric reconstructive surgery justified? *Plast Reconstr Surg* 1997;99:1184–1191.
40. Kass LR. Ageless bodies, happy souls: biotechnology and the pursuit of perfection. *The New Atlantis* Spring 2003;Volume 1.
41. Strauss RP. Ethical and social concerns in facial surgical decision making. *Plast Reconstr Surg* 1983;72:727–730.
42. Little MO. Cosmetic surgery, suspect norms and ethics of complicity. In: Parens E, ed. *Enhancing Human Traits.* Washington, DC: Georgetown University Press, 1998:162–175.
43. Geller J. (G)nos(e)ology: the cultural construction of the other. In: Eilberg-Schwartz H, ed. *People of the Bod—Jews and Judaism from an Embodied Perspective* Albany: State University of New York Press, 1992.
44. American Society of Plastic Surgery. Teens should be 18 for Breast Augmentation [transcript]. ASPS Recommends. December 22, 2004.
45. Hilhorst MT. Philosophical pitfalls in cosmetic surgery: a case of rhinoplasty during adolescence. *Medical Humanities* 2002;28:61–66.

Chapter 19

Professional and Legal Considerations in Cosmetic Surgery

Mark Gorney, MD

Unfortunately, in the lengthy process of postgraduate surgical education, the vast majority of candidates for certification by the American boards of plastic surgery, otolaryngology, or dermatology typically fail to acquire any real feeling for the interface between cosmetic surgery and mental health. Virtually all professionals enter the early part of their careers filled with knowledge of the latest techniques on the cutting edge of their specialty, but have only the vaguest sense of the critical importance of appropriate patient selection criteria for cosmetic procedures—an absolute essential in the building of a successful career.

There is little disagreement between cosmetic surgeons and mental health professionals that patients who display symptoms of severe psychopathology constitute poor candidates for aesthetic surgery. However, many psychiatric diagnoses, including body dysmorphic disorder and eating disorders (as discussed in Chapters 14 and 15) come in several shades of gray. Patients who present with mild forms of psychopathology likely present the greatest challenge to the surgeon's psychological assessment skills. To make matters even more confusing, most experienced cosmetic surgeons can point to patients in their practices who presented with minimal to moderate deformity but excessive concern with their appearance, but who, after a well-executed procedure, displayed psychological improvement.

How should the surgeon treat the patient who presents with significant psychological distress? As suggested in Chapter 16, learning to say "no" to a patient's requests for surgery may seem easy, but it is far more complicated then it appears. Referral to a psychiatrist or psychologist often results in an angry patient who walks out and will likely, sooner or later, have the procedure performed by another professional. Perhaps the most reasonable course left to the surgeon is to learn, as early as possible in his or her career, to carefully select patients among the shades of gray, and, where uncertainty exists, to fall back on the counsel of more experienced colleagues or a trusted mental health professional. Failure to do so universally produces headaches for the surgeon and his or her staff far beyond the value of any surgical fee. In its ultimate (but thankfully rare) form, ignoring these red flags has cost at least five surgeons their lives in the past two decades. All were shot to death by a disturbed patient dissatisfied with his or her results.

The issue of patient selection is further compounded by at least two factors. The first is the unending love affair between the mass media and the universe of cosmetic surgery and related treatments. As discussed by Sarwer and Magee in Chapter 3, cosmetic surgery is an incredibly popular topic for both the print and electronic media. The avalanche of publicity is inevitably accompanied by the usual ballyhoo promising improvements as dramatic as they are trouble-free. This mass media attention likely contributes to increasing numbers of women and men who seek cosmetic procedures each year. The second factor is political. In the late 1980s, the United States

Federal Trade Commission embarked on a misguided attempt to reduce the cost of medical care by forcing specialty societies to rescind their traditional prohibition of public advertising. It was their theory that advertising would create greater competition and lower medical costs. The first of these premises resulted in a flood of deceptive advertisements that made the distinction between authentic specialists and self-designated individuals difficult, if not impossible, for the typical consumer to comprehend. The second premise, lowering costs, was a dismal failure, as evidenced by the dramatic rise in medical costs. These outcomes further confused the definition of adequate surgical training qualifications and quickly added a carnival midway patina to the universe of cosmetic surgery.

To those whose primary responsibility is the maintenance of the highest quality in surgical competence, the continuous dramatic changes in medicine have added a steadily growing challenge and an increasingly heavier burden. As a result, the interface between elective cosmetic surgery and the specter of medical liability is as complex as perhaps at any previous time in history. Of all medical specialists, the plastic surgeon's exposure to professional liability is unique in at least two respects. First, the plastic surgeon who performs elective aesthetic surgery is not assuming the care of a sick or injured patient to make him or her *well*. Rather he or she is treating a well patient with the goal of making him or her *better*. Second, the patient judges the results of the treatment according to standards that are entirely subjective. The actual result may be good, but if it does not meet the patient's expectations, the procedure may be judged a failure.

This chapter discusses both professional and legal considerations in cosmetic surgery. Building on related discussions in Chapters 2 and 16, the chapter begins with an overview of issues related to patient selection, particularly as they related to the specter of legal actions against the surgeon. Legal principals such as "standards of care," "warranty," and "disclosure" as they apply to cosmetic surgery, are reviewed. Chapter 18 discussed informed consent from a bioethical prospective. This chapter discusses issues related to informed consent with a more concentrated focus on the relationship between the cosmetic surgeon and patient. The chapter concludes with an overview of the most common causes of legal actions related to specific cosmetic procedures.

PATIENT SELECTION

Contemporary plastic surgeons practicing in the United States will find it virtually impossible to end their careers unblemished by a claim of malpractice. Well over half of these claims, however, are likely preventable. Most, at least indirectly are based on failures in patient selection, not on technical faults with the specific procedure. Patient selection in cosmetic surgery is the ultimate inexact science. It is a mixture of surgical judgment and experience, ego strength and gut feelings, personality interactions, and regrettably, often economic considerations (1–2). Regardless of technical ability, a surgeon who appears cold, arrogant, or insensitive is more likely to be sued than one who relates to the patient on a "personal" level. Obviously, a person who is warm, sensitive, naturally caring, with a well-developed sense of humor, is less likely to be the target of a malpractice claim. The ability to communicate clearly is probably the most outstanding characteristic of the claims-free surgeon. Communication is the *sine qua non* of building a successful doctor–patient relationship. Decades ago, communications skills training and other courses on "doctoring" were absent from most, if not all, medical school curriculum. Today, an increasing number of medical schools not only offer such courses as electives, but also have them as part of the required curriculum. While basic communication skills can be taught, the most effective communicators likely have incorporated these skills into their personality (1).

Perhaps the greatest challenge for the practicing surgeon is to communicate effectively with the "difficult" patient. As discussed in Chapter 2, these patients can present in many different forms and are often dealing with significant psychological issues. As a result, they can represent a management problem for the surgeon and staff. The discussion in this chapter will focus on the types of patients, who as a result of their interactions with the surgeon or experiences postoperatively, may be more likely to threaten or bring legal action against the surgeon (1–2).

Unrealistic Patients

Some patients have unrealistic and idealized, but also vague, conceptions of what cosmetic surgery is going to do for them. Some anticipate that they will undergo "Cinderella-like" transformations in their appearance, perhaps fueled by the atypical results regularly depicted on television programs such as *The Swan* and *Extreme Makeover* (3). Other patients may bring with them photographs or drawings, either of themselves or Hollywood celebrities, depicting the desired changes in appearance. These patients should be managed with great caution. They typically have little comprehension that the surgeon is dealing with human flesh and blood, not wood or clay.

Others may expect that surgery will improve their employment or social status, anticipating a major change in lifestyle with immediate recognition of their newly acquired attractiveness. These patients have an unrealistic concept of where their surgical journey is taking them and, more often than not, are likely setting themselves up for significant postoperative disappointment. Such patients show little flexibility in accepting any failure on the part of the surgeon to deliver what was anticipated. As discussed below, this disappointment of unmet expectations can play an important role in the issue of informed consent.

Indecisive Patients

In contrast to the patient with unrealistic expectations, the indecisive patient may experience great difficulty in articulating appearance concerns to the surgeon. In turn, he or she may consider the surgeon to be a "beauty expert" and rely on that expertise, rather than his or her own sense of dissatisfaction with a specific appearance feature, to direct the course of treatment. This patient may say to the surgeon, "You are the expert, what would you suggest I do?" or "Do you think I ought to have this done?" The prudent surgeon should respond, "This is a decision that I cannot make for you. It is one you have to make yourself. I can tell you what I think we can achieve, but if you have any doubt whatsoever, I recommend strongly that you think about it carefully before deciding whether or not to accept the risks that I have discussed with you." The more the decision to undergo surgery is motivated from within and not "sold," the less likely legal recrimination will follow an unfavorable result.

Some patients may present as indecisive as a function of specific life circumstances. Some, regardless of their chronological age, may have rather immature, excessively romantic, and a highly unrealistic concept of what the surgery will achieve. Often when confronted with the mirror postoperatively, they are prone to react in disconcerting fashion if the degree of change achieved does not coincide with their preconceived notions. Others may be indecisive as a result of familial disapproval. A less-than-ideal postoperative result may produce a "See, I told you so!" reaction from family members, which deepens the guilt and dissatisfaction. Patients with an excessive need for secrecy, such as those who request the use of aliases or require appointments at unusual times, also may be experiencing some indecisiveness about the procedure. Such accommodations, while not only difficult to achieve, likely hint at a degree of indecisiveness, if not excessive paranoia, about cosmetic surgery.

"Surgiholic" Patients

Also referred to as the "insatiable patient" (4), the "surgiholic" patient typically has had a variety of plastic surgery procedures performed either on the same or different physical feature. As discussed in Chapters 14 and 16, as well as in other work by Sarwer et al. (3,5–10), many of the historical descriptions of these patients are consistent with the present-day diagnosis of body dysmorphic disorder (BDD). In these situations, not only is the surgeon likely confronted by a severe psychiatric illness, but, in the case of repeated procedures on the same feature, must also deal with a difficult anatomical situation. Often, these patients will make unfavorable comparisons to the previous surgeries and surgeons. No matter how much the surgeon may be tempted to play the role of the "White Knight" who finally "saves" the troubled patient, the percentage of achievable improvement isn't worth the risk of the procedure. As discussed in Chapter 16, these individuals are likely better treated by a qualified mental health professional than by another cosmetic procedure.

Unlikable Patients

Regardless of the surgeon's personality, in life there are people whom you simply do not like or who do not like you. An experienced surgeon knows within minutes of entering the examining room whether or not he or she will be operating on a given patient. Accepting a patient who is disliked is a serious mistake. A clash of personalities, for whatever reason, is bound to affect the outcome of the case, regardless of the actual quality of the postoperative result. Furthermore, such a relationship is likely to make dealing with an unanticipated result even more difficult. No matter how interesting such a case may appear, it is far better to decline the patient.

General Considerations

The diagram in Figure 19-1 historically has been used to assist in the patient selection process (1,11). The patient's objective deformity, as judged by the surgeon, is represented along the horizontal axis. The patient's degree of concern over that deformity is represented on the vertical axis. When considered together, two opposite extremes emerge.

1. The patient with major deformity but minimal concern (lower right corner). This is a patient with an obvious major deformity in whom any degree of improvement likely will be regarded with satisfaction.
2. The patient with the minor deformity but extreme concern (upper left corner). This, in contrast, is the patient with a deformity that the surgeon perceives to be minor, but who demonstrates an inordinate degree of concern and emotional turmoil. Most individuals with BDD will fall here. These are the patients who are most likely to be dissatisfied with any outcome.

Most patients who seek aesthetic surgery fit somewhere on a diagonal between the two extremes. The closer the patient comes to the upper left corner, the more likely an unfavorably perceived outcome (as well as a potential threat of legal action) may be.

For some individuals, the physical deformity really *is* at the center of the patient's psychological fragility. There are many examples of beneficial change wrought through successful aesthetic surgery. Nonetheless, the odds for an unfavorable result and subsequent legal action are much greater when the comparison between the objective deformity and the distress it creates in the patient is out of proportion. The surgeon is cautioned to search for appropriate psychological balance and lean strongly against surgery in those cases were there is doubt.

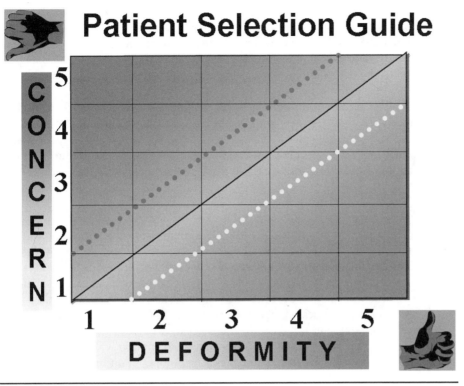

FIGURE 19-1. Patient selection guide.

Generally speaking, there is a clear risk-benefit ratio to every surgical procedure. If the risk-benefit ratio is favorable, the surgery should probably be encouraged. If the risk-benefit ratio is unfavorable, the reverse not only applies, but the unintended consequences of the unfavorable outcome may turn out to be disproportionate to the surgical result. The only way to avoid this debacle is to learn how to distinguish those patients whose personality characteristics make them unsuitable for cosmetic surgery.

As the marketing of cosmetic surgery grows worldwide, there is greater probability that increasing numbers of persons who are psychologically inappropriate for surgery will, nevertheless, see the surgeon's scalpel as an answer to their problem. With the rising number of practitioners in many specialties now offering cosmetic procedures, competitive and economic pressures likely influence patient selection criteria. Since patients with BDD and other significant psychiatric problems rarely admit these problems during the initial consultation with the plastic surgeon, the onus of determining patient appropriateness falls exclusively on the surgeon. In these cases, the surgeon should strive to reduce the influence of competitive and economic factors (let alone pure ego) in the decision to proceed with surgical treatment.

LEGAL PRINCIPLES APPLIED TO PLASTIC SURGERY

Several legal principles apply to the successful practice of plastic surgery (1,11). Of particular importance are issues related to standard of care, warranty, and disclosure.

Standard of Care

Malpractice generally means treatment that is contrary to accepted medical standards and that produces injurious results to the patient. Most medical malpractice actions are based on laws governing negligence. Thus, the cause of action is usually the failure of the defendant–physician to exercise that reasonable degree of care ordinarily possessed by others of the same profession in the community. Whereas in the past, the term *community* was accepted geographically, it is now based on the supposition that all doctors keep up with the latest developments in their field. Community, then, is generally interpreted as a "specialty community." The standards are now generally those of the specialty as a whole without regard to geographic location. This series of norms is commonly referred to as "standard of care."

Warranty

By merely engaging to render treatment, a doctor warrants that he or she has the learning and skill of the average member of that specialty and that he or she will apply that learning and skill with ordinary and reasonable care. This warranty is one of due care. It is legally implied—it need not be mentioned by the physician or the patient. The warranty, however, is one of service, not cure. If, for example, a surgeon removes a malignant lesion that is demonstrated to be completely excised by pathological exam, but later it recurs, this does not mean that he or she is guilty of negligence. Thus, the doctor does not imply that the operation will be a success, or that results will be favorable, or that he or she will not commit any medical errors *not* caused by lack of skill or care.

Disclosure

Disclosure involves informing a patient of the aspects of a given procedure before they provide informed consent. While attempting to define the yardstick of disclosure, the courts divide medical and surgical procedures into two categories. The first involves common procedures that carry minor or remote serious risk (including serious bodily harm or death), such as the administration of antibiotics. The second encompasses procedures involving serious risks for which the doctor has an "affirmative duty" to disclose the potential of serious harm or death and is bound to explain in detail the complications that might possibly occur.

Affirmative duty means that the physician is obliged to disclose risks on his or her own, without waiting for the patient to ask. The courts have long held that it is the patient, not the physician, who has the prerogative of determining what is in his or her best interests. Thus, the surgeon is legally obligated to discuss with the patient therapeutic alternatives and their particular hazards in order to provide sufficient information to allow the patient to determine his or her own best interest.

A balance of legal requirements and medical judgment dictates the level of detail in the explanation of a procedure. It is simply not possible to tell a patient "everything" without unnecessarily dissuading him or her from appropriate treatment. Rather, the law holds that the patient must be told the most probable of known dangers and the percent likelihood that they may occur. More remote risks may be disclosed in general terms, while placing them in a context of suffering from any unusual event. Does the patient have the legal right to make a bad judgment because he or she fears a possible complication? Increasingly, the courts answer affirmatively. In a case where breast reconstruction is indicated, for example, the patient often faces the choice between the uses of breast prostheses or autonogolous transplanted tissue. If the physician has provided the patient with information on the difference in both modalities of treatment, and consequences as well as anticipated possible complications results have been fully explained and documented, then he or she has fully discharged his or her responsibility of disclosure. The weighing of risks is usually not a medical judgment, but is, instead, reserved for the patient.

Obviously, the most common complications should be volunteered frankly and openly. Their probability, based on the surgeon's personal experience, also should be discussed. Finally, a discussion of any or all of this information is essentially meaningless unless it is documented in the patient's record. For legal purposes, if it is not in the record, it never happened.

Informed Consent

For many decades, the practice of medicine has required that the doctor acquire documented evidence of the patient's consent to treatment. The evolution of medical–legal requisites has also come to require that this document not only prove consent, but that the patient has received sufficient information as to nature, purposes, and risks of such treatment so as to allow him or her to make an appropriate decision about treatment (1,11).

"Prudent Patient" Test

In many states, and in any medical treatment, the issue of appropriate, informed consent revolves around the "prudent patient" test. The judge will inform the jury that there is no liability on the doctor's part if a prudent person in the patient's position would have accepted the treatment had he or she been adequately informed of all significant perils. Although this concept is subject to re-evaluation in hindsight, the prudent patient test becomes most meaningful where treatment is lifesaving or urgent.

The concept also may apply to simple procedures where the danger is commonly appreciated to be remote, such as in many cosmetic procedures. For example, a patient who undergoes a correction of the upper eyelids under local anesthesia as an outpatient procedure is not expected to develop a pulmonary embolism postoperatively. Therefore, this needs no specific mention in the preoperative consultation. In such cases, disclosure need not be extensive, and the prudent patient test will usually prevail.

As part of medical counseling, many state laws mandate that physicians warn patients of the consequences involved with failing to heed medical advice by refusing treatment or diagnostic tests. Obviously, patients have a right to refuse medical care. Such refusals and their consequences to the patient should be carefully documented.

Except in urgent situations, treating minors (defined as those under the age of 18) without consent from a parent, legal guardian, appropriate government agency, or court carries a high risk of legal or even criminal charges. There are statutory exceptions, such as for an emancipated adolescent or a married minor. Cosmetic surgeons should be familiar with their statutory provisions in the states where they practice. As discussed in Chapter 16, adolescents may, as a function of their cognitive development, be unable to comprehend the relatively permanent changes that they are requesting and appreciate the effects of a cosmetic procedure on their subsequent adult lives.

The Five Elements of Informed Consent

The law requires the following five elements of a valid informed consent to be fulfilled (1,11).

1. The diagnosis or suspected diagnosis. In cosmetic surgery, this typically is straightforward.
2. The nature and purpose of the proposed treatment or procedure, as well as its anticipated benefits.

3. The risks, complications, or side effects of the treatment.
4. The probability of success, based on the patient's condition.
5. Reasonable available alternatives to the proposed treatment or procedure.

As in cosmetic surgery, where the nature of the treatment is purely elective, the disclosure of risks, complications, and potential side effects often needs to be expanded. Pre-prepared office literature, readily available through the American Society of Plastic Surgeons and other professional associations, can provide additional information about a given procedure. In addition, an expanded discussion should take place regarding the foreseeable risks, possible untoward consequences, or unpleasant side effects associated with treatment. This discussion is particularly important if the procedure is new, experimental, hazardous, or capable of altering sexual capacity or fertility.

Documentation

In an increasing number of circumstances, state laws now require the completion of specifically designed informed consent documents. In malpractice cases, the absence of an informed consent form from the medical record places the burden of demonstrating legally sufficient reasons for such absence on the surgeon (1,11). No permit or form will absolve the doctor from responsibility if there is negligence; nor can any form guarantee that he or she will not be sued. These forms may vary from simple to incomprehensibly detailed. Most medical legal authorities agree that a middle ground exists. A well-drafted informed consent document is proof that the surgeon tried to give the patient sufficient information on which to base an intelligent decision. Such a document, supported by a handwritten note and entered in the patient's medical record, is often the key to a successful malpractice defense when the issue of consent to treatment arises. Written verification of consent to diagnostic or therapeutic treatment is crucial. At a minimum, a simple entry of several lines in the patient's chart might suffice: "Have discussed in detail objectives, technique, and potential complications of procedure. Have also discussed location and possible appearance of scars and sources of dissatisfaction. All questions answered. Patient understands and accepts."

Nevertheless, studies indicate that physicians often overestimate the patient's ability to understand the risks associated with cosmetic surgery (12–13). Patients are significantly better at recalling written warnings regarding possible complications as compared to verbal warnings (12). Nevertheless, one week after surgery, patients are able to recall no more than 50% of the written warnings of likely complications. Therefore, for cosmetic procedures, a second consultation shortly before the procedure is highly recommended, not only as a reinforcement exercise for the patient, but also as a prudent precaution for the surgeon. This interview gives the physician the opportunity not only to reinforce the crucial points of disclosure, but if properly documented, proves beyond doubt that the intention to assure the patient fully understands the risks of the procedure was always present.

The Therapeutic Alliance

Obtaining informed consent need not be an impersonal legal requirement. When properly conducted, the process of obtaining informed consent can help establish a "therapeutic alliance" and reinforce a positive doctor–patient relationship. If an unfavorable outcome occurs, that relationship can be crucial to maintaining patient trust.

A patient's usual psychological response to uncertainty is to endow his or her doctor with an aura of omnipotence. By weighing how something is said, as much as what exactly is actually said, an anxiety-ridden ritual can be turned into an effective claims prevention mechanism. The psychology literature refers to this as the "sharing of uncertainty." Rather than shattering a patient's inherent trust by presenting an insensitive approach, the surgeon's dialogue should be empathetic to the patient's particular concerns or tensions and should project believable reactions to an anxious and difficult situation.

Consider, for example, the different effects that the following two statements to a prospective patient might have:

1. "Here is a list of complications that could occur during surgery. Please read the list and sign it."
2. "I wish I could guarantee you that there will be no problems during or after surgery, but that wouldn't be realistic. Sometimes there are problems that cannot be foreseen, and I want you to know about them. Please read about the possible problems, and let's talk about them."

By using the second statement, the surgeon can reduce the patient's omnipotent image to that of a more realistic and imperfect human being, who is facing, and thus sharing, the same uncertainty. The implication to the patient is clear: "You (the patient) and I (the surgeon) are going to cooperate in doing something to your body that we hope will improve your appearance, but you must assume some of the responsibility."

The surgeon may seek to reassure the anxious patient. In so doing, the surgeon must be wary of creating unwarranted expectations or implying a guarantee. Consider the different implications of these two statements:

1. "Don't worry about a thing. I've had hundreds of cases like yours. You'll do just fine."
2. "Barring any unforeseen problems, I see no reason why you shouldn't do well. I'll certainly do everything I can to help you."

If the surgeon uses the first statement and the patient does not do "fine," he or she is likely to be angry. The second statement gently deflates the patient's fantasies about surgery to realistic proportions. This statement simultaneously reassures the patient and helps him or her to accept reality.

The therapeutic objective of informed consent should be to replace some of the patient's anxiety with a sense of participation in the procedure, which, ultimately, strengthens the therapeutic alliance. Instead of seeing each other as potential adversaries if an unfavorable outcome results, the surgeon and patient are drawn closer by sharing acceptance and understanding of the uncertainty of clinical practice (1,11).

Effective Communication

Most litigation in cosmetic surgery has the common denominator of poor communication (1,11). The doctor–patient relationship can be shattered by the surgeon's arrogance, hostility, coldness (real or imagined), or simply by the fact, at least in the patient's eyes, that "he or she didn't care." There are only two ways to avoid such a debacle: (i) make sure that the patient has no reason to feel that way; and (ii) avoid a patient who is going to feel that way no matter what is done.

Although the doctor's skill, reputation, and personality contribute to a patient's sense of confidence, rapport between the surgeon and patient is based on forthright and accurate communication. Effective communication can be easily jeopardized in the presence of a postoperative complication or, particularly from the patient's perspective, a less than "perfect" aesthetic result. In these instances, the patient may feel anxious, disappointed, and even angry. The surgeon may react to this with defensiveness, hostility, and arrogance. This response can further deepen the patient's anger and, ultimately, may provoke a lawsuit.

Anger is most likely the root cause of most malpractice claims. A patient may feel both anxious and bewildered when cosmetic surgery does not go smoothly. The line between anxiety and anger is tenuous, and the conversion of one to the other often is uncertainty—fear of the unknown. A patient frightened by a postoperative complication or disappointed with an aesthetic result may surmise: "If it is the doctor's fault, then the responsibility for correction falls on the doctor." The patient's perceptions may clash with the physician's anxieties, insecurities, and wounded pride. The patient blames the physician, who, in turn, becomes defensive. At this delicate juncture, the physician's reaction can set in motion or prevent a chain reaction. The physician must put aside feelings of disappointment, defensiveness, and hostility to understand that he or she is probably dealing with a frightened patient who is coping with uncertainty through the expression of anger.

The patient's perception that the physician understands that uncertainty, and will join with him or her to help to overcome it, may be the deciding factor in preserving the therapeutic relationship. One of the worst errors in dealing with an angry or dissatisfied patient is to try to avoid him or her. It is necessary to actively participate in the process rather than attempting to avoid the issue.

LEGAL CLAIMS IN COMMON PROCEDURES

It should come as no surprise that the overwhelming majority of all malpractice claims lodged against plastic surgeons are concentrated in a handful of aesthetic procedures. As noted above, the surgeon treating a patient who seeks aesthetic improvement is not trying to make a sick patient well, but rather a well patient better. This not only places a much heavier burden of responsibility on the surgeon, but also subjects him or her to a much broader range of possible reasons for unhappiness. Sources of dissatisfaction can range from a catastrophic result to something as unpredictable as a patient's unrealistic expectations. Given the incredible growth of cosmetic surgery and related procedures over the past decade, the steadily upward trend in the frequency of claims against plastic surgeons is not surprising.

The Doctor's Company has surveyed the genesis of patient complaints in approximately 1,000 plastic and reconstructive surgeons (The Doctor's Company, data on file). The loss experience in plastic surgery is notable for its frequency, rather than its severity. In other words, there are a large number of claims alleging relatively minor damages. Although severity has never characterized plastic surgery's loss experience in the past, the clear trend is toward ever-larger awards, particularly in those cases where an elective procedure has resulted in a fatal outcome. A significant example of this is the number of claims arising out of "large volume" suction-assisted lipectomy.

A detailed discussion of the most common legal claims can be organized around the type of surgical procedure.

Breast Surgery

As reviewed in Chapter 12, breast reduction patients typically report extremely high rates of postoperative satisfaction, even in the presence of less-than-ideal aesthetic results. When women are dissatisfied, it is most often the result of an unsatisfactory scar, loss of the nipple or additional breast skin requiring significant revision, or cosmetic asymmetry. Litigation involving breast augmentation is far more common. Approximately 44% of all elective aesthetic surgery claims involve augmentation (The Doctor's Company, data on file). Setting aside litigation related to silicone–gel filled breast implants and autoimmune as well as other systemic diseases, the most frequent causes of dissatisfaction and related litigation are encapsulation with distortion and firmness, infection, nerve damage with sensory loss, repetitive surgery and attendant costs, and incorrect size.

Rhytidectomy and Blepharoplasty

Rhytidectomy and blepharoplasty account for approximately 11% of legal claims against cosmetic surgeons (The Doctor's Company, data on file). The most common allegations include excessive skin removal resulting in a "starry" appearance of the face, inability to close the eyes/dry eyes, nerve damage resulting is a distorted expression, and skin slough resulting in excessive scarring. Plastic and ophthalmologic surgeons have received a warning advisory regarding the necessity of monitoring blepharoplasty patients for at least 3 hours after surgery. Since then, The Doctor's Company has seen no claims related to these conditions. Nevertheless, in 2004 two highly publicized deaths in New York raised new concerns about the safety of these procedures. Similarly, in the last several months of 2004 there were several mass media reports of botulism poisoning following botulinum toxin injections. As these and other anti-aging treatments continue to swell in popularity, not only in terms of the number of patients who seek them but also in terms of the number of physicians who offer them, an increase in legal claims is likely.

Rhinoplasty

Cosmetic rhinoplasty and septoplasty procedures constitute approximately 8% of claims. The most common reasons for these claims are dissatisfaction with the cosmetic result, continued breathing difficulties, and asymmetry. Of all the operations performed by plastic surgeons, this is the one with the highest degree of unpredictability. The problem is greatly aggravated by ignorance of patient selection criteria discussed earlier. In legal claims, there is almost universally a gap between the patient's expectations and results obtained, even when the surgical outcome appears excellent. The inappropriate use of imaging devices during the initial consultation often causes the patients to have unrealistic expectations, as does the use of photo albums that contain only excellent results. In many cases the actual result falls short of the promise, often setting legal proceedings into motion.

Abdominoplasty

Abdominoplasty, with or without suction-assisted lipectomy, represents approximately 3% of claims. Skin loss, scarring, nerve damage, mismanagement of a postoperative infection, use of an inappropriate surgical technique are the most common allegations. There is little question that the combination of suction-assisted lipoplasty prior to abdominoplasty has significantly increased the morbidity of this operation and doubled the number of claims in this category. These claims are typically related to skin sloughs. As bariatric surgery for extreme obesity continues to grow in popularity, an increasing number of patients who experience the resulting massive weight loss will likely present to plastic surgeons requesting abdominoplasty, lipectomy, or related procedures. This increase will likely bring with it a concurrent increase in claims again plastic surgeons who perform these procedures.

Suction-assisted Lipectomy

Suction-assisted lipectomy procedures, whether conventional or ultrasonic, have now become the single most requested elective aesthetic procedure in the United States. However, the rising popularity of this procedure has brought with it a host of problems. To begin with, since this is not a surgical procedure in the "traditional" sense, it is being performed by a wide variety of practitioners, some of them with no surgical background or clear understanding of the surgical anatomy involved. Additionally, with the advent of "tumescent" techniques, an unseemly race has developed to see who can suction out the most fat. The net result has been a dramatic rise in severe morbidity and fatal outcomes from "high volume" (greater than 5,000 cc of extracted fat) liposuction.

To make matters even worse, these procedures are often combined with other prolonged operations. Our experience clearly indicates that when a patient has been under anesthesia for over 6 hours while undergoing multiple procedures, the percentage of complications and/or fatal outcome, rises dramatically (The Doctor's Company, data on file). In a number of venues in the United States, the state medical regulatory authorities have begun to take notice. Regulatory intervention may be forthcoming unless there is a significant downturn in the morbidity of this procedure.

Skin Resurfacing

Chemical peels and laser resurfacing constitute roughly 3% of all claims. The principal allegations here typically revolve around blistering and/or burns with significant scarring, infection (often with medical mismanagement), and permanent discoloration. Because of the unpredictability of individual healing characteristics, it is probably a good idea to do a "test patch" in an area that can be hidden (for example, the back of the neck). Certainly, the documentation preceding this operation should contain clear warnings that quality of healing is linked to the individual's genetic makeup and, therefore, cannot be predicted. The surgeon must make it clear to the patient that final color and texture determination cannot be guaranteed and heavy makeup may be needed for an indeterminate period of time.

Scarring

Most plastic surgeons assume the patient understands that healing entails the formation of a scar. Unfortunately, scarring is seldom discussed in the preoperative consultation. In cosmetic surgery, the appearance of the resulting scar can be the major genesis of dissatisfaction. It is imperative that the surgeon obtains from the patient clear evidence of comprehension that without the creation of a scar, there is no healing. The patient must understand that healing qualities are as individualized as eye color and hair texture. Documentation of such conversations in the preoperative chart can go a long way in making any resulting legal claim more defensible.

Miscellaneous Claims

Approximately 5% of all complaints against plastic surgeons have to do with miscellaneous allegations. These include untoward reaction to medications or anesthesia, improper use of preoperative or postoperative photos, and sexual misconduct.

CONCLUSIONS

This chapter was written with the goal of providing an overview of the relevant professional and legal considerations in cosmetic surgery. Consistent with the overall theme of this book, consideration of the relevant psychological aspects of cosmetic surgery is a critical aspect of developing positive surgeon–patient relationships. Selecting a patient who is appropriate for surgery, and identifying one who is not, is the first step in this process. Once a patient has been selected for surgery, the surgeon must remain aware of the relevant legal considerations, particularly those that apply to the informed consent process. Open communication between the surgeon and patient, coupled with thorough documentation of all interactions, plays a central role in the maintenance of positive relationships and likely insulates surgeons from potential litigation when things go wrong. Nevertheless, despite all of the possible safeguards, litigation is a real, if not likely, possibility in the current medical climate. As cosmetic surgery continues to grow in popularity, litigation is an unfortunate certainty for most surgeons over the course of a career. However, the increasing popularity will also provide more opportunity to learn ways to reduce the likelihood of these unpleasant experiences.

REFERENCES

1. Gorney M. Claims prevention for the aesthetic surgeon: preparing for the less-than-perfect outcome. *Facial Plast Surg* 2002;18:135–142.
2. Gorney M, Martello J. Patient selection criteria. *Clin Plast Surg* 1999;26:37–40.
3. Sarwer DB, Crerand CE, Gibbons LM. Body dysmorphic disorder. In: Nahai F, ed. *The Art of Aesthetic Surgery*. St. Louis, MO: Quality Medical Publishing. In press.
4. Knorr NJ, Edgerton MT, Hoopes JE. The "insatiable" cosmetic surgery patient. *Plast Reconstr Surg* 1967;40:285–289.
5. Sarwer DB. Psychological considerations in cosmetic surgery. In: Goldwyn RM, Cohen MN, eds. *The Unfavorable Result in Plastic Surgery*. Philadelphia: Lippincott Williams & Wilkins, 2001:14–23.
6. Sarwer DB, Crerand CE. Body image and cosmetic medical treatments. *Body Image: An International Journal of Research* 2004;1:99–111.
7. Sarwer DB, Crerand CE, Didie ER. Body dysmorphic disorder in cosmetic surgery patients. *Facial Plast Surg* 2003;19:7–17.
8. Sarwer DB, Didie ER. Body image in cosmetic surgical and dermatological practice. In: Castle D, Phillips KA, eds. *Disorders of Body Image*. Stroud, England: Wrighton Biomedical Publishing, 2002:37–53.
9. Sarwer DB, Pertschuk MJ, Wadden TA, Whitaker LA. Psychological investigations of cosmetic surgery patients: a look back and a look ahead. *Plast Reconstr Surg* 1998;101:1136–1142.
10. Sarwer DB, Wadden TA, Pertschuk MJ, Whitaker LA. Body image dissatisfaction and body dysmorphic disorder in 100 cosmetic surgery patients. *Plast Reconstr Surg* 1998;101:1644–1649.
11. Gorney M. Medical malpractice and plastic surgery: the carrier's point of view. In: Goldwyn RM, Cohen MN, eds. *The Unfavorable Result in Plastic Surgery*. Philadelphia: Lippincott Williams & Wilkins, 2001:38–43.
12. Armstrong AP, Cole AA, Page RE. Informed consent: are we doing enough? *Br J Plast Surg* 1997;50:637–640.
13. Goin MK, Burgoyne RW, Goin JM. Face lift operation: the patient's secret motivations and reactions to "informed consent." *Plast Reconstr Surg* 1976;58:273–279.

INDEX

Testicles, undescended, 208, 211
Testosterone, 24, 25–26
Therapeutic alliance between physician
and patient, 322–323
Therapy, cosmetic surgery as, 302–303
Thompson, J. K.
body image disturbances, 48
contemporary perspectives of body
image, 39
Timing of procedures
breast reconstruction, 182, 183
ethical issues in craniofacial
reconstructive surgery, 291, 292
genital reconstruction, of, 210
pediatric burn patients, 96
surgical care for congenital
craniofacial conditions, 67–68
Tissue considerations for genital
reconstruction, 208–209
Topolski, T. D., 65
TRAM (transverse rectus abdominus
musculotaneous) flaps, 182
Transgender Identity Survey, 219
Transgender/transexual patients, 207,
212–222
Transplants for hair loss, 241–242
Transsexual patients, 4, 223–225
Transverse rectus abdominus musculotaneous (TRAM) flaps, 182
Trauma
brain injury with facial trauma,
127–130, 139q
facial, 125, 126–130, 131–135, 136–138,
139–141q
genital reconstruction, 207
Trazodone, 112
Treatment, nature of, and informed
consent, 321
Treatment plan for dissatisfied patients,
20
Tumescent liposuction, 326
Turner's Syndrome, 207, 211

U
Ultraviolet A light, 240
Undercontrolled children, 72–73
Understanding by patients, for informed
consent, 322
United States Federal Trade
Commission, 316
United States Public Health Service, 306
University of Louisville, 307
University of Texas, 305
Unlikable patients, 318
Unrealistic patient expectations, 317, 325
Uteruses, 209

V
Vaginal dilation, 209, 222
Vaginoplasties, 209, 217, 218t
Valence as attitude toward one's body,
236
Value as attitude toward one's body, 236
Van Steenbergen, E., 163
Veale, D., 243
*Venus Envy: A History of Cosmetic
Surgery* (Haiken), 5
Violence
body dysmorphic disorders, 244
dissatisfied patients, 315
orofacial injury patients, 126
psychological assessment, 267
VIP patients, 14–15
Visibility
burn scars, 109
hand injury disfigurement, 145
Vitiligo, 240
Vogele, C., 177
Volunteer therapy, 177

W
Waist-to-hip ratios, 25–26, 27
Ward, C., 290
Wardle, J., 44
Warranties of service, 320

Weight, body
body image dissatisfaction, 40–41, 44
breast augmentation, 252
breast hypertrophy, 191, 192
breast reduction changes, 195–196
eating disorders, 260–261
Weight training with muscle
dysmorphia, 262
Width, facial, 238–239
Wilkins, E. G., 182
Winder, A. E., 174
Winder, B. D., 174
Women. *See also* Gender differences
body image, 38, 40–41
cosmetic surgery patients, 27
femininity, 24, 26, 197t, 234
romantic relationships, 30
Work-related injuries, 146, 147
Workers Compensation, 147
World Health Organization, 214t
Wound healing
breast reconstruction, 178
breast reduction, 196, 200, 201
genital reconstruction, 208–209, 211
improved care, 5
skin resurfacing, 326

X
XX patients, 209, 211, 222
XY male infants, 209, 210, 211

Y
Yalom, Marilyn, 5
Young families and breast cancer
treatment, 180
Youthfulness and physical attractiveness,
24, 27
Yurek, D., 181

Z
Zaleplon, 112
Zolpidem, 112